W0043672

NEW FRONTIERS IN MAMMARY PATHOLOGY 1986

CCM
"NON PROFIT"

DEVELOPMENTS IN ONCOLOGY

Recent volumes

NEW FRONTIERS IN MAMMARY PATHOLOGY 1986

edited by

K.H. Hollmann and J.M. Verley
*International Society against Breast Cancer, Contra Cancrum Mammarium
and Marie-Lannelongue Hospital, Le Plessis Robinson, France*

Springer-Science+Business Media, B.V.

Library of Congress Cataloging in Publication Data

New frontiers in mammary pathology, 1986.

(Developments in oncology)
Papers presented at the Third Symposium of the
International Society against Breast Cancer held in
Paris, France, on Dec. 9-12, 1985.
Includes index.
1. Breast--Cancer--Congresses. I. Hollmann, K. H.
II. Verley, J. M. III. International Society against
Breast Cancer. Symposium (3rd : 1985 : Paris, France)
IV. Series.
RC280.B8N476 1986   616.99'449   86-28593

ISBN 978-94-010-7980-8   ISBN 978-94-009-3297-5 (eBook)
DOI 10.1007/978-94-009-3297-5

Copyright

© 1986 Springer Science+Business Media Dordrecht
Originally published by Martinus Nijhoff Publishers, Dordrecht in 1986
Softcover reprint of the hardcover 1st edition 1986

All rights reserved. No part of this publication may be reproduced, stored in a
retrieval system, or transmitted in any form or by any means, mechanical,
photocopying, recording, or otherwise, without the prior written permission of
the publishers, Springer-Science+Business Media, B.V.

V

PREFACE

The Third Symposium of the International Society against Breast Cancer CONTRA CANCRUM MAMMARIUM was held in Paris, at UNESCO, on December 9-12, 1985.

Scientists and physicians came from all over the world to attend this meeting. They came from Japan, Brazil, the United States and the Middle East, from Belgium, Finland, Germany, Greece, Italy, the Netherlands, Norway, Portugal, Spain, Sweden, Switzerland, Yugoslavia, and from all over France. They all contributed to the success of the Symposium and my cordial thanks go to all of them and particularly to the invited speakers and chairmen of the sessions, to the free-paper contributors, and to the contributors to the Slide Seminar.

Warm personal thanks go to two friends: to Professor Dan H. Moore from Hahnemann University, Philadelphia, who was always there to help in many ways, and to Professor Pietro Gullino from the National Cancer Institute, Bethesda, and now Torino, Italy, who consistently gave invaluable advice. Special thanks are also due to those who assisted in the preparation and organization of the Symposium: the UNESCO officers, the interpreters, the secretaries and hostesses, the BEBA Company with the help of Dr.Bernard Martin and Mrs.Jacqueline Bouchy, the WILD-LEITZ-France S.A. for projection facilities and microscope arrangements for the workshop on mammary cytology which was successfully conducted by Dr.Colette Marsan.

During the four days, three main topics were discussed:

1. Epidemiology, genetics and oncogenes, related subjects of great actuality.

2. Hormone receptors and monoclonal antibodies. Recent fundamental advances in the identification of tumors and metastases were discussed and the value of MABs as a promising tool in diagnosis and treatment was pointed out.

<u>**3.**</u> **<u>The process of metastasis</u>**. New and interesting results were reported: periodic growth cycles of primary tumors synchronized with nodal changes, facilitating progressive growth and the spread of tumors. The role of tumor markers in the detection of primary and secondary tumors. The spontaneous and experimental modifications of cell surface properties and their implications in the metastatic process were, among other subjects, the focus of the discussion.

I hope that the limited number of participants facilitated contacts and exchanges and made this Third Symposium again intimate and cordial.

It is hoped that the present volume truly reflects the efforts of the contributors and editors and will provide stimuli for continuing contacts and future collaboration in the struggle against this insidious disease.

K.H. Hollmann

NEW FRONTIERS IN MAMMARY PATHOLOGY

CONTENTS

EPIDEMIOLOGY, GENETICS AND ONCOGENES

HORMONE RECEPTORS, MONOCLONAL ANTIBODIES

Selected Free-Papers

METASTASIS

SELECTED FREE PAPERS

PRESENT TRENDS IN MAMMARY PATHOLOGY

K.H. Hollmann

Surgical Center Marie Lannelongue,
F-92350 Le Plessis-Robinson, France.

What is new in Breast Cancer? This is the question that is often asked by young and old people of all walks of life as well as by physicians who must daily face patients with breast problems. The same question brought together clinicians and scientists representing different specialities from many countries in the Third Symposium of the International Society against Breast Cancer CONTRA CANCRUM MAMMARIUM.

In the past few years tremendous advances have been made in all fields of breast cancer research as well as in diagnosis and treatment. In diagnostic radiology, X-ray mammography has gained in resolution, the radiation dose has been reduced and complementary techniques such as thermography, echography, diaphanoscopy and other methods have been developed. Today, mammography is on the way to providing digital results, improving early breast cancer detection and further reducing the radiation dose. NMR-imaging of the breast is already under clinical trial and promises to be harmless to the tissues and to resolve details even at the cellular level.

Under the stimulating influence of the French school, radiotherapy has been shown to be a very effective means of sterilizing primary breast cancer as well as metastatic involvement.

As a result of the classical concepts of Halsted and his successors, breast surgery has for decades been a radical, extended and mutilating operation. During the past few years, however, under the influence of immunological and other patho-physiological considerations, a more limited and tissue-sparing trend has emerged, improving esthetic, functional and, finally, psychological results.

There have been constant new developments and improvements in hormonetherapy and chemotherapy which have gained an undeniable place in the management of breast cancer.

Almost all of these advances were supported by the development of refined histo- and cytopathological methods which have facilitated the diagnosis and improved the prognosis of breast cancer. Whithout these methods, a logical treatment strategy could not be envisaged.

Advanced and refined diagnostic and therapeutic procedures have contributed to longer survival. Today, in many countries breast cancer patients rarely die from their primary tumors, which can now be detected early and easily controlled, but succumb instead to metastases. Early in the disease, breast cancer cells spread to other organs and give rise to secondary tumors. These secondary spreads are called metastases, if separate from the primary growth and arising from detached transported fragments of it. Thus, tumor cell embolism is not defined as metastasis, since emboli in lymphatics or blood vessels may be destroyed. We deal with metastasis only when the arrested tumor cells survive, multiply and extend into the perivascular tissues. The understanding of the factors involved in the metastatic process will be a fundamental step toward further improvement in the patient's survival.

But the definite prevention or eradication of breast cancer will probably not be achieved as long as we do not know the cause of the disease.

In the last decades it was thought that a mammary tumor virus (MTV) played an important role as a causal agent, at least in the mouse model, but also in human breast cancer. More recently, research has shown that this was erroneous and that the hope of vaccinating women against breast cancer can not be realized in the near future.

Nevertheless, the work on the MTV and other tumor viruses was not in vain. The study of retroviruses and their interrelations with the host genome led to the discovery of oncogenes, i.e. genes that are present in healthy animal and human cells which, in addition to normal functions, have the potential for inducing cancer. This recently discovered class of genes will result in a better understanding of the process of cancerogenesis.

The role of hormones in the promotion of breast cancer has been known for some time, but it is through the work on estrogen receptors (ER) under the leadership of Jensen that a more precise identification of hormone-dependent tumors has been made possible. The initial biochemical methods using in vitro radio-immuno-assays have been supplemented by enzyme-immuno-assays and anti-estrogen receptor immunocytochemical assays using polyclonal, and more recently, monoclonal antibodies (MABs). A technological revolution has been achieved by Kohler and Milstein (1976) who devised a technique for the production of "immortal" cell clones making monovalent antibodies by fusing antibody-producing plasma cells, isolated from the spleen of mice, with cultured myeloma cells from the same strain of mice that can be kept indefinitely in culture. These so-called hybridomas are then selected out in tissue cultures and by appropriate techniques single clones can be established. Whereas so-called (polyclonal) "specific antibodies" represent a whole spectrum of polyvalent molecules directed against different determinants (epitopes) on the antigen, the monoclonal antibodies produced by a given hybridoma are made of identical molecules. They have the same Ig class, the same structures and the same variable regions, affinities and specificities. The most important is that they provide the possibility to all laboratories through the world to use the same antibodies. Furthermore, the cell lines are, at least theoretically, "immortal". Monoclonal antibodies (MABs) have aroused considerable interest in breast cancer research and treatment. Different groups of MABs have been used according to the immunogens selected for their production; e.g., MABs against breast tumor cell lines, MABs against milk fat globule membranes, MABs against membrane-enriched extracts of breast cancer metastasis, or against gross cystic disease fluid protein (GCDFP-15), a marker for apocrine carcinoma. The "monoclonals" allow the identification of hormone receptor proteins (e.g. ER and PR), of all kinds of tumor markers, intracytoplasmic (intermediate) filaments etc., as well on fixed tissue sections as on cryostat material. They are therefore of greatest help for the diagnosis of primary tumors and their metastases. Coupled to cytotoxic agents, monoclonal antitumor-antibodies will play an important role in therapy by recognizing specifically their target cells.

One of the major drawbacks in the application of monoclonal antibodies in the detection and treatment of breast cancer and its metastases is the heterogeneity of tumor cell populations. The existence of distinct morphologies in different areas of a single mammary tumor is well known to histopathologists. Similar heterogeneities are observed at the ultrastructural level. Quantitative electron microscopy has shown that the mitochondrial volume, the ergastoplasmic surface and the development of the Golgi elements vary significantly in cells from different areas of spontaneous mouse mammary tumors. After grafting the same tumor into different organs such as the brain, the liver, the spleen, the uterus, or under the skin, there were quite different ultrastructural differentiations concerning the amount of mitochondria, ergastoplasm and Golgi elements in the different transplantation sites (personal observations). These structural heterogeneities, accompanied by a wide range of antigenic phenotypes of a tumor cell population are, among other, limiting factors for the useful application of monoclonal antibodies.

   The problem of cellular heterogeneity within a tumor
has not only theoretical interest but great clinical
implications. It is well known that patients who are
initially responsive to hormonetherapy have recurrencies at
variable intervals of time. These therapeutic failures may
be explained by the existence of heterogeneous cell
populations. Thus, a hormone responsive subpopulation may
be depleted after hormone deprivation and be replaced by
another, hormone-nonresponsive subpopulation. The understanding of factors regulating different stages of cellular
differentiation and expression or repression of hormone
receptors and thus responsible for cellular heterogeneities, will help to manipulate the growth characteristics
of a tumor and to develop better treatment strategies.

EPIDEMIOLOGY, GENETICS
AND
ONCOGENES

SYNERGISMS IN BREAST CANCER ETIOLOGY

DAN H. MOORE

Department of Microbiology and Immunology
Hahnemann University
School of Medicine
Broad and Vine
Philadelphia, PA 19102-1192, U.S.A.

Since breast cancer is the leading cause of cancer deaths* in women of North America and most of Europe and the incidence rate is three times the death rate and rising in all world populations, it would be helpful to recognize the most significant factors that place a woman in a position of high risk. The manifestation of this disease does not usually result from a single cause, but instead from a combination of causes which most probably exert their influences over a long period of time.

Data showing that the incidence is increasing in populations throughout the world are provided by "Cancer Incidence in Five Continents," Volume 4 (Waterhouse et al., 1982). The incidence is increasing not only in countries undergoing rapid changes such as China and Japan, but also in North America and Europe. In countries where the incidence is high, the greatest increase is in postmenopausal women, whereas in the areas with lower rates, the rise tends to be more in premenopausal women.

In consideration of preventative measures, it is important to recognize that there are strong indications that early life may be the most sensitive period to breast cancer-causing elements; or at least, early life seems to be important in setting the stage for the eventual development of the disease. In studies of atomic bomb survivors in Japan, it was found that those irradiated during early life were at highest risk and that the

---

*Lung cancer death rate is now overtaking breast cancer in the United States.

increased risk extended throughout their lifetimes (Tokunaga et al., 1979). It has also been reported that the use of radium ^{224} in the treatment of childhood tuberculosis of the bone increases risk and that the minimal latent period ranges from a few years to half the normal lifespan (Miller, 1982). In contrast to the high sensitivity of the adolescent breast to irradiation is the apparent low sensitivity of older women. Levitt and Mandel (1983) and Basco et al. (1985) found no increased risk of a second primary cancer in the contralateral breast from radiation therapy of breast cancer patients, and many investigators have reported no ill effects from diagnostic irradiation for women over 40 years of age. However, undergoing general anesthesia, appendectomies, tonsillectomies, and other sources of trauma during the pre- and perimenarchal period has been reported to significantly increase the risk of cancer (Meyer and Gelman, 1983). In extensive experiments carried out on rats, Ross and Bras (Ross and Bras, 1971; Ross et al., 1982) have shown that the important age for dietary influence on eventual development of cancer is the early life. After the animals reached maturity, diet was ineffectual. Furthermore, the induction of mammary tumors in rats by DMBA and other carcinogens is most effective at the beginning of reproductive life, which is around 50 days of age, depending on strain.

Another evidence that human breast cancers take a long time to become perceptible has been derived from studies of growth rates of the tumor cells in vitro. It was found that the doubling time for cells from various tumors ranged from 81 to 900 days (Gershon-Cohen and Ingleby, 1959), which means that it would take from 10 to 100 years for a tumor to reach one centimeter in diameter. Although in vitro studies may not portray in vivo conditions, they do emphasize the relatively long time required for a single cancerous cell to produce an easily detectible mass. It is concluded, therefore, that most breast cancers start in early life; otherwise, they would not be detected in a lifetime. The rate of growth may change for any given tumor, but even so, many years are usually required for it to become large enough to be detected by standard methods. Its growth is exponential, however, and once it reaches a size of one centimeter, with a constant doubling time of 10 days (about average), it would reach a diameter of two centimeters in less than one year.

FAMILY HISTORY

Probably the most important factor in determining whether or not a woman is at high risk is family history, i.e., whether or not she has a close relative who has had the disease. Mother, daughter, or sister constitute what is called first-degree relatives, and grandmothers and aunts, either maternal or paternal, constitute second-degree relatives. It is not yet established how familial breast cancer is transmitted or which relative has the greatest influence on risk or what the risk is in any particular situation because risk depends on synergistic action among several factors. In determining the significant factors in any population, it is necessary to collect data on many factors and then segregate them into different groups for analytical purposes. For example, it seems that some of the factors involved in the etiology of the disease in women with a family history are often different from those for women without a family history. In a study of 166 breast cancer patients, 53 with a family history, and 332 matched controls, Macera et al. (1982), using the Mantel-Haenszel method to obtain an odds ratio, found that the two groups (the breast cancer women with and without family history) showed consistently different risk profiles on various reproductive, hormonal, and environmental factors known to be associated with the disease. Furthermore, those breast cancer women with menstrual activity in excess of 37 years had an odds ratio of 12.3 for the family history group vs 1.1 for the group without a family history. For the family history group, more than 12 years from menarche to first childbirth, use of thyroid medication, and for post-menopausal women, a Quetelet index score, a measure of fatness (wt/ht), greater than 3.33 were associated with a significantly elevated risk. For women without a family history, the only significant risk factors were large breasts and childhood spent in an urban area. The authors state that no risk factor was significant in both groups, indicating that breast neoplasia in the two groups may have different etiologies. These data show the remarkable synergy between certain risk factors such as family history, ages at menarche and menopause, and parity.

In a comparison made in Sweden by Adami et al. (1981) on 1,330 women with breast cancer and an equal number of matched controls, a first-degree familial history of breast cancer was found in 149 of the patients and in 90 of the controls, giving a standardized relative risk (SRR) of 1.7. The figures for second-degree relatives were 115 and 81, respectively (SRR=1.5). For women with unilateral disease, the SRR for breast cancer in first-degree relatives was 1.7 and for those with bilateral cancer, it was 2.2. A slightly higher, but nonsignificant relative risk was found for women diagnosed before 50 years of age (SRR=2.4) compared with a SRR of 1.7 for those older than 50 years.

Why do the risk values seem to be so different in these two surveys? Certainly, we do not know precisely and completely, but the ways in which the data were analyzed are different. In addition, the studies are on two different populations with possibly many subtle differences in heredity and lifestyle. The subjects of the Macera et al. study were divided into more subgroups, such as those who had a menstrual activity under or over 37 years, and length of menstrual life is dependent on age at menarche and age at menopause. Macera et al. also considered time span from menarche to first childbirth and used the Mantel-Haenszel method, which takes into account age differences of the subjects. Further, they took into account Quetelet index scores and use of thyroid medication. However, neither survey included pre- and perimenarchal stress or trauma, or dietary and other factors that sometimes seem to influence risk.

Another extensive study of the effect of family history on the incidence and age of occurrence was made by Black et al. (1983), who reported that risk depended to some extent on which particular relative had had the disease. The effect of use of oral contraceptives (OC) also depended on family history (FH). Of 1,541 cases studied, 324, or 21%, were under 45 years of age and 370 were FH-positive; of these, 125 (34%) were under 45 years of age. The proportion of cases under 45 years old had breast cancer relatives in the following order: grandmother (most common) > aunt > mother > no relative > sister. A similar FH relation sequence occurred with regard to current (during two years prior to diagnosis) OC use in the <45 yrs age group. It also appeared that current OC usage increased the risk of invasive breast cancer among grandmother- or aunt-positive women, while decreasing risk among family-history negative women. The effect of OC seemed to depend on which relative had had the disease. Furthermore, in FH-negative, OC-negative women, the menarche and parity features of patients with nonmalignant breast lesions are the same as those of age-matched breast cancer patients.

The age distribution of the breast cancer patients according to family history in this study is also interesting. The distribution of patients under 45 years of age was: family-history negative, 17%; paternal-grandmother positive, 65%; maternal-grandmother positive, 57%; maternal-aunt positive, 48%; paternal-aunt positive, 38%; mother-only positive, 28%; sister, not grandmother, positive, 11%. Many reports have indicated that a FH increases risk, but I have seen no other report that has attempted to quantitate the effect of the various relatives. Of more practical import- ance, however, is the apparent association between previous use of oral contraceptives by a breast cancer patient and the occurrence of breast cancer in second-degree relatives. The data of Black et al. (1983) show that "among those women whose grandmothers or aunts-only had breast cancer, OC usage was associated with an increased relative risk (RR) of breast cancer; viz., RR 2.7 for total users and RR 4.9 for current users. On the other hand, OC usage by FH-negative women was associated with a significant reduction in risk; viz., RR 0.4 for current users and 0.58 for total users." The authors state that "if such effects can be shown to be universally true, it should be possible to significantly reduce the incidence of premenopausal breast cancer by limiting OC usage to FH-negative women."

These data of Black et al. emphasize the need to evalu- ate the many risk factors in various combinations in order to determine synergistic actions. A particular factor, e.g. OC use, in combination with one factor may increase risk, while ·in combination with a different factor, it may decrease risk.

A recent report by Zhang et al. (1983) also demon- strates the strong effect of synergism between factors. A case-control study of 516 breast cancer cases in the area of Tianjin, Peoples Republic of China, where the incidence of breast cancer is rapidly increasing, showed that only about 4% of women who now have the disease have a family history of breast cancer. The usual factors, early age at menarche, late age at first birth, nulliparity, low parity, high family income, good education, occupation with a high level of skill, family history of breast cancer, etc., considered separately, seemed to have little effect on risk. However, a combination of some unfavorable factors were associated with greatly increased risk. For example, a combination of higher education and a family history gave a relative risk of more than 8.

Risk among sisters and mothers of a population-based series of 1,137 breast cancer patients diagnosed before age 55 in Metropolitan Detroit was compared with risk to the same relatives of 1,001 age-matched population-based controls by Schwartz et al. (1985). The odds ratio for women with affected sisters was 2.2; for women with affected daughters, 3.2; and for those with affected mothers and daughters, it was 9.9.

Sometimes the type of breast cancer is associated with a particular family history. In a survey of 1,024 breast cancer patients at Memorial Sloan-Kettering Hospital, Rosen et al. (1982) found that a maternal breast cancer history was significantly ($p<0.006$) more frequent among patients with medullary carcinoma, especially among those patients who were pre- or perimenopausal at the time of diagnosis ($p>0.001$). Additionally, of the 727 patients who had one or more sisters, 12% had a sister who had been treated for breast cancer. The highest frequency of carcinoma in at least one sister occurred in the group of patients who had lobular carcinoma, while the medullary carcinoma group had the lowest number of patients with an affected sister ($p<0.03$). Occurrence of the disease in a sister was almost twice as common in patients who were postmenopausal at the time of diagnosis as in those who were premenopausal ($p<0.005$). Thus, pre- and perimenopausal patients had more medullary carcinomas and a mother-associated history, while postmenopausal patients had more lobular carcinomas and a sister-associated history. This might be interpreted to mean that some factor or combination of factors is not usually transmitted to other daughters.

In a comparison of women with and without a family history, Lynch et al. (1984) conclude that hereditary breast cancer shows a distinctive natural history with character-istics different from those found in the non-familial dis-ease. Familial breast cancer is characterized by an earlier age of onset, excessive bilaterality, heterogenous tumor associations, and improved survival, as well as vertical transmission. Early first full-term pregnancy did not alter the frequency of the disease nor the age at diagnosis for those with a family history. This was contrary to the find-ings in their general breast cancer population, as well as to the findings reported in many other studies.

Wolke et al. (1984) have reported a relationship between biliary cirrhosis and breast cancer. The incidence of breast cancer in 208 primary biliary cirrhosis patients in New York was found to be 4.4 times greater than that expected, but the incidence in sites other than the breast and of primary hepatocellular tumors was not significantly increased.

Sometimes there is a negative relationship between breast cancer and other cancers. In a series of 17,756 breast cancer patients and 4,817 cervical cancer patients in England, Prior and Waterhouse (1981a) found no etiological relationship between the two diseases, although in the breast series, a small deficit of cervical tumors was observed (observed, 16; expected, 22.19), and in the cervical series, a small excess of breast cancers was found (observed, 29; expected 23.38).

These same authors (Prior and Waterhouse, 1981b), in the analysis of a series of 22,000 breast cancer patients, found that the risk of a second primary tumor in the contralateral breast depended on age. The risks for three age ranges (at the time of diagnosis of the first primary) were 5.3 (ages 15-34), 3.3 (ages 35-59), and 1.5 (ages >60 yrs). A maximal risk of 5.0-fold was observed in the series as a whole during the third year after diagnosis of the first primary.

More recently, in a comprehensive study of correlations between incidence rates in Canada, Howe et al. (1984) found a notable correlation between female lung and breast cancer; and from an evaluation of breast and thyroid multiple primary cancers using the Connecticut Tumor Registry, Ron et al. (1984) found a significant (SIR=1.89) elevation of primary breast cancers following thyroid cancer. Women under age forty with follicular or mixed papillary-follicular thyroid cancer had a 10-fold increased risk of developing breast cancer.

In an earlier survey of genetic and environmental factors involved in the etiology of several cancers associated with smoking, Lynch et al. (1982) found that a cohort trend found for lung cancer was also apparent among relatives of breast cancer probands (i.e., relatives of breast cancer patients had elevated lung cancer incidence), but not for relatives of colon cancer probands. This was interpreted to suggest the possibility of an intrinsic association of carcinomas of the breast and lung.

Ciambellotti et al. (1985) report the occurrence of lung carcinomas in four women who had undergone mastectomies and suggest that certain histochemical factors induced by the lung tumors may somehow become pathologically transformed to simulate a new primary malignant tumor in the breast.

Another report indicating a linkage between hereditary factors and premenopausal breast cancer is found in a study of cerumen type (wet or dry). Petrakis (1983) reported that a significantly greater proportion of premenopausal but not postmenopausal Caucasian women who had cerumen of the wet type had dysplastic epithelial cells in the aspirates of their breast fluid, and that the presence of dysplastic cells was associated with a 6- to 8-fold increase of risk for breast cancer. Thus, dysplastic cells in nipple aspirates and/or wet type cerumen appear to be indicators of elevated risk.

Papatestas et al. (1979) found a strong association between age at tumor diagnosis and serum levels of immune globulin A. Hypo-IgA was associated with early tumor appearance, and the association was greater if the patient had a family history of breast cancer. Papatestas et al. (1980) also found an association between estrogen receptors and weight in breast cancer women. Overweight women had fewer or absent receptor proteins.

Still another possible marker which may indicate a genetic susceptibility to breast cancer is being found in dermatoglyphic patterns. Upon examining ten-digit fingerprints of 200 women with breast cancer, Bierman et al. (1979) found that 42 (21%) of the patients had one or more of a configuration called composite "accidentals," which occur in <0.63% of the "normal" population on any finger; 36 (83%) of the patients with the "accidentals" were premenopausal. Family histories were available on 175 of the patients, and 34 (82%) of the patients with "accidentals" had a family history of breast cancer as compared to 60% of the remaining patients. The authors conclude that certain rare dermatoglyphic patterns may serve as a reliable predictor of increased risk..

These authors also state that dermatoglyphic patterns are inherited under complex polygenic influences and can be developmentally altered by intrauterine stimuli (viruses, chemicals, radiation, etc.) prior to the fifth fetal month. Is it not possible, therefore, that in addition to true hereditary factors, fetal exposure to one or more of those elements could increase the propensity for breast cancer as well as alter the fingerprints?

In another report, Seltzer et al. (1982) examined fingerprints of 119 Caucasian women, 34 of whom had breast cancer, and 11 (32.4%) of these had specific patterns (6 or more whorls) that were seen in only 3.1% of the controls. If all the women considered to be at high risk for breast cancer (53) were included, 95% of those whose fingerprints contained 6 or more whorls would either have had breast cancer or were at high risk. Women considered at high risk were those with either a first-degree relative with the disease, a history of nulliparity, or severe bilateral fibrocystic mastopathy.

It is now apparent that human as well as other animal cells contain specific cancer genes. Biologically active DNAs of various tumors can induce oncogenic transformation in cultured cells by a process called transfection. The infecting DNA is known as cellular transforming genes (Cooper, 1982). The ability to transfer a selectable phenotype to a recipient cell has made it possible to transfer specific cancer genes. Transforming genes from the human mammary carcinoma cell line MCF-7 as well as nonviral-induced mouse mammary tumor genes have been used by Lane et al. (1981) to transform NIH3T3 mouse cells. The mouse mammary tumor cells were from a BALB/c CRGL mouse, a strain that has no demonstrable mammary tumor virus, and the carcinoma was chemically (dimethylbenzanthracene) induced. Furthermore, the NIH3T3 cells transformed by the DNAs, mouse and human, did not contain exogenous mouse mammary tumor virus DNA sequences.

Later, Becker et al. (1982) were able to identify an 86,000-dalton glycoprotein antigen that was associated specifically with the transforming genes of mammary carcinoma, both human and mouse. Sera from tumor-bearing mice immunoprecipitated the glycoprotein from extracts of the NIH cells transformed by human mammary carcinoma DNA and by mouse mammary carcinoma DNA, but sera from mice bearing many kinds of tumors except mammary carcinomas did not precipitate the glycoprotein antigen. From many tests, the authors concluded that this glycoprotein antigen was specifically associated with expression of the transmissible transforming genes of human and mouse mammary carcinomas.

In other studies, Murray et al. (1981) obtained foci of transformed mouse cells after transfection of human DNA from colon and bladder carcinoma cell lines and a promyelocytic leukemia cell line. These foci were shown to contain a large number of human DNA sequences by using highly repetitive human DNA sequence probes. Cellular DNA from the primary foci was then used in a subsequent cycle of transfection, which resulted in secondary foci that contained relatively

little human DNA. These secondary foci appeared to contain
only the human sequences proximal to those responsible for
the transformed phenotype, and comparison of the common DNA
fragments found in the secondary foci derived from the three
different human tumor cell lines indicates that these three
cell lines (colon carcinoma, bladder carcinoma, and promyelocytic leukemia) contained three different transforming
genes.

MENARCHE, PARITY, AND MENOPAUSE

Age at menarche, age at first birth, marital status,
age at menopause, and total time span of menstrual life have
been considered to be important factors in the etiology of
breast cancer (MacMahon et al., 1973).

More recent publications, however, have not always
confirmed this conclusion. In a study of 179 consecutively
detected breast cancer patients and age-matched controls
selected from a computerized population register in an area
of Sweden northwest of Stockholm, Adami et al. (1978) found
no signif_icant difference in age of menarche, age at first
birth, age at menopause, or number of children. These
investigators also concluded that a subdivision into pre-
and post-menopausal women yielded no further information.
The authors suggested that their results are at variance
with most earlier reports, possibly because their controls
were selected from the whole female population instead of
hospitalized patients.

Najem et al. (1982), in a survey of 60 breast cancer
patients and 125 controls matched for race, age, place of
birth (New Jersey), marital status, education, and annual
family income, found no difference in any of these variables
between the two groups.

Most reports, however, do show significant differences
in reproductive life between breast cancer and control
groups. In a study of 1,038 breast cancer patients and
1,791 matched controls in the San Francisco Bay area,
Paffenbarger et al. (1980) found a gradual increase in risk
with age at first birth, rising from an RR of 1.0 at ages
≤20 yrs to 2.7 at 30 yrs for the premenopausal disease, but
to only about 1.7 for postmenopausal; parity had a lesser
effect. A late age at menarche reduced risk, but only when
it occurred after age 15. The effect of child-bearing was
greater for premenopausal breast cancer. However, this

study did not take into account family history or use of
exogenous estrogens.

In an analysis of 236 breast cancer patients and 937
controls, Hunt et al. (1980) showed that late age at first
birth increased risk and also that there was a strong
interaction between age at first birth and age at last
birth, and that the association of age at first birth with
low breast cancer incidence was stronger for women whose
last delivery occurred before she reached 35 years. This
was true even after adjustment for parity (relative odds:
4.1; p<0.001). Furthermore, having a child after age 35
significantly increased risk.

In a study of 362 urban breast cancer patients and 694
matched controls in the Estonian Republic, MacMahon et al.
(1982a) concluded that women whose first birth occurred
before age 20 had a risk less than one-third that of nulliparous women. They also concluded that risk increased
with increase in age at first birth (AFB) but remained below
1.0 (relative to nulliparity) even in the highest of AFB
categories. This was also the conclusion reached by
MacMahon et al. (1970, 1973) from studies conducted in
several different populations throughout the world. Thus,
it was believed that an early first birth reduced risk, but
additional births had little or no effect. However, in a
re-analysis of these extensive data, Trichopoulos et al.
(including MacMahon) (1983) conclude that age at any birth
after the first is also an independent and statistically
significant risk indicator. They found that it was associated with a 0.9% increase of risk for every year of increase
in age at any and every birth. Furthermore, they found that
the age of approximately 35 years is a critical one: before
35 years, any childbirth confers some degree of protection,
but after this age, every full-term pregnancy is associated
with an increase in risk.

From the data taken in the Estonian Republic by
MacMahon et al. (1982a), it was observed that for women who
had only two children, the age at the time of the second
birth was a determinant of the amount of further decrease in
risk. Compared to nulliparous women, the odds ratio for
uniparous women who had their child before age 25 was 0.62,
but was only 0.18 for duoparous women who had both their
children before age 25. Thus, data from this Estonian
survey indicate that having two full term pregnancies before
age 25 confers considerable protection, which is an observation not previously reported from surveys in other popula-

tions. Age at menarche was not found to be a risk factor in this population.

In a hospital-based case control study of 1,185 women with breast cancer and 3,227 controls (90% from the USA, 4% from Canada, and 6% from Israel), Helmrich et al. (1983) found that a history of menarche at age 15 or later was related to a lower risk, but there was no evidence of a trend of increasing risk with decreasing age at menarche. This effect was also restricted primarily to premenopausal breast cancer, as has been found in most other published surveys (MacMahon et al., 1973; Staszewsky, 1971; Stavraky and Emmons, 1974).

In a study of 714 premenopausal and 130 postmenopausal breast cancer cases matched with 8,440 controls in Boston, MA, Lipnick et al. (1984) found that a first birth before age 25 yrs gave a relative risk of 0.7 compared to nulliparous women for both pre- and postmenopausal cases. However, in the premenopausal cases, a history of breast cancer in a sister gave an RR of 3.0, and in a mother, 1.9, whereas for the postmenopausal women, the RR's were 1.4 and 1.3, respectively.

In a population-based study of 23,511 women 50-67 years of age at the time of first screening, de Waard et al. (1981) found a striking relationship between parity and age at first childbirth, on the one hand, and two radiologic aspects of Wolfe's breast parenchymal pattern (dysplasia and prominent duct pattern) (Wolfe, 1976) on the other. These relationships appeared to be causal. This report shows the increase in information that can be obtained by combining procedures and the resulting data. Risk based on Wolfe's xerographic parenchymal breast patterns alone have been continuously questioned, but when Wolfe's patterns were combined with age of subject, age at first birth, parity, and Quetelet's index, selection of high-risk women became much more definite.

Although most studies show that early marriage and childbearing decrease risk of breast cancer, late childbearing, over the age of approximately 35, increases risk. Another effect of parity is on the age at which the breast cancer occurs. Age-incidence studies have usually shown that parity increases risk of early breast cancer over nulliparity (Lilienfield, 1963). Data from the New York State Registry showed a lower rate for the never married up to age 40, and it was suggested by Janerich (1979) that early breast cancer may be pregnancy-related. Juret et al. (1974) in France reported that parous women present breast cancer at a significantly earlier age than nonparous; that early menarche was associated with a poorer prognosis, and that more than five deliveries was associated with marked decline in prognosis (Juret et al., 1980). From the 1961 and 1971 censuses of England and Wales, Alderson (1981) estimated the breast cancer age distribution of women of various parities. From age-specific incidences, it was shown that the highest average age (65.9 years) occurred in nulliparous women and that the lowest average age (60.4 years) for the presentation of the disease occurred in women who had borne two children. Janerich and Hoff (1982) report that married women of New York State have a higher risk before age 40 than unmarried women and that this is especially true for non-white women. Mortality rates show a similar pattern, except that the cross-over age is about 45 instead of 40 years.

A word of caution concerning the effect of early menarche and early parity has been sounded by Wang et al. (1985) on the grounds that some studies have not included a control population and therefore the relationships could be the result of temporal changes in the general population. They simultaneously compared the reproductive histories of 739 breast cancer patients with those of 1,989 unaffected women. Age at menarche and age at first baby increased, while the average number of children declined, with increasing age in both patients and controls. The change in the average number of children was largely due to the fact that 15% of those women aged 41-50 years were nulliparous compared with 30% in those older than 60. They conclude that these reproductive events do not alter the time of onset of disease and that the association between the two parameters can be explained by temporal changes in reproductive patterns which occur in both cancerous and control women.

Woods et al. (1980) in a study of 341 unselected breast cancer patients presenting to a clinic in Birmingham, England, found that the mean age at presentation was 5.2 years younger in parous than in nulliparous women (p<0.001) and fell with increasing parity. Thirty-nine percent of the women who had 3 or more childbirths presented at or below 50 years of age.

Breast cancer patients under the age of 30 have been found by Tabbane et al. (1985) in Tunis, Tunisia, to have more often a rapidly progressing inflammatory breast cancer than older premenopausal patients (age 45-49). The prognosis is usually poor in the young patients, especially in those who are pregnant or lactating.

Hardy et al. (1983) in Brazil reported that nulliparity increases risk significantly only for postmenopausal breast cancer and that becoming parous at age 30 or later increased risk four-fold for postmenopausal, but did not affect pre-menopausal, breast cancer.

The evidence seems to indicate that in most populations early parity decreases risk only of the postmenopausal dis-ease; late parity increases this risk; and early first childbirth increases risk of the premenopausal disease.

HORMONES

The possibility that hormones, acting synergistically with other factors, constitute an important influence on the occurrence of breast cancer has been recognized by many investigators. Endocrine hormones are responsible for the development and function of the mammary gland, and their concentrations vary greatly with age and reproductive func-tion. It seems that prolactin and possibly growth hormone may condition cells of the mammary epithelium to make them more susceptible to malignant transformation. This condi-tioning may also be effected by estrogens. Progesterone, however, seems to oppose such action.

Rose and Pruitt (1981) found that the plasma prolactin levels of 98 healthy women showed a strong inverse correla-tion with age, whereas there was no correlation with age in a wide age range of 110 breast cancer patients. The women whose cancers were in their earlier stages had prolactin levels that were significantly higher than those of the cor-responding control groups (p<0.001 in all cases, pre- and postmenopausal). In advanced breast cancer, however, ele-vated plasma prolactin concentrations were found only in the postmenopausal patients.

Recently, Wang et al. (1984) reported that prolactin levels were inversely related to parity in both pre- and postmenopausal women and that a life-long effect of reduced prolactin levels as a result of childbearing was implied because an average of 33 years had elapsed in their post-menopausal group since the birth of the last child.

Murphy et al. (1984) report that although hypophysectomy is of therapeutic benefit in some patients with
advanced breast cancer, agents that lower serum prolactin
are of little value, and this suggests that other pituitary
hormones may be important. Therefore, the effect of human
growth hormone and human prolactin was tested on two
cultured human breast cancer cell lines, T-470 and MCF-7,
with the conclusion that human growth hormone is a patent
ligand for the lactogenic hormone receptor in human breast
cancer cells and may be important in the pathogenesis,
growth, and metastasis of human breast cancer.

Henderson and Pike (1981) found little difference in
the plasma prolactin level of Catholic nuns and their nulliparous sisters, but sisters who were parous had lower
levels that were highly significant. Adjusting for possible
effects of age and weight did not significantly change the
differences in levels, which were 24% to 35% higher in
nulliparous over their parous sisters. Furthermore, the
levels were not significantly different in the parous women,
irrespective of the number of deliveries. However, Kwa et
al. (1981) found that the decrease in plasma prolactin at
parturition was transitory and rose with increasing time
after each delivery.

In summary, it is reported that in healthy women, prolactin levels decrease with age, that Catholic nuns have
higher levels than their parous sisters, that levels were
inversely related to parity, and that childbearing permanently lowered prolactin levels, but that agents which
lowered prolactin levels in breast cancer patients were
ineffective.

The effectiveness of cyclic hydrocarbons in mammary
tumorigenesis in rats is increased by prolactin (Nagasawa et
al., 1976; Yanai and Nagasawa, 1976). Nagasawa (1979) later
hypothesized that one of the functions of prolactin is to
create conditions in the mammary gland favorable to the
action of carcinogens via its stimulation of the rate of
mammary gland DNA synthesis. It is not presumed by Nagasawa
that prolactin is a carcinogen, but that it can prepare the
tissue for a carcinogen and act as a growth promoter. To
test this hypothesis, Nagasawa and Morii (1981) gave rats
daily s.c. injections of 0.5 mg of 2 bromo-alpha-
ergocryptine mesylate, a potent suppressor of pituitary prolactin secretion, beginning at 4 weeks of age and continuing
for 7 weeks. This treatment resulted in almost complete
prevention of mammary tumor appearance by 20 months of age:

only 1 in 30 rats developed mammary tumors vs 10 of 21 controls. However, treatment given between 11 and 18 weeks of age decreased the incidence to a lesser extent.

Progesterone deficiency is often associated with increased risk. Miller and Bulbrook (1980) suggested that estrogen action unopposed by progesterone during critical periods such as menarche and menopause may be a significant etiological factor. In a study of 400 breast cancer patients and 400 matched controls, Choi et al. (1978) found that the members of the breast cancer group were less fertile, and concluded that estrogenic stimulation without sufficient cyclic progestrone secretion may have provided a favorable setting for breast cancer. Tramier (1979) compared the etiology of breast and endometrial cancer and concluded that the contribution of endogenous and exogenous estrogens and the lack of progesterone were the most marked elements common to cancer development in both of these organs.

The effect of progesterone deficiency (PD) was evaluated by Cowan et al. (1981) on 1,083 women who were studied for involuntarily delayed first birth at the Lipid Research Clinic, Oklahoma City. After 13 to 33 years, those with endogenous PD had a risk of premenopausal breast cancer 5.4 times greater than those whose infertility was due to non-hormonal causes. This excess risk could not be explained by differences between the two groups in ages at menarche or menopause, history of oral contraceptive use or benign breast disease, or age at first birth. The incidence of postmenopausal breast cancer, however, did not differ significantly between the two groups, but deaths from all malignant neoplasms were ten-fold greater in the PD group than in the group whose infertility was nonhormonally caused.

Moore et al. (1982) reported that in premenopausal women the serum level of nonprotein bound estradiol (E2) was significantly higher in breast cancer patients than in matched controls, although the total serum concentrations of E2 were normal. These authors speculate that premenopausal women with breast cancer may have been exposed to elevated levels of biologically active E2.

In order to determine whether anovular menstrual cycles are responsible for the increased breast cancer risk sometimes associated with early menarche, MacMahon et al. (1982b) made pregnanediol measurements on 8-hr urine accumulations from 681 women aged 15 to 19 taken 11 to 3 days prior to onset of a subsequent menstrual period. A concentration <1 mg/l was taken as evidence of an anovular cycle. The probability of a cycle's being anovular was inversely (significantly) related to the numbers of years since menarche, and with years since menarche held constant, was positively (not significantly) associated with age at menarche. This observation was interpreted to indicate that women with early menarche do not have a longer duration of exposure to anovular cycles than those whose menarche is delayed, and that variation in the duration of exposure to postmenarcheal anovular cycles does not explain the association of breast cancer risk with early age of menarche. Anovular cycles were not more common in high-risk groups. Women in the lowest risk category had the highest proportion of anovular cycles.

According to Clark et al. (1983), the synthesis of progesterone receptors (PgR) is dependent on estrogen stimulation in normal reproductive tissue and in human breast cancer cell lines in culture. Estrogen receptors (ER) are predictive of improved patient survival and longer disease-free periods. Absence of ER manifestation may be due to nonfunctional ER or to absence of estrogen. However, survival in patients whose breast cancers were ER+ and PgR+ was much improved over those with ER+ and PgR-. The latter were almost as poor as those with ER- and PgR-. Also those with >50 fmol/mg PgR had a much better survival rate than those with 5-49 fmol/mg. Those with <5 fmol/mg had the worst survival rate.

Urine levels of estrone, estradiol, and pregnanediol were found by Trichopoulos et al. (1981) to be higher in 76 nulliparous daughters of breast cancer patients than in 115 matched daughters of non-breast cancer mothers. There was no difference in the estriol ratios (estriol/estrone+estradiol) of the two groups.

Trichopoulos et al. (1984) have compared urinary levels of estrone (E1) and estradiol (E2) in endogenous Chinese, Hawaiian Chinese, and American Chinese (Boston). The breast cancer rates of the Hawaiian Chinese were 3 times those of the endogenous Chinese, but 35% lower than those of Whites in Hawaii or on the mainland, while the American Chinese of Boston were the same as the Whites. Levels of E1 and E2 increased greatly from the low to the high risk groups. However, the decrease in estriol (E3) was more modest. These researchers conclude that the results are compatible

with the hypothesis that high levels of estrone and estradiol are important to breast cancer carcinogenesis; nevertheless, it has not been shown that the estriol quotient,
E3/E1+E2, is very helpful in selecting individual women at
high risk.

Use of conjugated estrogens was associated with a 40%
elevation in breast cancer risk in a study by Hoover et al.
(1981) of 345 women with breast cancer and 611 healthy controls. The relative risk rose to about 2.0 for women with
10 or more prescriptions, for those with 5 or more years
between their first and last prescription, and for those
with a usual daily dose of 1.25 mg or more. The RR associated with having ever used conjugated estrogen and with
long-term use was highest among those women with a family
history of breast cancer.

From these and many other reports, it seems that several of the endocrine hormones must be involved in synergistic actions among themselves and with other factors to
influence the manifestation of breast cancer. Prolactin,
growth hormone, and estrogen may, by increasing growth rate,
make cells more susceptible to carcinogens. After transformation, however, an incipient cancer may require many
years to become large enough to be recognized, with hormones
influencing its growth rate. Progesterone seems in some way
to interfere with those hormones promoting growth. Hormones
of the adrenal cortex, the pancreas, and the pineal gland,
among others, may also be involved.

Seasonal variation in breast cancer detection has
recently been reported by two groups of investigators
(Kirkham et al., 1985, and Mason et al., 1985), one located
in England and the other in New Zealand. Both found the
peak season to be late spring and early summer (June in
England and December in Australia). Kirkham et al. state
that the premenopausal age group accounted for almost all of
the seasonality. The New Zealand group found that the
cyclic trend was similar in patients above and below age 50,
but in the under-50 age group, the seasonal variation was
mainly restricted to those having progesterone receptor-
positive or estrogen receptor-positive tumors.

In a monograph on breast cancer etiology, Boyd (1984)
suggests that sexual conflict may be a significant factor.
Boyd has composed an instrument by which she may detect a
woman's attitude toward her body, her degree of satisfaction
with her sexual partners, and her ability to accept the way

becoming a woman has affected her life. These factors may possibly exert their influence through hormones and the immune system.

GROSS CYSTIC DISEASE

Breasts of premenopausal women frequently contain microscopic cysts of benign nature, but only those larger, macroscopically detectable will be considered here. Breasts containing cysts larger than 3 mm in diameter are defined by Haagensen et al. (1981) as affected by gross cystic disease. The etiology of these lesions is not understood, but their presence may increase the risk of breast cancer. A familial history of breast disease, exposure to X-rays, mastitis, and breast injury have been suggested as causative factors. The development of carcinoma in cystic breasts is usually slow (7-20 yr). According to Haagensen et al. (1978), it may take up to 25 years after diagnosis of gross cystic disease for a clinical carcinoma to develop. Ismailov and Bakhtina (1980) reported that dyshormonal hyperplasia and carcinomas developed in the majority of women 20 to 25 years after recording mastitis or breast injury, and DeSanso et al. (1980) found that the highest percentage of carcinomas occur 10 to 14 years after diagnosis of fibrocystic disease.

A synergy between cysts and family history has been reported by Dupont and Page (1985). They found that cysts alone do not substantially elevate risk of breast cancer, but women with both cysts and family history had a risk 2.7 times higher than women without either.

Black and Kwon (1980) concluded from a New York study that oral contraceptives favor the development of cancer in cystic diseased breasts in women whose grandmother and/or aunts had breast cancer, but impaired this evolution in women who had no family history of the disease.

It has been reported by Lees et al. (1978) that the relative risk of breast cancer is increased by use of oral contraceptives in women who have had prior breast biopsies, and it has been hypothesized by Fasal and Paffenbarger (1975) that pre-existing subclinical breast cancers may be promoted by oral contraceptives, but if the cysts were not already neoplastic, oral contraceptives did not increase risk.

Tokuhata (1969) has reported a marked increase in benign breast tumor and breast cancer in daughters of breast cancer women and has speculated on a causal relationship between benign and malignant breast tumors. Data on breast feeding give no indication of a milk-transmitted influence.

In a review of the literature, Boyd and Webber (1985) found 22 publications that reported an increase in risk in subjects with benign breast disease, 11 that reported no increase, and three that drew no conclusions. Boyd and Webber set up standards by which to judge the quality of the publications and concluded that the positive association studies met each of the standards more often than the negative and for eight of the fifteen standards, the difference was statistically significant.

DIET

Diet in all of its aspects may constitute one of the most significant factors in the etiology of breast cancer, yet it does not seem possible at present to select any high risk women in a population from their lifetime record of diet. Over-nutrition, high fat, and several vitamin and mineral deficiencies are most often accused of increasing risk. High family income and higher education have often been correlated with increased risk. Income and education may exert their influence through richer, more nutritious diets as well as delayed and decreased parity and possibly increased stress. Diet and other factors in several populations have been reviewed by Moore et al. (1983a, 1983b)

The breast cancer death rate in Japan has doubled in the last quarter century, and diet change has been considered as an important factor in this rapid increase (Hiriyama, 1978).

In the Beijing-Tianjin area of the Peoples Republic of China, the breast cancer death rate has risen from sixth place in the list of cancer death sites in 1963 to first place in 1983 (Dr. LiPing, Vice-director, Cancer Institute, Beijing, personal communication). Food production and distribution during the last 40 years has markedly improved, and life expectancy has increased from under 40 years to more than 60 years. There seems to be little question that high nutrition in populations correlate with breast cancer death rate, but selecting high risk individuals via diet records is not yet feasible.

Consumption of methylxanthine (in coffee, tea, chocolate, etc.) has been reported to increase risk of fibrocystic diseases (Minton et al., 1979; Minton et al., 1981), but these reports of fibrocystic disease have been criticized by Heyden (1980) on the grounds that clinically palpable breast cysts are known to wax and wane, and on the grounds that the number of patients involved in some of the findings was not specified. Also criticized was the referral to epidemiologic findings of the low incidence of breast cancer among Mormons and Seventh Day Adventists who abstain from drinking coffee and tea, because other factors in their lifestyle were not accounted for in the reports (Ernster et al., 1982).

Obesity may be an influential factor, especially in the postmenopausal disease. Many publications have given support to the view that being overweight increases risk, and a lesser number report no effect (Moore et al., 1983b). De Waard et al. (1981), in a survey of 23,500 women (258 were breast cancer patients) over 50 years of age, found evidence that obesity promotes but does not initiate cancerous growth. Tests for estrogen receptors were made on 180 of the patients, and 117 were positive. The authors conclude that the effect of overweight and obesity is extra-ovarian, probably mediated through a menopausal extra-ovarian estrogen mechanism and that weight reduction could probably be a means of controlling some breast cancers in their preclinical stages.

Frisch and MacArthur (1974), Murayama (1983), and many others have found evidence that fatness may be a factor also in premenopausal breast cancer.

ACKNOWLEDGMENT

This review was supported in part by the American Cancer Society Research Professors Grant #RDP-34.

SUMMARY

Relative risk values depend on many factors and combinations of factors, many of them probably unknown or uninvestigated. It is, therefore, difficult to assign numerical values to specific items of risk. However, for convenience, the following list is given.

	Nominal relative risk values
Family history plus menstrual activity in excess of 37 years.	12
Family history (grandmother or aunt) in combination with use of oral contraceptives.	2.7 - 4.9
Use of oral contraceptives by family-history negative women.	0.4 - 0.58
Family history in combination with higher education (China).	8
Mother-associated history increases risk of pre- and perimenopausal breast cancer of the medullary type.	>1
Sister-associated history increases risk of postmenopausal breast cancer of the lobular type.	>1
Breast cancer in one breast increases risk for a second primary in the contralateral breast according to age at first diagnosis:	
For ages 15-34	5.3
35-59	3.3
>60	1.5
Dysplastic cells in breast fluid aspirates	6 - 8
Wet-type cerumen	>1
Dermatoglyphic patterns:	
Composite accidentals	>1
6 or more whorls on 10 fingers	>1
Age at menarche: over 15 yrs.	0.88
under 15 yrs.	little effect
Age at first birth <20 yrs.	1
Age at first birth >20 yrs.	increases with age
for premenopausal breast cancer	>2.7
for postmenopausal breast cancer	>2.7
Parity greater than 4:	
premenopausal breast cancer	>1
postmenopausal breast cancer	<1
Childbirth after age 35 yrs.	>1
(Late childbearing nullifies effect of early childbearing.)	
Two births before age 25 yrs. may confer considerable decrease in risk.	0.18
Early menopause decreases risk.	0.4
Late menopause increases risk.	1.3
Normal menopause (age 45-49 yrs.)	1.0

	Nominal relative risk values
High levels of plasma prolactin	>1
Low levels of plasma progesterone	>1
High levels of estradiol (E2)	>1
Conjugated estrogen use	>1

ABSTRACT

Risk of breast cancer depends on synergistic actions among many factors. A review of the recent literature shows that any single factor does not greatly increase or decrease risk, but a combination of certain factors may yield relative risks in excess of the summation of individual relative risk values. Furthermore, a risk factor may in one situation increase risk, while in another, it may decrease risk. Family history or heritage seems to be a most important factor. A history of breast cancer in first- or second-degree relatives in combination with certain other factors can in some cases greatly increase risk. Second-degree relatives may have a greater influence than first degree when combined with other influencing factors, such as use of oral contraceptives. A combination of family history and higher education greatly increased risk in some populations. The early life, particularly the period around menarche, seems to be especially amenable to influences that affect breast cancer. At that time, the breast seems to be especially sensitive to radiation and probably to stressful events such as hospitalization and to dietary factors such as overnutrition and to chemical mutagens, carcinogens, and pollutants. The overt manifestation of these neoplasms may require a half-lifetime or more, depending on other synergistic events that influence tumor growth rate. Dysplastic epithelial cells in nipple fluid aspirates, wet cerumen, and specific dermatoglyphic patterns may sometimes be associated with high risk. An early full-term pregnancy may decrease risk of postmenopausal, but increases risk of premenopausal, breast cancer. Multiple early births may further increase risk of early cancer, and a delivery after age 35 increases risk. Unmarried women have a lower premenopausal rate but a higher postmenopausal rate. A late menopause increases risk. A high blood level of prolactin and/or nonprotein-bound estrogen and a low level of progesterone are associated with increased risk. Overnutrition, high fat diet, and obesity have often been associated with increased risk, but it is difficult to select high-risk individuals from diet records.

REFERENCES

Adami, H.O., Rimsten, A., Stenkvist, B., Vegelius, J. Reproductive history and risk of breast cancer. A case-control study in an unselected Swedish population. Cancer 41:747-757, 1978.

Adami, H.O., Hansen, J., Jung, B., Rimsten, A. Characteristics of familial breast cancer in Sweden: Absence of relation to age and unilateral versus bilateral disease. Cancer 48:1688-1695, 1981.

Alderson, M. Parity and breast cancer. British Med. J. 283:9-10, 1981.

Basco, V.E., Coldman, A.J., Elwood, J.M., Young, M.E. Radiation dose and second breast cancer. Br. J. Cancer 52:319-325, 1985.

Becker, D., Lane, M.A., Cooper, G.M. Identification of an antigen associated with transforming genes of human and mouse mammary carcinomas. Proc. Natl. Acad. Sci. USA 79:3315-3319, 1982.

Bierman, H.R., Faith, M.R., Hammarstedt, P., Holmes, B. Prediction of susceptibility to mammary carcinoma by dermatoglyphic patterns. Proc. Am. Assoc. Cancer Res. 20:109, 1979.

Black, M.M., Kwon, S. Precancerous mastopathy: Structural and biological considerations. Pathol. Res. Pract. 166:491-514, 1980.

Black, M.M., Barclay, T.H.C., Polednak, A., Kwon, C.S., Leis, H.P. Jr., Pilnik, S. Family history, oral contraceptive usage, and breast cancer. Cancer 51:2147-51, 1983.

Boyd, N.F., Webber, W. A critique of the methodology used by studies investigating breast cancer risk in benign breast disease (Meeting abstract). Biennial Int. Breast Cancer Res. Conf., 1985. Imperial Cancer Research Fund, p. 221.

Boyd, P. The Silent Wound. Addison-Wesley Publishing Co., Reading, Mass., 1984; pp. 1-179.

Choi, N.W., Howe, G.R., Miller, A.B., Matthews, V., Morgan, R.W., Munan, L., Burch, J.D., Feather, J., Jain, M., Kelly, A. An epidemiologic study of breast cancer. Am. J. Epidemiol. 107:510-521, 1978.

Ciambellotti, E., Moro, G., Lanza, E., Coda, C., Cartia,
     G.L. Lung cancers synchronous and metachronous with
     primary malignant neoplasms in other sites. Minerva
     Med. 76:1693-1697, 1985.
Clark, G.M., McGuire, W.L., Hubay, C.A., Pearson, O.F.,
     Marshall, J.S. Progesterone receptors as a prognostic
     factor in stage II breast cancer. New England J. Med.
     309:1343-1347, 1983.
Cooper, G.M. Cellular transforming genes. Science
     217:801-806, 1982.
Cowan, L.D., Gordis, L., Tonascia, J.A., Seegar, A.,
     Jones, G. Breast cancer incidence in women with a
     history of progesterone deficiency. Am. J. Epidemiol.
     114:209-217, 1981.
DeSanso, G., Ferraiis, E., Crovella, U. Mastopathy:
     Etiopathogenetic indications for medical treatment.
     Minerva Chir. 35:177-182, 1980.
deWaard, F., Poortman, J., Collette, B.J. Relationship of
     weight to the promotion of breast cancer after
     menopause. Nutr. Cancer 2:237-240, 1981.
Dupont, W.D., Rogers, L.W., Vander Zwaag, R., Page, D.L.
     The epidemiologic study of anatomic markers for
     increased risk of mammary carcinoma. Pathol. Res.
     Pract. 166:471-480, 1980.
Dupont, W.D., Page, D.L. Risk factors for breast cancer in
     women with proliferative breast disease. New Engl. J.
     Med. 312:146-151, 1985.
Ernster, V.L., Mason, L., Goodson, W.H. III, Sickles, E.A.,
     Sacks, S.T., Selvin, S., Dupuy, M.E., Hawkinson, J.,
     Hunt, T.K. Effect of caffeine-free diet on benign
     breast disease: A randomized trial. Surgery
     91:263-267, 1982.
Fasal, E., Paffenbarger, R.S. Oral contraceptives as
     related to cancer and benign lesions of the breast. J.
     Natl. Cancer Inst. 55:767-773, 1975.
Frisch, R.E., MacArthur, J.W. Menstrual cycles: Fatness as
     a determinant of minimum weight necessary for their
     maintenance and onset. Science 185:949-951, 1974.
Gershon-Cohen, J., Ingleby, H. The rate of growth and
     progression in three principal types of breast cancer.
     Acta Un. Int. Contra Cancrum 15:1093-1096, 1959.
Haagensen, C.D., Lane, N., Lattes, R., Bodian, C. Lobular
     neoplasia (so-called lobular carcinoma in situ) of the
     breast. Cancer 42:737-769, 1978.
Haagensen, C.D., Bodian, C., Haagensen, Jr., D.E. Breast
     Carcinoma. Risk and Detection. W.B. Saunders Co.,
     Philadelphia, Pa., 1981.
Hardy, E.E., Pinotti, J.A., Brenelli, H.B., and Faudes, A.
     Risk factors of breast cancer in postmenopausal and

premenopausal women in Campinas, Brazil. In: New Frontiers in Mammary Pathology, Vol. 2 (K.H. Hollman and J.M. Verley, Eds.) Plenum Press, New York, 1983, pp. 85-98.

Helmrich, S.P., Shapiro, S., Rounberg, L., Kaufman, D.W., Slone, D., Bain, C., Mietlinen, O., Stolley, P.D., Rosenshien, N.B., Knapp, R.C., Leavitt, T. Jr., Schollenfeld, D., Engle, R. Jr., Levy, M. Risk factors for breast cancer. Amer. J.. Epidem. 117:35-45, 1983.

Henderson, B.E., Pike, M.C. Prolactin--an important hormone in breast neoplasia? In: Banbury Report 8. Hormones and Breast Cancer. (M.C. Pike, P.K. Siiteri, C.W. Welsch, Eds.) Cold Spring Harbor Laboratory, 1981. pp. 115-130.

Heyden, S. Coffee and fibrocystic breast disease. Surgery 88:741-742, 1980.

Hiriyama, T. The epidemiology of breast cancer with special reference to the role of diet. Prevent. Med. 7:173-195, 1978.

Hoover, R., Glase, A., Finkle, W.D., Azevedo, D., Milne, K. Conjugated estrogens and breast cancer risk in women. J. Natl. Cancer Inst. 67:815-820, 1981.

Howe, G.R., Sherman, G.J., Malhotra, A. Correlations between cancer incidence rates from the Canadian National Cancer Incidence Reporting System, 1969-78. J. Natl. Cancer Inst. 72:585-591, 1984.

Hunt, S.C., Williams, R.R., Skolnick, M.H., Lyon, J.L., Smart, C.R. Breast cancer and reproductive history from genealogical data. J. Natl. Cancer Inst. 64:1047-1053, 1980.

Ismailov, AKh., Bakhtina, N.N. Role of mastitis and injury in the genesis of dyshormonal diseases and mammary carcinoma. Khirurgiia (Mosk) 10:8-10, 1980.

Janerich, D.T. Pregnancy, breast-cancer risk, and maternal-fetal genetics (Letter to the Editor). Lancet 1:1240-1241, 1979.

Janerich, D.T., Hoff, M.B. Evidence for a crossover in breast cancer risk factors. Amer. J. Epidemiol. 166:737-742, 1982.

Juret, P., Couette, J.E., Brune, D., Vernhes, J.C. Parous women present breast cancer at significantly earlier age. Eur. J. Cancer 10:591-594, 1974.

Juret, P., Couette, J.E., Brune, D., Vernhes, J.C. Age at Menarche and Age at First Delivery as Prognostic Factors in Breast Cancer. In: Proc. Int. Symp Detect. Prev. Cancer Vol. 2, 1980; pp. 1539-1549.

Kirkham, N., Machin, D., Cotton, D.W., Pike, J.M. Seasonality and breast cancer. Eur. J. Surg. Oncol. 11:143-146, 1985.

Kwa, H.G., Cleton, F., Bulbrook, R.D., Wang, D.Y., Hayward, J.L. Plasma prolactin levels and breast cancer: Relation to parity, weight and height, and age at first birth. Int. J. Cancer 28:31-34, 1981.

Lane, M-A., Santen, A., Cooper, G.M. Activation of related transforming genes in mouse and human mammary carcinomas. Proc. Natl. Acad. Sci. USA 78:5185-5189, 1981.

Lees, A.W., Burns, P.E., Grace, M. Oral contraceptives and breast disease in premenopausal Northern Albertan women. Int. J. Cancer 22:700-707, 1978.

Levitt, S.H., Mandel, J. Breast irradiation and future risk of carcinogenesis. Front. Radiat. Ther. Oncol. 17:131-142. 1983;

Lilienfeld, A.M. The epidemiology of breast cancer. Cancer Res. 23:1503-1513, 1963.

Lipnick, R., Speizer, F.E., Bain, C., Willett, W., Rosner, B., Stamfer, M.J., Belanger, C., Hennekens, C.H. A case-control study of risk indicators among women with premenopausal and early postmenopausal breast cancer. Cancer 53:1020-1024, 1984.

Lynch, H.T., Fairn, P.R., Albano, W.A., Tuma, T., Block, L., Lynch, J., Shomka, M. Genetic/epidemiological findings in a study of smoking-associated tumors. Cancer Genet. Cytogenet. 6:163-169, 1982.

Lynch, H.T., Albano, W.A., Layton, M.A., Kimberling, W.J., Lynch, J.F. Breast cancer, genetics, and age at first pregnancy. J. Med. Genet. 21:96-98, 1984.

Macera, C., Leung, R., King, M.C. Comparison of risk factors associated with familial and nonfamilial breast cancer. (Meeting abstract) Amer. J. Epidemiol. 116:563, 1982.

MacMahon, B., Cole, P., Lin, T.M., Lowe, C.R., Mirra, A.P., Ravnihar, B., Salber, E.J., Valaoras, V.G., and Yuasa, S. Age at first birth and breast cancer risk. Bull. World Health Org. 43:209-221, 1970.

MacMahon, B., Cole, P., Brown, J. Etiology of human breast cancer: A review. J. Natl. Cancer Inst. 50:21-42, 1973.

MacMahon, B., Purde, P., Cramer, D., Hint, E. Association of breast cancer risk with age at first and subsequent births: A study in the population of the Estonian Republic. J. Natl. Cancer Inst. 69:1035-1038, 1982a.

MacMahon, B., Trichopoulos, D., Brown, J., Anderson, A., Aoki, K., Cole, P., deWaard, F., Kauraniemi, T., Morgan, R.W., Purde, M., Ravnihar, B., Stormby, N., Westlund, K., Woo, N.C. Age at menarche, probability of ovulation and breast cancer risk. Int. J. Cancer 29:13-16, 1982b.

Mason, B.H., Holdaway, I.H., Mullins, P.R., Kay, R.G., Gillman, J.C. Seasonal variation in breast cancer detection: Correlation with tumor progesterone receptor status (Meeting abstract). Biennial Int. Breast Cancer Res. Conf., 1985, Imperial Cancer Research Fund, p. 95.

Meyer, K.K., Gelman, R.S. Increased risk of malignancy and uterine disease following perimenarchal hospitalization. Surgery 94:548-553, 1983.

Miller, A.B., Bulbrook, R.D. The epidemiology and etiology of breast cancer. New England J. Med. 303:1246-1248, 1980.

Miller, R.W. Radiation effects: Highlights of a meeting. J. Pediatr. 101:887-888, 1982.

Minton, J.P., Foecking, M.K., Webster, D.J.T., Matthews, R.A. Response of fibrocystic disease to caffeine withdrawal and correlation of cystic nucleotides with breast disease. Amer. J. Obstet. Gynecol. 135:157-158, 1979.

Minton, J.P., Abou Issa, H., Reiches, N., Roseman, J.M. Clinical and biochemical studies on methylxanthine-related fibrocystic breast disease. Surgery 90:299-304, 1981.

Moore, D.H., Moore, D.H.II, Moore, C.T. Breast carcinoma etiological factors. In: Advances in Cancer Research, Vol. 40. Academic Press, Inc., 1983a. pp. 189-253.

Moore, D.H., Moore, C.T., Moore, D.H.II. Factors implicated in breast cancer risk. In: New Frontiers in Mammary Pathology, Vol. 2 (K.H Hollman and J.M. Verley, eds.) Plenum Publishing Corp., 1983b. pp. 29-84.

Moore, J.W., Clark, G.M., Bulbrook, R.D., Hayward, J.L., Murai, J.T., Hammond, G.L., Siiteri, P.K. Serum concentration of total and nonprotein-bound oestradiol in patients with breast cancer and normal controls. Int. J. Cancer 29:17-21, 1982.

Murayama, Y. Plasma sex hormone binding globulin (SHBG) and obesity in breast cancer patients. Cancer Detect. Prev. 6:425-433, 1983.

Murphy, L.J., Vrhovsek, E., Sutherland, R.L., Lazarus, L. Growth hormone binding to cultured human breast cancer cells. J. Clin. Endocrinol. Metab. 58:149-156, 1984.

Murray, M.J., Shilo, B.-Z., Shih, C., Cowing, D., Hsu, H.W., Weinberg, R.A. Three different human tumor cell lines contain different oncogenes. Cell 25:355-361, 1981.

Nagasawa, H., Yanai, R., Taniguchi, H. Importance of mammary DNA synthesis on carcinogen-induced mammary tumorigenesis in rats. Cancer Res. 36:2223-2226, 1976.

Nagasawa, H. Prolactin: Its role in the development of mammary tumors. Medical Hypothesis 5:1117-1121, 1979.

Nagasawa, H., Morii, S. Prophylaxis of spontaneous mammary tumorigenesis by temporal inhibition of prolactin secretion in rats at young age. Cancer Res. 41:1935-1937, 1981.

Najem, G.R., Rush, B.E., Miller, F.W., Dimarco, P.E., Roellke, S.E., Grobstein, N., Levitt, J.W. Pre- and postmenopausal breast cancer. Prev. Med. 11:281-290, 1982.

Paffenbarger, R.S., Kampert, J.B., Chang, H.G. Characteristics that predict risk of breast cancer before and after the menopause. Am. J. Epidemiol. 112:258-268, 1980.

Papatestas, A. E., Bramis, J., Aufses, A.H. Serum immunoglobulins in women with breast cancer. J. Surg. Oncol. 12:155-163, 1979.

Papatestas, A. E., Panveliwalla, D., Pertsembidis, D., Mulvihill, M., Aufses, A.H. Association between estrogen receptors and weight in women with breast cancer. J. Surg. Oncol. 13:177-180, 1980.

Petrakis, N.L. Cerumen phenotype and epithelial dysplasia in nipple aspirates of breast fluids. Amer. J. Anthropol. 62:115-118, 1983.

Prior, P., Waterhouse, J.A. The incidence of bilateral breast cancer: II. A proposed model for the analysis of coincidental tumors. Br. J. Cancer 43:615-622, 1981a.

Prior, P., Waterhouse, J.A. Multiple primary cancers of breast and cervix uteri: An epidemiological approach to analysis. Br. J. Cancer 43:623-631, 1981b.

Ron, E., Curtis, R., Hoffman, D.A., Flannery, J.T. Multiple primary breast and thyroid cancer. Br. J. Cancer 49:87-92, 1984.

Rose, D.P., Pruitt, B.T. Plasma prolactin levels in patients with breast cancer. Cancer 48:2687-2691, 1981.

Rosen, P.P., Lesser, M.L., Siene, R.T., Kinne, D.W. Epidemiology of breast carcinoma. III. Relationship of family history to tumor type. Cancer 50:171-179, 1982.

Ross, M.H., Bras, G. Lasting influence of early caloric restriction on prevalence of neoplasms in the rat. J. Natl. Cancer Inst. 47:1095-1113, 1971.

Ross, M.H., Lustbader, E.D., Bras, G. Dietary practices of early life and spontaneous tumors of the rat. Nutrition and Cancer 3:150-167, 1982.

Schwartz, A.G., King, M.C., Belle, S.H., Satariano, W.A., Swanson, G.M. Risk of breast cancer to relatives of young breast cancer patients. J. Natl. Cancer Inst. 75:665-668, 1985.

Seltzer, M.H., Plato, C.C., Engler, P.E., Fletcher, H.S.
Digital dermatoglyphics and breast cancer. Breast
Cancer Res. Treat. 2:261-265, 1982.

Staszewski, J. Age at menarche and breast cancer. J. Natl.
Cancer Inst. 47:935-940, 1971.

Stavraky, K., Emmons, S. Breast cancer in premenopausal and
postmenopausal women. J. Natl. Cancer Inst.
53:647-654, 1974.

Tabbane, F., el May, A., Hachiche, M., Bahi, J., Jaziri, M.,
Cammoun, M., Mourali, N. Breast Cancer Res. Treat.
6:137-144, 1985.

Tokuhata, G.K. Morbidity and mortality among offspring of
breast cancer mothers. Amer. J. Epidemiology
89:129-153, 1969.

Tokunaga, M., Norman, J.E., Asano, M., Tokuoka, S., Ezaki,
H., Nishimore, I., Tsuji, Y. Malignant breast tumors
among atomic bomb survivors, Hiroshima and Nagasaki,
1950-74. J. Natl. Cancer Inst. 62:1347-1359, 1979.

Tramier, D. Cancer of the endometrium. The evaluation of
high risk cases. J. Gynecol. Obstet. Biol. Reprod.
(Paris) 8:223-228, 1979.

Trichopoulos, D., Brown, J.B., Garas, J., Papaioannou, A.,
MacMahon, B. Elevated urine estrogen and pregnanediol
levels in daughters of breast cancer patients. J.
Natl. Cancer Inst. 67:603-606, 1981.

Trichopoulos, D., Hsieh, C.C., MacMahon, B., Lin, T.M.,
Lowe, C.R., Mirra, A.P., Ravnihar, B., Salber, E.J.,
Valaoras, V.G., Yuasa, S. Age at any birth and breast
cancer risk. Int. J. Cancer 31:701-704, 1983.

Trichopoulos, D., Yen, S., Brown, J., Cole, P., MacMahon, B.
The effect of Westernization on urine estrogens,
frequency of ovulation, and breast cancer risk. Study
of ethnic Chinese women in the Orient and the U.S.A.
Cancer 53:187-192, 1984.

Wang, D.Y., Sturzaker, H.E., Kwa, H.G., Verhofstad, F.,
Hayward, J.L., Bulbrook, R.D. Nyctohemeral changes in
plasma prolactin levels and their relationship to
breast cancer risk. Int. J. Cancer 33:629-632, 1984.

Wang, D.Y., Rubens, R.D., Allen, D.S., Millis, R.R., Bulbrook, R.D., Chaudary, M.C., Hayward, J.L. The effect
of breast cancer risk factors on age at onset of disease (Meeting abstract). Biennial Int. Breast Cancer
Res. Conf., 1985, Imperial Cancer Research Fund,
p. 107.

Waterhouse, J.A., Muir, C., Shanmugaratnam, K., Powell, J.
Cancer Incidence in Five Continents. Vol. IV. International Agency for Research on Cancer, Lyons, France,
1982.

Wolfe, J.N. Breast patterns as an index of risk for developing breast cancer. Am. J. Roentgenol. 126:1130-1139,
1976.

Wolke, A.M., Schaffner, F., Kapelman, B., Sacks, H.S.
Malignancy in primary biliary cirrhosis. High incidence of breast cancer in affected women. Am. J. Med.
76:1075-1078, 1984.

Woods, K.L., Smith, S.R., Morrison, J.M. Parity and breast
cancer: Evidence for a dual effect. Br. Med. J.
281:419-421, 1980.

Yanai, R., Nagasawa, H.J. Effects of pituitary grafts and
2-bromo-α-ergocryptine on DNA synthesis in relation to
mammary tumorigenesis. J. Natl. Cancer Inst.
56:1055-1056, 1976.

Zhang, A.Y., Ma, F.G., Ma, S.M., Geng, G.Y., Jin, X.Z. Risk
factors associated with development of female breast
cancer in Tianjin. (Meeting abstract). International
Assoc. for Breast Cancer Research, Mar. 20-24, 1983.
Denver, Colorado.

FAMILIAL HETEROGENEITY OF BREAST CANCER RISK

Henry T. Lynch,[1] William J. Kimberling,[2] and Jane F. Lynch[1]

1. Department of Preventive Medicine/Public Health,
    Creighton University School of Medicine, and the
    Hereditary Cancer Institute, Omaha, Nebraska 68178, USA
2. Department of Otolaryngology, Boystown National Institute
    for Hearing and Speech Disorders in Children, and The
    Hereditary Cancer Institute, Omaha, Nebraska 68178, USA

INTRODUCTION

The family history is one of the most neglected aspects in the workup of cancer patients. This is paradoxical in that familial breast cancer, characterized by early age at onset, excess of bilaterality, and tumor heterogeneity, poses a significant public health problem in much of the world. It is therefore surprising that screening strategies for breast cancer often ignore this fact in that they are almost invariably based upon general population age-adjusted rates for this disease, with more or less arbitrary guidelines for their initiation somewhere between ages 40 and 50 years (Lynch, 1981a).

Perhaps more attention would be given to familial breast cancer risk if physicians had a better appreciation of its magnitude in the general population. There is abundant literature dealing with descriptive phenomena about the natural history of familial breast cancer; i.e., its tumor heterogeneity, autosomal dominant mode of genetic transmission (Lynch, 1981a), and empirical risk estimates (Anderson and Badzioch, 1985a and b), but in contrast, there is only a paucity of information dealing with its incidence among breast cancer affected individuals (Lynch et al, 1981b, 1984).

Our purpose was to study family histories of cancer among a series of consecutively ascertained breast cancer probands, with attention to its heterogeneity, the influence of age at onset and histology, and its interaction with several common environmental factors (smoking, alcohol, and caffeine consumption). This was performed in concert with its occurrence in context with cancers of differing anatomic sites, as found in a cohort of cancer patients analyzed under similar conditions, so that relatively unbiased internal comparison of the respective parameters could be critically evaluated.

METHODS

Over the past 5 years, we have ascertained 1777 patients with histologically verified cancer at any site who were being treated in oncology clinics at two Omaha medical schools. The sample used in the analysis for this report included 1056 patients whose family histories have been computerized. The distribution of these 1056 cancers is given in Table 1 and includes all cases of smoking related cancers, all cases of colon and ovarian cancers, and over one-half of the breast cancer families ascertained in this series. The number of families analyzed in the permutation test was less than that shown in Table 1. Since the permutation test (discussed below) was sensitive for family size, any families with 2 or fewer female primary relatives were not incorporated in the analysis. All families, regardless of size, were evaluated to estimate lifetime risk. All analyses were limited to primary family members.

Cancer	Number of Families
Lung	256
Bladder	49
Larynx	34
Colon	182
Breast	283
Ovary	38
Other	
Lip	5
Palate	5
Sinus	4
Tonsil	11
Epiglottis	1
Mouth	16
Nasopharynx	5
Pharynx	13
Esophagus	21
Tongue	19
Throat	2
Prostate	20
Cervix	1
Uterus	2
Skin	9
Kidney	3
Leukemia	5
Hodgkins lymphoma	1
NonHodgkins lymphoma	12
Thyroid	3
Parotid	4
Penis	1
Appendix	1
Anus	1
Other nonspecified	4

Table 1. Distribution of 1056 cancers, including all smoking related cancers, all colon and ovarian cancers, and more than one-half of breast cancers in this series.

Each patient was interviewed in a standardized manner by a trained interviewer. Next of kin were also interviewed when they accompanied the patient. Detailed information was obtained on general medical and cancer history for first and second degree relatives. Detailed questionnaires were sent to these relatives. 4.8% of all living primary relatives returned a questionnaire, while 9.8% of all living second degree relatives (grandparents, aunts, uncles) returned a questionnaire. Every attempt was made to verify cancer status in relatives. Pathology confirmation was vigorously sought in relatives of each proband. Death certificates were utilized only when all other methods for documentation had been exhausted. Of all relatives with cancer, 45.3% were verified through pathologic report, 16.2% through death certificates, and the remainder were taken as affected on the basis of family report. All probands were interviewed personally, as were 5% of their primary relatives. Data was entered into the Medical Genetics Acquisition and Data Transfer (MEGADATS) System (Gersting, 1976).

We determined the cumulative risk in primary relatives by the formula

$$\text{Risk} = R_t = \prod_{i=0}^{t} (1-q_i)$$

$$\text{where } q_i = x_i/m_i - \sum_{j=1}^{w_i} y_{ij}/10$$

(x_i = number of persons with cancer in the ith decade of life; m_i = number of persons under observation and unaffected at the beginning of the ith decade; w_i = number of individuals during the ith decade; y_{ij} = number of years remaining in the ith decade for the jth withdrawal) (Kalvin et al, 1985).

The permutation test evaluates whether the hypothesis that empiric cancer probabilities, estimated from the sample, are homogeneous and independent of family membership. Rejection of this null hypothesis is evidence for the presence in the sample of families at a distinctly higher risk for the specific cancer. Details for the use of this approach to detect heterogeneity of genetic risk are described elsewhere (Lynch et al, 1981b; Kalvin et al, 1985).

The combination of these two tests - risk analysis and permutation analysis - allowed the evaluation of two questions: 1) what is the magnitude of breast cancer in relatives?; and 2) is the risk heterogeneous between families? Answers to these two questions would further our understanding about any underlying familial liability, and if an underlying liability is found, allow preliminary assessment of whether or not it is qualitative and therefore megaphenic.

RESULTS

Table 2 shows the results of the analyses of breast cancer in relatives by cancer type in the proband. Families of breast cancer probandds showed significant heterogeneity with regard to breast cancer risk. A lifetime risk for breast cancer (through age 80) of 11% was observed in the primary relatives of breast cancer probands. The

Cancer	N	Permutation Test		Families with P(z) < 0.05		Cumulative Risk to Age 80 (N=1056 families)
		s2	P	N	%	
Colorectal	131	0.81	.92	2	1.53	0.04
Lung	168	1.21	.21	3	1.78	0.07
Pancreas	30	0.81	.96	0	0.0	0.01
Bladder	33	0.88	.91	0	0.0	0.02
Larynx	21	1.74	.14	1	4.76	0.08
Ovary	24	2.79	.05	1	4.18	0.10
Breast	206	1.51	.02	12	5.82	0.11
Other	127	0.91	.81	1	0.79	0.04
TOTAL	740	1.24	.01	20	2.70	0.07
Nonbreast	534	1.13	.19	8	1.50	0.06

Table 2. Proportion of families showing significantly elevated Z scores

other group showing significant heterogeneity for breast cancer in primary relatives were those families ascertained through an ovarian carcinoma proband. While the ovarian cancer families showed a lifetime risk of 10% for breast cancer among primary relatives, this was not significantly elevated over the other nonbreast cancer groups. Heterogeneity of breast cancer in relatives of families ascertained through nonbreast cancer probands was not significant. The cumulative lifetime breast cancer risk for this group was estimated at 6%.

Also shown in Table 2 is the proportion of families in each group that showed a significantly elevated (p < 0.05) Z score. 5.8% of the families of breast cancer probands had significantly elevated Z scores, whereas only 1.5% of the nonbreast cancer group were in the same category. This is a highly significant difference (p < 0.05).

Analysis of age at onset in the breast cancer probands is provided in Figure 1. There was a highly significant relationship between mean Z score and its variance with age at diagnosis of breast cancer in the proband. A negative correlation in both cases is observed graphically in Figure 1, where both variance and mean are shown to decrease with increasing age.

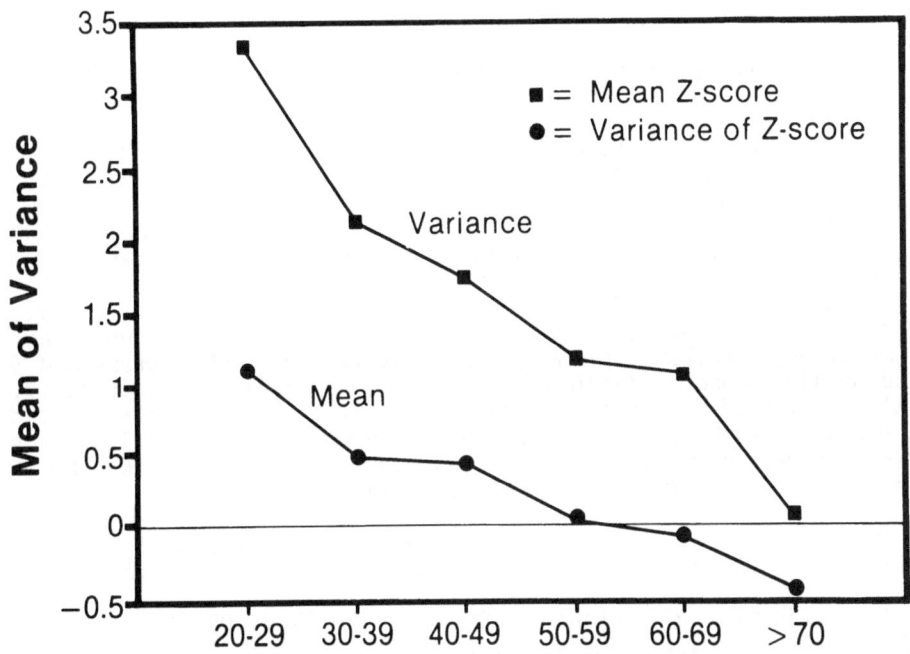

Figure 1. Means and variances of Z scores by age at diagnosis of proband. These results show a negative regression of both parameters with age indicating both greater heterogeneity and risk in the families of early breast cancer onset probands. Z scores measure the deviation of actual number of cancers from expected.

There was no effect of family size on mean Z score or its variance when the analysis was limited to families with three or more female relatives. There was no relationship observed between the number of primary cancers and mean Z score, its variance, or cumulative risk.

Heterogeneity of the Z score was analyzed in relation to three environmental parameters in the proband; namely, smoking, alcohol, and caffeine use (Table 3). In all three cases, there was no significant effect on mean Z score or breast cancer risk. While we did not find any significant difference with respect to variance for smoking and caffeine use, we did observe a significantly increased variance among families of probands who used alcohol.

Proband		YES	NO	F	df	
Smoking	Z score	0.025	-0.138	0.75	1,114	NS
	variance	1.184	0.854	1.39	52,64	NS
Alcohol	Z score	0.096	-0.179	2.15	1,114	NS
	variance	1.344	0.741	1.81	48,68	$P < 0.05$
Caffeine	Z score	-0.036	-0.125	0.20	1,114	NS
	variance	1.124	0.761	1.48	78,38	NS

Table 3. Heterogeneity in relation to three environmental parameters.

A similar analysis was also performed with respect to histology of breast cancer in the probands (Table 4). We did not observe any significant difference between the groups for mean Z score. We did, however, observe heterogeneity of the Z score variances. The histologic category, which included medullary (6 cases), lobular (3 cases), and papillary (5 cases) carcinoma of the breast, showed significantly increased variance. The number of families with significant Z scores was 2.7%, 3.4%, and 14.3% for adenocarcinoma, ductal, and other (medullary, lobular, papillary), respectively. It is of interest that 5 out of the 38 unclassifiable histologic breast cancer types, or 13.2%, also had a significant Z score. In the medullary, lobular, and papillary breast carcinoma group, of the two significant families which we observed, both were of the medullary type. Thus, 2 out of 6 (33%) of medullary carcinomas had a significantly elevated Z score.

Histologic Type	N	z	Sz	Families with $P(z) < 0.05$ N	%	Risk to Age 80
Adenocarcinoma	37	-0.075	0.85	1	2.70	0.08
Ductal	117	0.031	1.30	4	3.42	0.09
Other*	14	0.048	2.50	2	14.29	0.15
TOTAL	168					

*Other includes 6 cases of medullary, 3 cases of lobular, and 1 case of papillary carcinoma of the breast.

Table 4. Analysis with respect to histology of breast cancer in probands.

DISCUSSION

Familial clustering of breast cancer had been recognized in the Roman medical literature since 100 A.D. (Lynch, 1981a). In spite of this long historical experience, surprisingly little knowledge has emerged with respect to its biological significance and its frequency in the general population. Elucidation of fundamental pathogenetic phenomena which might be modulating its distinctive natural history when compared to its sporadic counterpart should be given high priority. Problems which clearly confound the search for those oncogenic events, both genetic and environmental, are the very common occurrence of breast cancer, its heterogeneity, particularly with respect to the potential for differing tumor combinations in certain breast cancer-prone families, and the present lack of any consistent biomarker(s) which have high sensitivity and specificity to breast cancer-prone genotype(s).

The search for biomarkers must be intensified, and should include the investigation of potential oncogenes and the mechanisms of their amplification in order to further elucidate etiology and carcinogenesis. Cancer-prone families have a powerful potential for the development of hypotheses for achieving some of the above objectives. With this in mind, Mulvihill recently stated (1985) "...clinicians can contribute to the national goal of reducing mortality from cancer by 50% by the year 2000 by asking each patient with or without cancer about his or her family history of cancer." This approach would unquestionably lead to a greater recognition of the importance of host factors in carcinogenesis and would provide ample resources for the study of genetics, environmental perturbations, and biomarkers.

Our results clearly indicate that there is heterogeneity of breast cancer risk between families of breast cancer probands (see Table 2). One would conclude therefore that some families have a higher risk than others. Some of this heterogeneity appears to be related to the histologic type (Table 4) of breast cancer found in the proband. In addition, age at diagnosis also appears to have a major effect (Fig. 1). Families of probands with an earlier age of onset show not only a greater risk but also greater heterogeneity. These findings are consistent with the hypothesis that at least two types of breast cancer exist: one with a strong familial component and one without.

The results in Figure 1 are more meaningful than having them presented as a pre- and post-menopausal classification. When defined by age only, this classification is too imprecise to be of any value. Certainly, our results do not conflict with the supposition that pre-menopausal breast cancer carries a higher familial risk.

Our results, with respect to histology, while involving relatively small numbers, are nevertheless intriguing. The association of medullary carcinoma with positive family cancer history has been previously noted by Mulcahy and Platt (1981).

In addition, the histologically unclassifiable group appears to be different from the adenocarcinoma and ductal carcinoma categories in that it has a higher frequency of high risk families. Further analysis of risk by histologic type may provide data which will allow at least partial identification of high risk families.

We found a trend towards greater heterogeneity of risk with respect to cigarette smoking and caffeine use (Table 3). In the case of alcohol use, the findings were statistically significant, indicating that those probands who consumed alcohol had families with greater heterogeneity of breast cancer risk.

There has been a paucity of studies dealing with cancer family history among large series of cancer patients. One recent noteworthy example of such a study was that of Ogawa et al (1985) in Japan. They evaluated 9131 cancer patients from the Aichi Cancer Registry in 1979-81, all of whom were over 20 years old at diagnosis. Concordance between a study patient and a family member with cancer was observed for cancer of the breast, colon and rectum, and stomach. Of interest was the finding that the rate of family history of breast cancer patients was 3.3 times higher than the rate for other cancer patients, findings which are in accord with our own, although not fully comparable because of differing methodologies as well as the distinctly different racial groups under study.

REVIEW OF PERTINENT LITERATURE ON BREAST CANCER GENETICS

Extended Breast Cancer-Prone Kindreds

Detailed medical-genetic studies of breast cancer-prone families with meticulous pathology correlation were initiated by Lynch and colleagues in the mid-1960s (Lynch, 1967; Lynch and Krush, 1966). These investigations have been continuous and now involve several hundred kindreds. They have aided in the comprehension of breast cancer genetics. This experience provides the basis for much of the material which follows.

Cardinal Clinical Features of Hereditary Breast Cancer

Lynch (1981a) has emphasized the distinctive natural history of hereditary breast cancer, which is characterized by an earlier age of onset, excess bilaterality, vertical transmission (consonant with an autosomal dominantly inherited factor), heterogeneous tumor associations, and improved survival when compared to its sporadic counterpart (Lynch, 1981a; Lynch et al, 1984a and b). The literature on hereditary breast cancer has been increasing at a remarkable rate during the past decade. Surprisingly, however, most investigators fail to recognize the clinical nuances of hereditary breast cancer when compared to its sporadic counterpart (Lynch, 1981a; Lynch et al, 1984a and b). This also includes those familial aggregations of this disease which fail to fulfill criteria for hereditary breast cancer

(Lynch et al, 1984a). In addition, there is a paucity of information dealing with interrelationships between environmental breast cancer risk factors and genetics.

Site-Specific Hereditary Breast Cancer

Site-specific breast cancer infers that the particular pedigree shows a predominance of breast cancer in the absence of other histologic varieties of cancer (Figure 2). This is an exceedingly difficult breast cancer genetic diagnosis since it is based primarily upon the exclusion of integral patterns of other forms of cancer. For example, if we are dealing with a relatively small kindred, it is then possible that other forms of cancer were not represented simply because of the limited number of at risk subjects. Similarly, if there were a disproportionately greater number of males than females in the pedigree, then it would decrease the likelihood of discovering associated tumors which might be integral to a particular hereditary breast cancer syndrome, such as association of carcinoma of the ovary in the breast/ovarian cancer syndrome.

One must therefore be cautious when designating a given family as fitting the so-called site-specific variant of hereditary breast cancer. As a general rule, we consider the possibility that all patients who are first degree relatives of breast cancer affecteds from so-called site-specific breast cancer-prone kindreds are vulnerable for cancer of differing anatomic sites, particularly in those kindreds wherein paternal transmission and/or limited numbers of at risk patients are present.

Breast/Ovarian Cancer

Based upon their evaluation of 12 breast/ovarian cancer-prone kindreds, Lynch et al (1978b) concluded that the findings did not allow discrimination of an exact mode of genetic transmission. However, the findings were compatible with the assumption that a genetic factor was transmitted from affected mothers to half of their daughters, "...thereby causing the predisposition to breast/ovarian carcinoma. The observed high rate of father-to-daughter transmission leaves open the possibility of X-linkage, at least in certain families. Thus, genetic heterogeneity must also be considered."

Additional studies of informative pedigrees, such as those seen in Figure 3, will be needed to more fully clarify the exact mode(s) of inheritance in this familial tumor association. More importantly, intensified cancer surveillance focusing upon the breasts and ovaries must be implemented in high genetic risk patients/families such as these for effective cancer control. Finally, biochemical, virological, and pathological study of individuals whose specific location in the pedigree marks them at high risk for cancer may provide important clues to carcinogenesis.

46

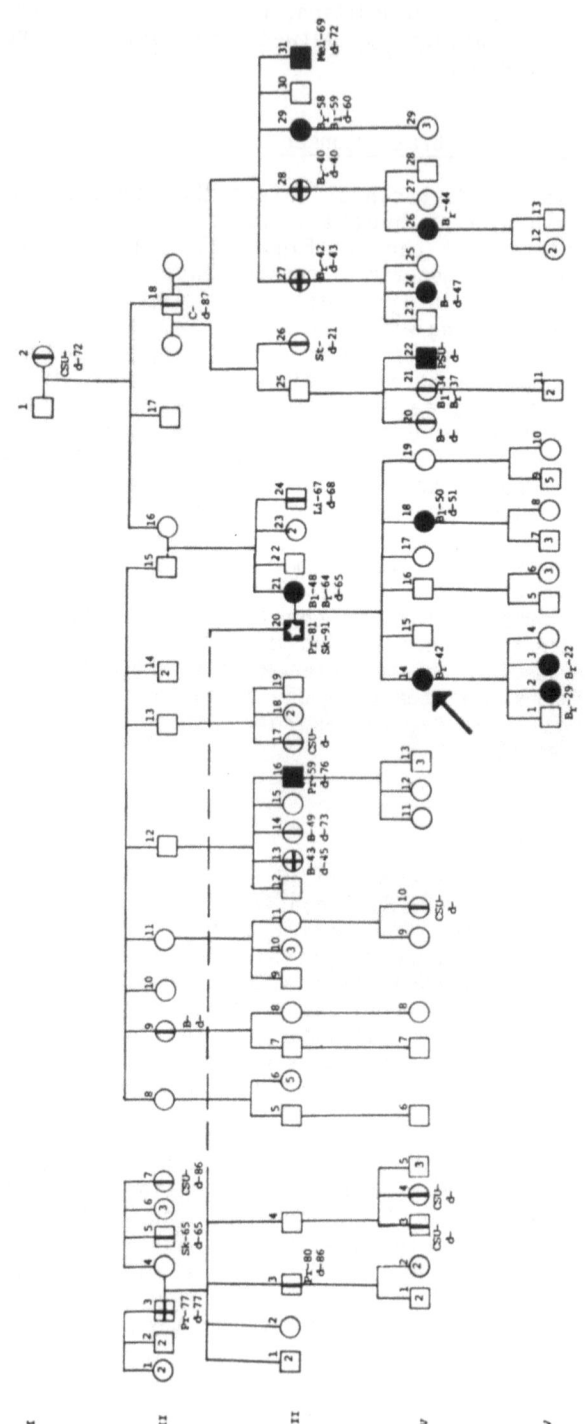

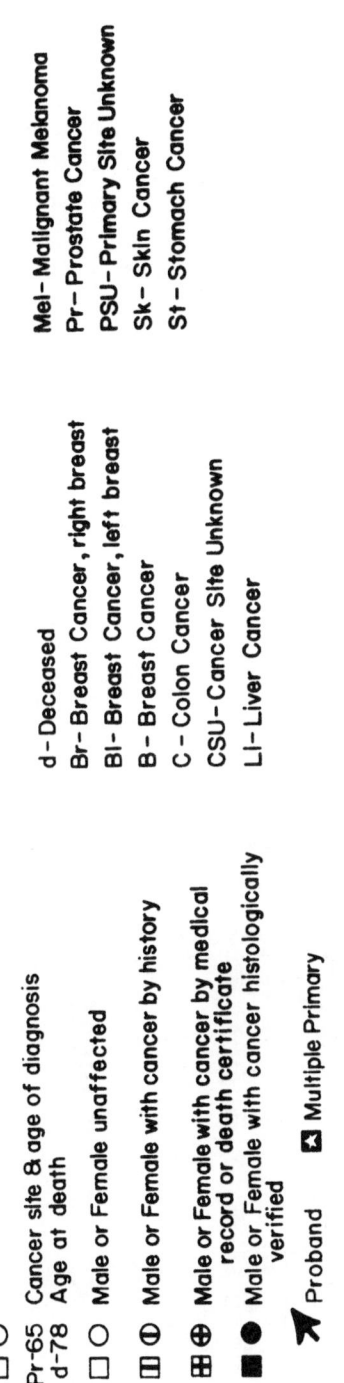

LEGEND

5 6 Code Number
□○

Pr-65 Cancer site & age of diagnosis
d-78 Age at death

□ ○ Male or Female unaffected

▨ ◐ Male or Female with cancer by history

⊞ ⊕ Male or Female with cancer by medical record or death certificate

■ ● Male or Female with cancer histologically verified

✦ Proband ▨ Multiple Primary

d – Deceased
Br – Breast Cancer, right breast
Bl – Breast Cancer, left breast
B – Breast Cancer
C – Colon Cancer
CSU – Cancer Site Unknown
Ll – Liver Cancer

Mel – Malignant Melanoma
Pr – Prostate Cancer
PSU – Primary Site Unknown
Sk – Skin Cancer
St – Stomach Cancer

Figure 2. Pedigree of a family showing site-specific breast cancer (from HT Lynch, et al; 1976, Arch Surg, 111, 126-131).

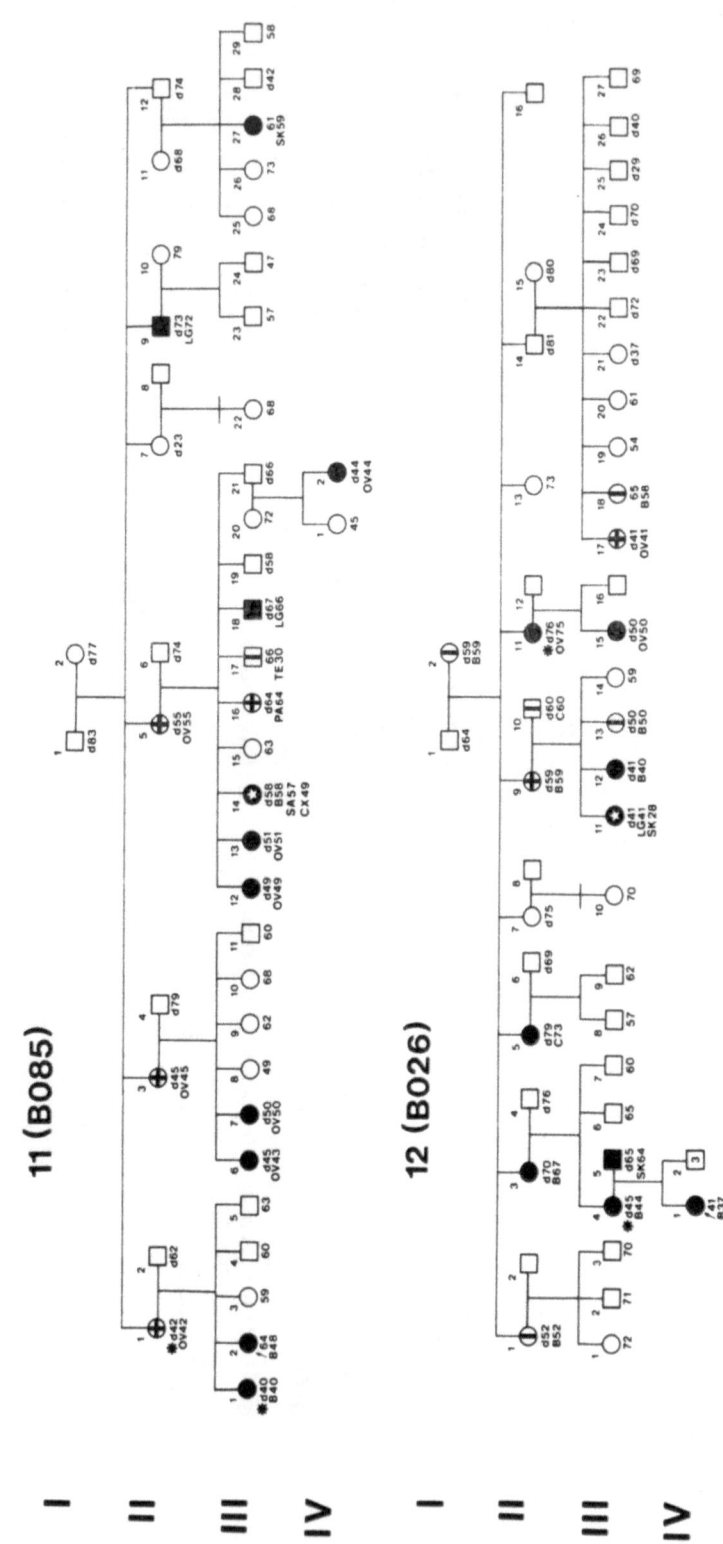

11 (B085)

12 (B026)

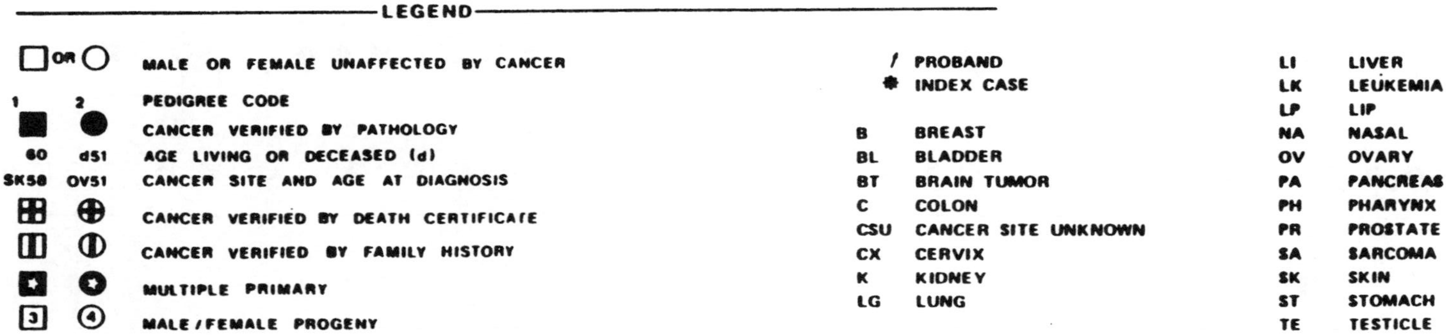

Figure 3. Pedigrees manifesting familial breast/ovarian cancer (from HT Lynch, et al; 1978, Cancer, 41, 1543-1548).

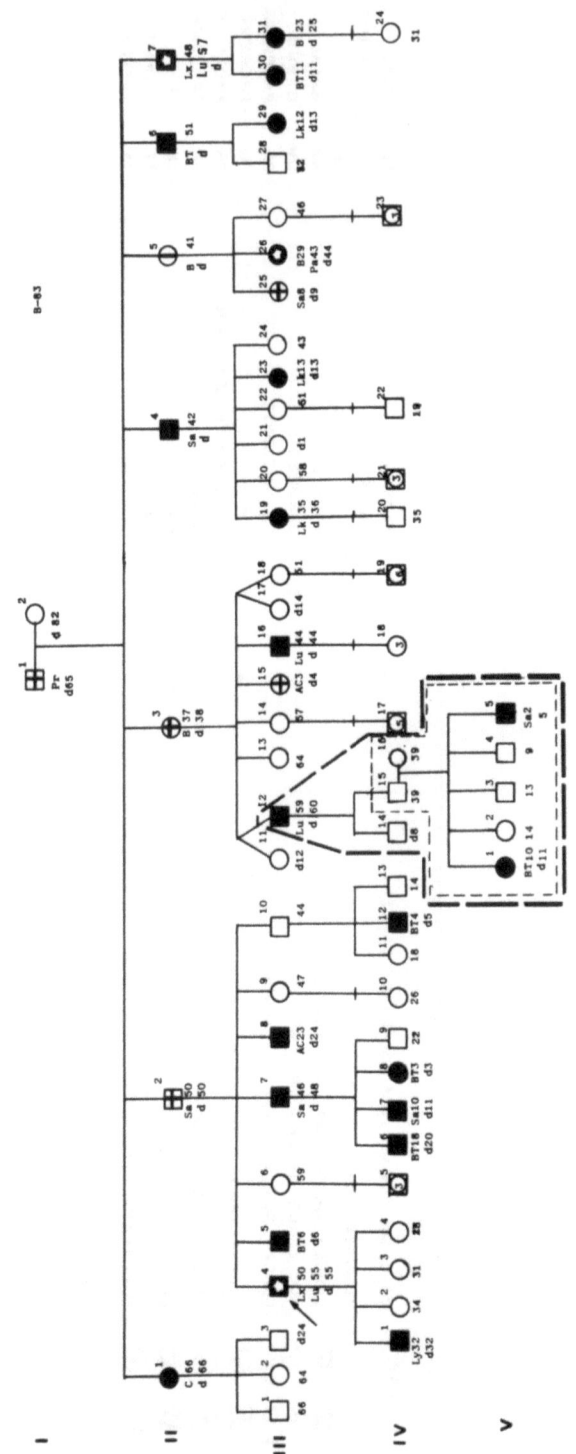

LEGEND

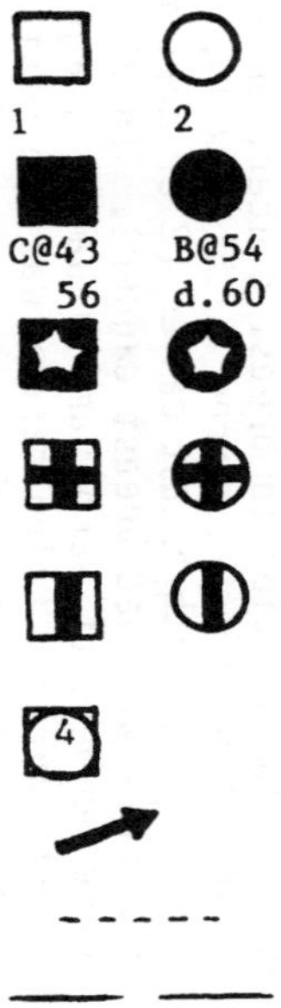

☐ Male or female unaffected

○

Pedigree Code

1
2

Cancer verified by pathology

■ ●

C@43 B@54   Cancer site and age when diagnosed
56 d.60   Age living or deceased

✪ Multiple primaries verified by pathology

⊕ Cancer verified by death certificate

⊖ Cancer reported by family history

④ Number of progeny

↗ Proband

- - - - - First degree relatives

———— Extended to include second degree relatives

AC Adrenal Cortical

B   Breast

BT Brain Tumor

C   Colon

Lk Leukemia

Lu Lung

Lx Larynx

Ly Lymphoma

Pa Pancreas

Pr Prostate

Sa Sarcoma

Figure 4. Pedigree of a family with the SBLA syndrome (from HT Lynch et al; 1985, AJDC, 139, 134-136).

The Sarcoma, Breast Cancer, Brain Tumor, Lung and Laryngeal Cancer, Leukemia, and Adrenal Cortical Carcinoma (SBLA) Syndrome

A remarkable familial cancer aggregation comprising sarcoma, breast cancer, brain tumors, leukemia, and adrenal cortical carcinoma was first reported by Bottomley and Condit (1968) and by Bottomley et al (1967, 1971). These investigators suggested that an autosomal dominant factor was of etiologic importance in this large kindred. In addition, they reported an increased percentage of aneuploid cells in cultured peripheral blood leukocytes in certain relatives. Li and Fraumeni (1969, 1975) subsequently proposed an interactive genetic etiologic hypothesis involving exogenous factors (putative oncogenic virus?) and the cancer-prone genotype to describe etiology for what we now refer to as the SBLA syndrome (Lynch et al, 1978a).

We studied this complex tumor aggregation in a large Nebraska kindred which showed the full complement of these tumors (Lynch et al, 1978a). The inheritance pattern was consonant with an autosomal dominantly inherited factor. This syndrome is mentioned in this particular context in that breast cancer is an integral tumor. In addition, some of the earliest ages of breast cancer onset which we have encountered in hereditary breast cancer settings have occurred in the SBLA syndrome. We subsequently updated this kindred (Lynch et al, 1985) when the first members of the fifth generation in the direct genetic lineage manifested syndrome cancers. This involved 2 affected siblings. One was a male child who developed rhabdomyosarcoma above the right eye at 2½ years. This child's sister developed a glioblastoma of the cerebral cortex at age 10 years (Figure 4).

Finally, it is of interest that Birch et al (1984) studied the health status or cause of death in the mothers of 143 children with soft tissue sarcomas. Interestingly, 6 of these mothers had premenopausal onset of breast cancer, 2 of whom had bilateral disease. This represented a 3-fold excess risk of breast cancer.

When considering the SBLA syndrome, it is clear that one must meticulously document cancer of all anatomic sites, inclusive of those in children, in order to elucidate etiology.

Breast Cancer and Gastrointestinal Tract Cancer

Breast cancer has also been associated with gastrointestinal tract cancer. The first significant report of familial breast cancer was that of Broca (1866). In addition to breast cancer, an excess of cancer of the gastrointestinal tract occurred in this family. Lynch et al (1972) studied 34 families with breast cancer (2 or more first or second degree relatives who had breast cancer). In 22 of these families, one or more members of each family had a diagnosis of gastrointestinal tract cancer. Colon cancer was the most frequent tumor followed by carcinoma of the stomach and pancreas. However, when interpreting this type of an association, it must be realized that carcinoma of the colon is the second most common visceral tumor affecting Americans. There is some question as to whether or not breast cancer may be an integral tumor in the Cancer Family Syndrome (Lynch syndrome II) (Figure 5). This disorder is characterized by significant early age of onset of nonpolyposis colorectal carcinoma with proximal predominance, carcinoma of the endometrium and ovary, multiple primary cancer excess, and autosomal dominant mode of inheritance. More work will be required in order to provide further documentation of this matter. Also, Lynch syndrome II may be heterogeneous from the standpoint of tumor combinations and therefore, there may well be heterogeneous forms of this disorder wherein breast cancer may be a prominent occurrence.

Family History and Bilaterality

Chaudary et al (1985) studied the family history in 54 women with bilateral, primary breast cancer and compared these with 208 women with unilateral breast cancer. Specifically, 44% of the 54 women with bilateral breast cancer had a positive family history of breast cancer as opposed to 23% of the 208 patients with unilateral disease. In addition, women with bilateral disease had almost twice the number of affected second degree relatives when compared to patients with unilateral disease. Thus, findings showed a significantly greater prevalence of family history of breast cancer in those women with bilateral breast cancer as opposed to those affected with unilateral breast cancer ($p < 0.01$). When compared with the unilateral cases, those individuals with bilateral breast cancer had a significantly ($p < 0.05$) greater proportion of first degree relatives with breast cancer. In turn, those affected relatives of probands manifesting bilateral breast cancer showed a significantly greater prevalence of bilateral breast cancer when compared with those affected with unilateral breast disease ($p = 0.04$). The affected relatives of the probands with bilateral disease showed an increased prevalence (16%) of bilateral breast cancer, which was 8 times that which was observed in the affected relatives of women with unilateral disease (2%), showing a statistical significance between the two groups ($p = 0.04$). The authors concluded that bilateral breast cancer was a characteristic of familial breast cancer. Their review of the literature showed familiality in individuals manifesting bilateral breast cancer to range from 11% to 45%. However, there were reports showing an absence of a significant difference of positive family history in patients with bilateral vs. unilateral disease.

Unfortunately, as has been almost the rule with reports of this type, Chaudary et al (1985) failed to evaluate cancer of other anatomic sites in his series of patients. Thus, we are not able to determine from their data whether bilaterality may be more frequently associated with specific heterogeneous breast cancer syndromes (such as site-specific breast cancer, breast/ovarian carcinoma, SBLA syndrome, and others).

It is important to note that Chaudary et al (1985) did not trace relevant hospital records and histopathologic reports as a basis for confirmation of the reported familial cases. The information was restricted to questionnaires and thereby relied solely on the patient's ability to recall.

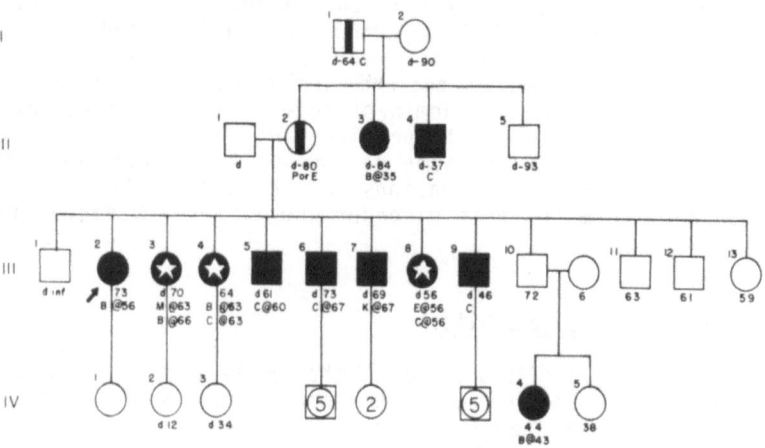

LEGEND

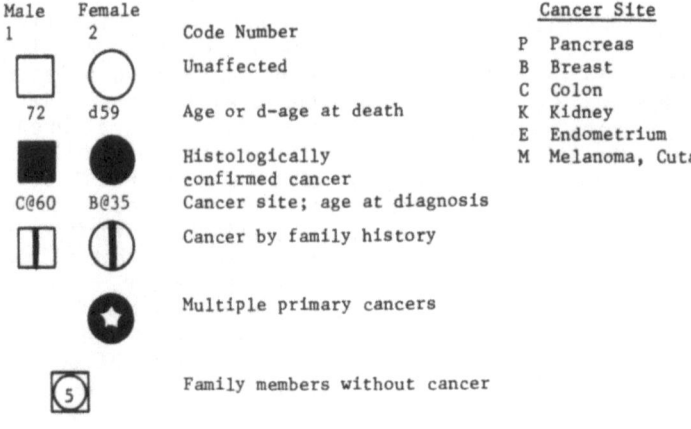

Male	Female		
1	2	Code Number	
□	○	Unaffected	
72	d59	Age or d-age at death	
■	●	Histologically confirmed cancer	
C@60	B@35	Cancer site; age at diagnosis	
▯	◑	Cancer by family history	
	★	Multiple primary cancers	
⑤		Family members without cancer	
↗		Proband	
		inf - infant	

Cancer Site

P Pancreas
B Breast
C Colon
K Kidney
E Endometrium
M Melanoma, Cutaneous

Figure 5. Pedigree showing breast cancer in association with the Cancer Family Syndrome (from HT Lynch, et al; 1973, Am J Gastroent, 59, 31-40).

Pathology reports of 198 familial breast cancer patients were reviewed by Harris et al (1978) to determine chronologic features of tumorigenesis in the breast contralateral to the site of initial mastectomy. Actuarial data revealed two major risk periods with a prolonged intervening postoperative gap in which no malignant tumors of the contralateral breast were detected. The cumulative cancer risk to the contralateral breast increased annually at 2.8% in the first 6 postoperative years, then showed no increase in the next 7 years, and finally resumed its upward climb at an accentuated annual rate of 6.8% between years 13 and 16 (inclusive). The corresponding annual rates of increase for second primary breast cancer in the two risk periods were 1.6 and 5.9%, respectively. A total of 37 patients manifested bilateral breast cancer, of whom 21 had pathologically confirmed second primary carcinomas; i.e., primary tumors of the contralateral breast. Of these patients, 27 exhibited a relatively short interval between mastectomies ($\bar{x}$ = 1.7 years), whereas 10 had a much longer disease-free period ($\bar{x}$ = 16.5 years). It is possible that tumors manifested in the contralateral breast within 6 years of the initial breast cancer were already developing but were not clinically discernible at the time of first mastectomy. In contrast, the extended disease-free period of many patients suggests that host defense mechanisms may have been stimulated by the first tumor, which in turn had a persisting suppressive effect on de novo carcinogenesis in the contralateral breast.

Genetics and Carcinoma of the Breast in Males

Carcinoma of the male breast is rare. Approximately 1 case of breast cancer occurs in men for every 100 cases occurring in women. Possibly because of its infrequency, examination of the male breast is a seriously neglected portion of the physical examination.

Patients with Klinefelter's syndrome harbor a substantially increased risk for the development of breast cancer (Jackson et al, 1965). Greater attention should therefore be given to examination of the male breasts in patients with Klinefelter's syndrome. Lynch et al (1974) described a patient with the classical habitus for Klinefelter's syndrome who had this diagnosis verified by cytogenetic investigation of cultured peripheral blood leukocytes which showed a consistent XXY chromosomal complement. In addition, skin fibroblasts were cultured and simian papovavirus (SV40) studies were performed. These studies showed a relatively high transformation rate, with an average of 3.55% transformation.

This individual, at age 54, showed a firm, fixed mass in the upper outer zone of the left breast that had overlying skin retraction and skin dimpling. Clinically, this lesion appeared to be a far advanced carcinoma of the breast. An excisional biopsy was performed and frozen sections disclosed invasive adenocarcinoma, both scirrhous and medullary. Consequently, radical mastectomy was performed on the left breast. The diagnosis was infiltrating carcinoma of the breast, ductal type, without demonstrable axillary lymph node metastases. This patient had a prolonged course, with many complications and was treated with chemotherapy and hormones, the details of which are the subject of a separate report (Miller and Lynch, 1986). It was of interest that one of the patient's sisters had breast cancer at age 62, another sister had carcinoma of the small bowel at age 66, and a third sister had carcinoma of the urinary bladder at age 51. The patient's father had gastric carcinoma.

Patients with Klinefelter's syndrome have approximately the same breast cancer risk as women in the general population (Jackson et al, 1965; Nadel and Koss, 1967). It is possible that breast cancer risks of XXY males are influenced by genetic variables for cancer diathesis in a manner similar to the breast cancer risk of XX females (Lynch et al, 1974).

LaRaja et al (1985) reported a family wherein 3 siblings, namely, a sister and her 2 brothers, manifested breast cancer. The paternal grandmother of the proband also manifested breast cancer. The sibship was of further interest in that the female sibling had bilateral breast cancer during her premenopausal years and one of her brothers who manifested breast cancer developed this disease at age 41 years. The authors state that their family study is the first one in which a sister and 2 brothers manifested breast cancer. The family was also noteworthy for other varieties of cancer in that 2 family members had gastric cancer, 1 had brain cancer, 1 had laryngeal cancer, 1 had a carcinoma of the colon, and 1 had skin cancer. There was no evidence in the men of clinical features consistent with Klinefelter's syndrome. The authors reviewed the literature for familial breast cancer occurring in male siblings and found only 4 reports (Everson et al, 1979; Marger et al, 1975; Teasdale et al, 1976).

BIOMARKERS

Lynch et al (1984b) reviewed the subject of biomarkers in hereditary cancer and have clearly shown that in spite of the importance of this subject to hereditary breast cancer diagnosis, control, and comprehension of pathogenesis, we remain in the dark so far as identification of biomarkers of sufficient sensitivity and specificity for clinical application is concerned. However, some clues have been provided and these are summarized in the table (Table 5) (Danes, 1976, 1981; Danes and Deschner (unpublished), Danes and Lynch, 1982, 1983; Fishman et al, 1978, 1979, 1983; Kasid et al, 1985; Lynch et al, 1983; Ohno et al, 1979; Petrakis, 1974, 1986; Petrakis et al, 1975; Pross et al, 1984; Tissot et al, 1984).

Table 5.   Biomarkers and breast cancer.

1.   Apocrine glands and secretory status - wet ear wax and increased breast secretion positively associated with breast cancer risk (Petrakis, 1974; Petrakis, 1975).

2.   Dysplastic epithelial cells in nipple aspirates of premenopausal white women with statistically significant correlation with wet cerumen (Petrakis, 1983).

3.   HLA - generally unrewarding; no single HLA antigen or haplotype found to associate with breast cancer (Lynch et al, 1984b).

4.   gp52 antigen - the envelope glycoprotein (gp52) of the murine mammary tumor virus (MMTV) shows cross-reactivity with human breast cancer and with patients showing positive family histories (Ohno et al, 1979).

5.   Endocrine profiles - premenopausal high familial breast cancer risk women.
     a.   low urinary estrone and estradiol glucuronides
     b.   plasma androsterone sulfate significantly low
     c.   genetic risk for breast cancer risk associated with an abnormality in estrogen conjugation (Fishman et al, 1978; Fishman et al, 1979; Fishman et al, 1983).

6.   In vitro hyperdiploidy - observed in affected high genetic risk and affecteds (Danes, 1976; Danes and Lynch, 1983; Danes, 1981; Danes, unpublished; Danes and Lynch, 1982; Lynch et al, 1983).

7.   Plasminogen activators (PA) - malignant transformation of breast and colon appeared to be accompanied by important changes in the production of urokinase (UK)-related PA and of an inhibitory activity directed against UK. The anti-UK activity was absent in extracts of normal breast or colon tissue (Tissot et al, 1984).

8.   Oncogene research - ras activation may be a mechanism by which breast cancer might alter its hormone dependent phenotype (Kasid et al, 1985).

9.   Natural killer cell activity (NK) - elevated NK activity may be a reaction to the hormonal factors in women with diffuse benign breast syndrome (Pross et al, 1984).

Segregation Analysis and Gene Linkage

Eighteen large kindreds from Creighton's Breast Cancer Family Resource were investigated in order to test the hypothesis that a single gene increased breast cancer susceptibility and that such a gene may segregate according to Mendelian laws in some families (Go et al, 1983). Sixteen of the pedigrees showed findings consistent with an autosomal dominant mode of inheritance, while the 2 remaining families fit an environmental hypothesis. Heterogeneity by tumor association was observed. Nevertheless, conclusive demonstration of the existence of an allele that increases susceptibilty to breast cancer in any family must rely on the detection of genetic linkage between the hypothetical allele and the marker locus. In a companion paper (King et al, 1983), in 7 families with primarily premenopausal breast cancer and 5 families showing the combination of breast and ovarian cancer, a dominant susceptibility allele was shown to be putatively linked to the genetic marker glutamic-pyruvic transaminase (GPT), with a lod score of 1.95 at zero recombination. Further investigation will be necessary in order to test the full significance of these linkage findings. Meanwhile, the data requires cautious interpretation. In any family with possible GPT linkage, women who carry the hypothetical susceptibility allele would be at high risk for breast cancer, whereas the relatives who do not carry that allele would not be at an increased breast cancer risk. GPT genotype, however, is not associated with breast cancer in the general population, and therefore, this cannot be used as a screening test. GPT has been assigned to the short arm of chromosome 16. Genes for a regulator of interferon production and a regulator of the antiviral state are believed to be located on this same chromosome. Hence, it would be interesting to investigate linkage between these loci and hereditary breast cancer.

We stress the potential value of linkage studies for research, as well as for clinical utility because it would be possible to: 1) detect genetically susceptible young women from high risk families prior to clinical symptoms; 2) counsel highly selected cases who would become candidates for surgical prophylaxis; 3) determine if more than one genetically influenced form of breast cancer exists, an assumption that we have confidence in on a clinical basis, but which we would like to confirm through further linkage studies; 4) investigate why some genetically susceptible women do not develop breast cancer; 5) scrutinize the role of environment in genetically susceptible women more critically; and 6) study biochemical and physiologic mechanisms by which a gene increases breast cancer susceptibility, by comparing young women who have not yet developed breast cancer with other young women in the same family who are at low risk (by linkage analysis). This would enable comparison of appropriate immunologic, biochemical, and endocrinological parameters among these high and low risk young women and would be potentially informative in understanding how breast cancer susceptibilty genes are expressed. The implications for prevention of familial breast cancer would then become legion.

CONCLUSION

We conclude that while the results from our Oncology Clinic do not unequivocally prove the existence of a distinct hereditary type of breast cancer, they nevertheless are not inconsistent with such an hypothesis. Our results do establish the fact that familial aggregations of breast cancer do not occur by chance alone. Whether or not the etiology of familial breast cancer is due to common family environment or common genetic makeup, the result is the same: some families have a higher risk than others and should be subject to a more intensive surveillance protocol.

The issue of genetics vs. common environment in the causation of breast cancer is vitally important, but still needs to be resolved. One approach, thus far unsuccessful, is to demonstrate a linkage between the familial type of breast cancer and a Mendelian marker. The possible linkage of breast cancer with GPT (Go et al, 1983; King et al, 1980, 1983) was encouraging, but its validity needs to be established to a scientific certainty. The highest priority must be given to the detection of a biomarker(s) which has acceptable sensitivity and specificity to the cancer-prone genotype(s) to allow for clinical application for risk status identification. This would also enable the testing of hypotheses dealing with genetic/environmental interaction in breast cancer etiology.

ACKNOWLEDGEMENTS

Support for this endeavor was provided by The Council for Tobacco Research, USA, Inc., Grant #1297B.

REFERENCES

Anderson, D.E. and Badzioch, M.D., 1985a, Risk of familial breast cancer. Cancer, 56, 383-387.

Anderson, D.E. and Badzioch, M.D., 1985b, Bilaterality in familial breast cancer patients. Cancer, 56, 2092-2098.

Birch, J.M., Hartley, A.L., and Marsden, H.B., 1984, Excess risk of breast cancer in the mothers of children with soft-tissue sarcomas. Br J Cancer, 49, 325-331.

Bottomley, R.H., Condit, P.T., Chanes, R.E., 1967, Cytogenetic studies in familial malignancy. Clin Resource, 15, 334.

Bottomley, R.H. and Condit P.T., 1968, Cancer families. Cancer Bull, 20, 22-24.

Bottomley, R.H., Trainer, A.L., and Condit, P.T., 1971, Chromosome studies in a "cancer family." Cancer, 28, 519-528.

Broca, P.P., 1866, Traite' des Tumeurs. Asselin, Paris, Vols 1 and 2.

Chaudary, M.A., Mills, R.R., Bulbrook, R.D., and Hayward, J.L., 1985, Family history and bilateral primary breast cancer. Breast Cancer Res Treat, 5, 201-205.

Danes, B.S., 1976, The Gardner syndrome: increased tetraploidy in cultured skin fibroblasts. J Med Genet, 13, 52-56.

Danes, B.S., 1981, Occurrence of in vitro tetraploidy in the heritable colon cancer syndromes. Cancer, 48, 1596-1601.

Danes, B.S. and Lynch, H.T., 1982, A familial aggregation of pancreatic cancer: an in vitro study. JAMA, 247, 2798-2802.

Danes, B.S. and Lynch, H.T., 1983, Increased in vitro tetraploidy in dermal monolayer cultures derived from normals. Cancer Genet Cytogenet, 8, 81-87.

Danes, B.S. and Deschner, E.E., Detection of in vitro tetraploidy in the heritable colon cancer syndromes: confirmation by 3 different assays (unpublished).

Everson, R.B., Li, F.P., Fraumeni, J.F., Fishman, J., Wilson, R.E., Stout, D., and Norris H.J., 1976, Familial male breast cancer. Lancet, i, 9-12.

Fishman, J., Fukushima, D., O'Connor, J., Rosenfeld, R.S., Lynch, H.T., Lynch, J.F., Guirgis, H., and Maloney, K., 1978, Plasma hormone profiles of young women at risk for familial breast cancer. Cancer Res, 38, 4006-4011.

Fishman, J., Fukushima, D.K., O'Connor, J., and Lynch, H.T., 1979, Low urinary estrogen glucuronides in women at risk for familial breast cancer. Science, 204, 1089-1091.

Fishman, J., Bradlow, H.L., Fukushima, D. O'Connor, J., Rosenfeld, R., Elston, R., and Lynch, H.T., 1983, Abnormal estrogen conjugation in women at risk for familial breast cancer is concentrated at the periovulatory stage of the menstrual cycle. Cancer Res, 43, 1884-1890.

Gersting, J.E., 1976, MEGADATS - a computer system for family data acquisition, storage, and analysis. In: A.E.H. Emery and J.R. Miller (eds), Registers for the Detection and Prevention of Genetic Disease. Stratton Intercontinental Medical Book Corp, New York.

Go, R.C.P., King, M-C., Bailey-Wilson, J., Elston, R.C., and Lynch, H.T., 1983, Genetic epidemiology of breast cancer and associated cancers in high risk families, Part I. J Natl Cancer Inst, 71, 455-462.

Harris, R.E., Lynch, H.T., and Guirgis, H.A., 1978, Familial breast cancer: risk to the contralateral breast. J Natl Cancer Inst, 60, 955-960.

Jackson, A.W., Muldol, S., Ockey, C.H., and O'Connor, P.J., 1965, Carcinoma of male breast in association with the Klinefelter syndrome. Br Med J, 1, 223-225.

Kalvin, S., Williams, P.T., Carmelli, D., and Cameron, E., 1985, Permutation methods for the structured exploratory data analysis (SEDA) of total cholesterol measured in five Israeli populations. Am J Epid, 122, 163-186.

Kasid, A., Lippman, M.E., Papageorge, A.G., Lowy, D.R., and Glemann, E.P, 1985, Transfection of v-ras$_H$ DNA into MCF-7 human breast cancer cells bypasses dependence on estrogen for tumorigenicity. Science, 228, 725-728.

King, M-C., Go, R.C.P., Elston, R.C., Lynch, H.T., and Petrakis, N.L., 1980, Allele increasing susceptibility to human breast cancer may be linked to the glutamate-pyruvate transaminase locus. Science, 208, 406-408.

King, M-C., Go, R.C.P., Lynch, H.T., Elston, R.C., Terasaki, P.I., Petrakis, N.L., Rodgers, G.C., Lattanzio, D., and Bailey-Wilson, J., 1983, Genetic epidemiology of breast cancer associated cancers in high risk families, Part II. J Natl Cancer Inst, 71, 463-467.

LaRaja, R.D., Pagnozzi, J.A., Rothenberg, R.E., Georgiou, J., Sabatini, M.T., and Hirschman, R.J., 1985, Carcinoma of the breast in three siblings. Cancer, 55, 2709-2711.

Li, F.P. and Fraumeni, J.F., 1969, Soft-tissue sarcomas, breast cancer, and other neoplasms. Ann Int Med, 71, 747-752.

Li, F.P. and Fraumeni, J.F., 1975, Familial breast cancer, soft-tissue sarcomas, and other neoplasms. Ann Int Med, 83, 833-834.

Lynch, H.T. and Krush, A.J., 1966, Heredity and breast cancer: implications for cancer detection. Med Times, 94, 599-605.

Lynch, H.T., 1967, Hereditary Factors In Carcinoma, Recent Results in Cancer Research, vol 12. Springer-Verlag, New York, pp186.

Lynch, H.T., Krush, A.J., Lemon, H.M., Kaplan, A.R., Condit, P.T., Bottomley, R.H., 1972, Tumor variation in families with breast cancer. JAMA, 222, 1631-1635.

Lynch, H.T., Kaplan, A.R., and Lynch, J.F., 1974, Klinefelter syndrome and cancer: a family study. JAMA, 229, 209-211.

Lynch, H.T., Mulcahy, G.M., Harris, R.E., Guirgis, H.A., and Lynch, J.F., 1978a, Genetic and pathologic findings in a kindred with hereditary sarcoma, breast cancer, brain tumors, leukemia, lung, laryngeal, and adrenal cortical carcinoma. Cancer, 41, 2055-2064.

Lynch, H.T., Harris, R.E., Guirgis, H.A., Maloney, K., Carmody, L., and Lynch, J.F., 1978b, Familial association of breast/ovarian cancer. Cancer, 41, 1543-1548.

Lynch, H.T., 1981a, Genetics and Breast Cancer. Van Nostrand Reinhold, New York.

Lynch, H.T., Fain, P.R., Goldgar, D., Albano, W., Mailliard, J.A., and McKenna, P.J., 1981b, Familial breast cancer and its recognition in an oncology clinic. Cancer, 47, 2730-2739.

Lynch, H.T., Fusaro, R.M., Danes, B.S., Kimberling, W.J., Lynch, J.F., 1983, Hereditary malignant melanoma, including biomarkers in the familial atypical multiple mole melanoma syndrome. Cancer Genet Cytogenet, 8, 325-358.

Lynch, H.T., Albano, W.A., Layton, M.A., Lynch, J.F., Costello, K.A., Tindall, S.L., Wagner, C.A., and Cheng, S.C., 1984a, Genetic predisposition to breast cancer. Cancer, 53, 612-622.

Lynch, H.T., Albano, W.A., Heieck, J.J., Mulcahy, G.M., Lynch, J.F., Layton, M.A., and Danes, B.S., 1984b, Genetics, biomarkers, and control of breast cancer: a review. Cancer Genet Cytogenet, 13, 43-92.

Lynch, H.T., Katz, D.A., Bogard, P.J., and Lynch, J.F., 1985, The sarcoma, breast cancer, lung cancer, and adrenocortical carcinoma syndrome revisited. Am J Dis Child, 139, 134-136.

Marger, D., Undaneta, N., and Fischer, B., 1975, Breast cancer in brothers. Cancer, 36, 458-461.

Miller, D.M. and Lynch, H.T., 1985, Klinefelter's syndrome and metastatic breast cancer. Breast, 11, 23.

Mulcahy, G.M. and Platt, R., 1981, Pathologic aspects of familial carcinoma of the breast. In: H.T. Lynch (ed), Genetics and Breast Cancer. Van Nostrand Reinhold Co, New York, pp65-97.

Mulvihill, J.J., 1985, Clinical ecogenetics: cancer in families. N Eng J Med, 312, 1569-1570.

Nadel, M. and Koss, L.G., 1967, Klinefelter's syndromme and male breast cancer. Lancet, ii, 366.

Ogawa, H., Kato, I., and Tominaga, S., 1985, Family history of cancer among cancer patients. Gann, 76, 113-118.

Ohno, T., Mesa-Tejada, R., Keydar, I., Ramanarayanan, M., Bausch, J., and Spiegelman, S., 1979, Human breast carcinoma antigen is immunologically related to the polypeptide of the group-specific glycoprotein of mouse mammary tumor virus. Proc Natl Acad Sci USA, 76, 2460-2464.

Petrakis, N.L., 1974, Association of genetically determined wet cerumen and breast fluid secretion (abstract). XI Int Cancer Cong (20-26 Oct 1974, Florence, Italy), Vol 2, p71.

Petrakis, N.L., Mason, L., Lee, R., Sugimoto, B., Pawson, S., and Catchpool, F., 1975, Association of race, age, menopausal status, and cerumen type with breast fluid secretion in nonlactating women, as determined by nipple aspiration. J Natl Cancer Inst, 54, 829.

Petrakis, N.L., 1983, Cerumen phenotype and epithelial dysplasia in nipple aspirates of breast fluid. Am J Phys Anthro, 62, 115-118.

Pross, H.F., Sterns, E., and MacGillis, D.R., 1984, Natural killer cell activity in women at "high risk" for breast cancer, with and without benign breast syndrome. Int J Cancer, 34, 303-308.

Teasdale, C., Forbes, J., and Baum, M., 1976, Familial male breast cancer. Lancet, i, 360-361.

Tissot, J.D., Hauert, J., and Bachmann, F., 1984, Characterization of plasminogen activators from normal human breast and colon and from breast and colon carcinomas. Int J Cancer, 34, 295-302.

ONCOGENES IN HUMAN CANCER

GEOFFREY M. COOPER

Dana-Farber Cancer Institute and Department of Pathology, Harvard Medical School, Boston, MA 02115

A variety of tumors, including mammary carcinomas, have been found to contain active oncogenes which have been detected by the ability of tumor DNAs to induce transformation upon transfection of NIH 3T3 cells. I will review here the basic observations leading to the identification of these oncogenes and discuss recent work involving the characterization of four examples of the genes detected by this approach.

These studies are based on the assay of transfection of NIH 3T3 cells. This particular cell line is used as a common recipient because of its ability to efficiently take up and integrate exogenous DNA when it is presented to the cells in the form of a calcium phosphate co-precipitate. A gene which induces transformation can then be detected by the appearance of foci of transformed cells in the DNA treated recipient cell population about two weeks after transfection, and these transformed foci can be picked and cultivated for further study.

There are two basic observations leading to the detection of transforming genes of cellular origin by this assay. First, if one takes DNA from a variety of normal cells, one finds that fragments of these normal cell DNAs induce transformation with a low efficiency, corresponding to about 0.003 transformants per microgram of DNA (Cooper et al., 1980; Schafer et al., 1984). If one picks cells transformed at this low efficiency by normal cell DNA and extracts DNA from these transformants, one then finds that their DNA induces transformation with high efficiency (0.1 to 1 transformants per microgram of DNA) in secondary transfection assays. These results indicate that normal cells contain latent transforming genes whose transforming potential can be activated by DNA rearrangements occurring during transfection and that the transformed cells then

contain active transforming sequences which can be efficiently transmitted to new cells in further rounds of
transfection. A recent example of this mechanism of activation of a cellular transforming gene (ret) is discussed
below.

In contrast to normal cell DNAs, many tumors (overall
30% to 50% of the neoplasms studied) contain activated
transforming sequences which can be detected by the ability
of those tumor DNAs to efficiently induce transformation of
NIH 3T3 cells in primary transfection assays (see Cooper and
Lane, 1984, for review). That is, a number of tumor DNAs
will induce transformation with efficiencies of 0.1 to 1
focus per microgram of DNA, and these genes can be serially
transmitted in subsequent transfection assays at similar
efficiencies. These results indicate that those tumors
which possess these activated transforming sequences have
undergone dominant genetic alterations, either by mutation
or DNA rearrangement, at some point during their
pathogenesis and suggest the hypothesis that the transforming genes detected in these tumor DNAs have contributed to
the development of the neoplasms from which they were
isolated. Such active transforming sequences have now been
detected in DNAs of a wide variety of neoplasms from several
different species including chicken, rodents, and man. In
terms of cell types, transforming genes have been detected
in a variety of different kinds of hematopoetic neoplasms, a
number of different carcinomas, sarcomas, neuroblastomas,
melanomas, and a teratocarcinoma. Neoplasms which contain
these transforming sequences include primary tumors as well
as tumor derived cell lines, so that activation of transforming genes is not an artifact of in vitro cultivation of
tumor cells. In addition, it has been possible in many
cases to test normal tissue from the same individual animal
or patient whose tumor DNAs possess transforming activity:
in these cases, DNAs of normal cells lack efficient transforming sequences, indicating that the events which resulted
in activation of transforming potential in the tumor DNAs
were somatic mutations that occurred during neoplasm development. Finally, neoplasms which possess these activated
transforming sequences include spontaneously arising tumors
in man and, in animal systems, tumors induced by a variety
of carcinogens including different chemicals, irradiation,
and viruses which do not contain their own oncogenes.

One approach which proved useful to characterizing the
transforming sequences activated in tumor DNAs was to
compare the tumor transforming genes to transforming genes

which were previously known as part of the genomes of
acutely transforming retroviruses. These are viruses
isolated from several different animal species which have
the biological properties by very efficiently inducing both
transformation of cells in culture and tumors in infected
animals. In all of these cases, the viruses possess this
transforming activity as a consequence of the presence of
transforming genes, for example the src gene of Rous sarcoma
virus, in the viral genome. These transforming genes are
not required for virus replication but are the determinants
of viral oncogenicity. Further, cells normally contain
genes which are closely related to the retroviral transforming genes. It was therefore reasonable to ask whether any
of the transforming genes detected by transfection of
non-virus induced tumor DNAs might be cellular homologues of
these known retroviral transforming sequences. This initially proved to be the case for the ras genes of Harvey and
Kirsten sarcoma virus (Der et al., 1982; Parada et al.,
1982; Santos et al., 1982). The ras genes comprise a family
of at least 3 human genes which have been implicated as ras^H
active transforming genes of a variety of neoplasms. Ras^H
is closely related to the transforming gene of Harvey
sarcoma virus and ras^K to that of Kirsten sarcoma virus.
The ras^N gene is not found in any virus but was first
isolated from a neuroblastoma and then found to be a member
of the ras gene family (Shimizu et al., 1983). Ras genes
have been found as active transforming sequences in human
neoplasms of a wide variety of cell types including
hematopoetic tumors, carcinomas, sarcomas, melanomas,
neuroblastomas, and a teratocarcinoma. However, the ras
genes are detected as active transforming sequences in only
a relatively small fraction (10%-20%) of neoplasms of any
particular cell type. This would appear to suggest that
activation of these genes can contribute to tumorigenesis of
many different types of cells but that activation of ras
genes is not a necessary event for the development of any
particular type of neoplasm. In addition, recent evidence
suggests that activation of ras genes may be a relatively
late event in tumor progression. For example, Albino et al.
(1984) were able to study five individual metastases of a
single patient with melanoma. They found that in one, but
only one, of these five metastases was there an active ras^N
gene. The other four metastases were negative for ras
activation. In this particular case, therefore, it is clear
that activation of ras was not required for formation of the
primary neoplasm nor was it required for formation of four
out of five metastatic lesions. Rather, it appeared to be a
late event occurring in only one of those metastases.

Nevertheless, the frequent and widespread activation of ras genes in human tumors suggests that they can contribute significantly to the development of several different kinds of neoplasms, although their activation may not be necessary for tumor formation.

The identification of some of the tumor transforming genes as human homologues of ras greatly accelerated their study because what was already known about the retroviral ras genes could be immediately applied to the analysis of the related genes activated in human neoplasms. In particular, it was known that the viral ras genes encoded proteins of 21,000 daltons, and monoclonal antibodies against these proteins were available which turned out to cross-react with the related human gene products (Furth et al., 1982),. Ras genes can be induced to transform cells by either of two mechanisms. Expression of the normal protein at levels about 100-fold above those found in non-transformed cells is sufficient to induce transformation of NIH cells (Chang et al., 1982). However, the mechanism by which activation of ras occurs in human neoplasms does not involve abnormal gene expression but instead involves structural mutations. These mutations are single amino acid substitutions which occur at one of three positions in the ras gene products, altering either amino acid 12, 13, or 61 (Tabin et al., 1982; Reddy et al., 1982; Taparowsky et al., 1982; Yuasa et al., 1983; Bos et al., 1985). At amino acids 12 and 61, a variety of different substitutions will confer transforming activity on the ras proteins, although the efficiency of transformation induced by these different mutant genes varies with the particular amino acid substitution (Seeburg et al., 1984; Der et al., 1986). The ras proteins are localized to the inner face of the plasmid membrane and are post-translationally modified by acylation, which is necessary for their membrane localization (Furth et al., 1982; Sefton et al., 1982). They have two known biochemical properties. They bind guanine nucleotides, GTP and GDP, with high affinity and specificity and they display a low level of hydrolysis of bound GTP (Scolnick et al., 1979; McGrath et al., 1984). These properties are similar to those of other cell membrane proteins, the G proteins, which are involved in transduction of signals from a variety of membrane receptors to second messengers (Gilman, 1984). Current hypotheses for function of the ras proteins draw on this analogy, suggesting that the ras proteins function as transducing agents between receptors involved in cell growth and putative second messengers which control this process. In their latent state, the G proteins are bound to GDP and associated with surface receptors. Activation of the receptor by ligand binding stimulates the exchange of GDP for GTP, and the activated GTP bound form of the alpha subunit of the G protein acts to affect target enzymes of second messenger metabolism. Deactivation of the G proteins is accompanied by hydrolysis of the bound GTP. The analogous biochemical properties of ras and the G proteins, then, are the GTP and GDP binding activity and the GRO hydrolysis exhibited by both ras and the G proteins. Mutations which activate the transforming activity of ras do not affect GTP or GDP binding although they do lead to about a 10-fold reduction in the rate of GTP hydrolysis (Finkel et al., 1984; McGrath et al., 1984; Der et al., 1986). This is again consistent with the G protein model. Since GTP hydrolysis is involved in deactivation of the G proteins, a lower rate of GTP hydrolysis would tend to keep the proteins more frequently in the active state. However, the situation is somewhat more complex, since certain mutations at position 61 reduce GTPase activity but do not increase ras transforming potential (Der et al., 1986). Therefore, although there is an association between transformation and reduction in GTPase, it would appear that reduced GTPase is not sufficient to convert a normal ras gene to an active transforming gene. Nevertheless, this analogy would appear to be a reasonable one and the major questions regarding ras function relate to identification of the receptors with which one believes the protein is associated and with identification of the putative second messengers which are potential targets for the ras transducing signal.

Another retrovirus related gene recently found to be activated as a transforming gene in human neoplasms is the human homologue of the raf/mil viral oncogene (Shimizu et al., 1985; Fukui et al., 1985). We have detected transformation by raf genes in NIH 3T3 cells transfected with DNAs of three human carcinomas: a mammary carcinoma, a renal cell carcinoma, and a lung carcinoid (Stanton and Cooper, manuscript submitted). Each of the three activated raf transforming genes was generated by a recombination event between other human sequences, which are different in each of the three transformants, and a raf locus which has been truncated in the vicinity of exon 6 or intron 7. The viral raf genes, compared to cellular raf, have also undergone recombination events which led to truncation, as has a raf gene activated by co-transfection of normal mouse DNA with LTR sequences (Molders et al., 1985). These observations suggest that truncation in this region is critical to raf activation, and this is substantiated by analysis of raf transcripts in the transformants. Each of the three transformants express raf transcripts of abnormal size as compared to the transcripts of normal human or mouse raf. In one case, the transforming gene derived from the breast carcinoma, the abnormal raf transcript is expressed at levels at least 100-fold greater than those of normal mouse or human raf RNAs. However, this abnormal expression is not critical to raf activation since in other cases, particularly the lung carcinoid, the abnormal raf transcripts from the recombined activated raf locus are expressed at levels which are no higher than that of the mouse transcript. Therefore, it would appear that raf is activated by recombination events, the critical effect of which is to lead to expression of a truncated protein lacking the amino terminal domain of normal raf. This truncation results in transforming activity, suggesting the hypothesis that the amino terminal domain normally functions to regulate raf activity and that deletion of regulatory sequences in this region leads to abnormal raf activity leading to cell transformation.

In addition to the ras and raf genes, related to retroviral oncogenes, a variety of other transforming genes have been detected by transfection of human DNA which are not related to previously known viral genes. At least a dozen such new transforming genes have at this point been identified by transfection of human tumor DNAs, and I will discuss two of these as examples. The first is the Blym-1 transforming gene which we first observed as a transforming sequence activated in DNAs of chicken bursal lymphomas (Cooper and Neiman, 1980). This gene was isolated as a molecular clone by sib selection in which a genomic library was screened for a biologically active transforming sequence using transfection as the assay (Goubin et al., 1983). Analysis of the isolated chicken Blym-1 revealed that it was a member of a small gene family which was present not only in chicken DNA but was also conserved in human DNA (Goubin et al., 1983). We had observed active transforming genes by transfection of DNAs of Burkitt's lymphomas, which represent a B-cell neoplasm of man which is pathologically quite similar to the chicken B-cell lymphomas from which chicken Blym-1 was isolated. We therefore attempted to isolate the Burkitt's lymphoma transforming gene using the chicken Blym-1 gene as a molecular hybridization probe (Diamond et al., 1983). A library of DNA of a Burkitt's lymphoma which contained a biologically active transforming sequence was screened not for biological activity but to isolate the family of human sequences which were homologous to chicken

Blym by plaque hybridization. One such human phage containing sequences homologous to chicken Blym-1 also proved to be
an active transforming gene in the transfection assay. In
addition, we could use this clone as a probe in the Southern
blots of DNAs of NIH cells transformed by genomic Burkitt's
lymphoma DNAs to demonstrate that this gene, designated
human Blym-1, was a transforming gene activated in DNAs of
these Burkitt's lymphomas (Diamond et al., 1983).

The distribution of Blym-1 activation in neoplasms is
significantly different from that of ras. We have only
detected Blym-1 transforming activity in these two B-cell
neoplasms: chicken bursal lymphomas and human Burkitt's
lymphomas. However, in these particular neoplasms, activation of Blym-1 is a highly reproducible event, such that we
have observed active Blym-1 transforming sequences in all of
the individual tumors of these types that have been analyzed
(Cooper and Neiman, 1980; Diamond et al., 1983). Thus,
Blym-1 activation appears to be, in contrast to ras, restricted to particular kinds of neoplasms but highly reproducible in the development of individual tumors of those
specific types.

Both the chicken and human Blym-1 transforming sequences are quite small, less than 1 kb, so by determination of
their nucleotide sequence, we could make a reasonable
prediction as to their coding potential. Both the chicken
and human Blym-1 sequences suggest that the genes encoded
related small proteins, 65 amino acids for the chicken gene
product and 58 amino acids for the human (Goubin et al.,
1983; Diamond et al., 1984). In order to begin to study the
protein encoded by the human Blym gene, we have prepared
antisera against a synthetic peptide predicted by the amino
acid sequence (Shipp et al., manuscript submitted). Rabbit
heterosera and monoclonal antibodies prepared against this
peptide identified a nuclear protein of 6.5 kd in the Raji
Burkitt's lymphoma cell line. The size of this protein is
in good agreement with the predicted molecular weight of the
Blym-1 product, 6.8 kd. Both the rabbit heterosera and the
monoclonal antibodies raised against this peptide also give
a clear pattern of nuclear fluorescence, substantiating its
nuclear localization by cell fractionation. The Blym-1
nuclear protein is expressed not only in Raji cells but also
in primary Burkitt's lymphomas, in EBV negative as well as
EBV positive Burkitt's lymphoma cell lines and in EBV
immortalized lymphocytes. It is not detected by the
immunofluorescence assay in normal resting B cells but, if
the B cells are stimulated to proliferate either by exposure

to Epstein-Barr virus or anti-IgM, then this mitogen stimulation results in expression of the nuclear Blym-1 protein.
The protein thus appears to be expressed in both normal and
neoplastic proliferating B cells, and its expression appears
to be related to mitogen stimulation or proliferation. This
is a similar behavior to that displayed by several other
oncogenes encoding nuclear proteins, including the myc gene,
which is activated by chromosomal translocations or viral
integration events in the same lymphomas in which Blym-1
transforming activity is detected.

The 6.5 kd nuclear protein thus appeared to represent
the Blym-1 gene product on the basis of molecular weight and
specific reactivity with immunological reagents prepared
against the predicted amino acid sequence. To further
demonstrate this, we introduced the Blym-1 gene in a tran-
sient over-expression vector into Cos-7 cells (Shipp et al.,
manuscript submitted). Cos cells transfected with the
Blym-1 gene and stained with anti-Blym sera gave a clear
pattern of nuclear fluorescence which was not detected with
control sera and was blocked by addition of the peptide. In
addition, they over-expressed the 6.5 kd Blym-1 nuclear
protein.

These observations thus identify a 6.5 kd nuclear
protein as the human Blym gene product. This cellular
localization is different from those of the ras or raf gene
products, which are membrane proteins, although similar to
several other oncogene products, including myc. The Blym-1
protein seems to be regulated in response to proliferation,
again like certain other oncogene products, and studies of
its potential biochemical activities and the regulation of
its expression in more detail are in progress.

Finally, I would like to discuss a fourth gene, ret,
which illustrates another type of oncogene detectable in the
transfection assay, namely one which we believe was activated not in the tumor from which it was obtained but rather by
rearrangement of a normal cell transforming gene during the
process of transfection (Takahashi et al., 1985). The
origin of ret was DNA of a T-cell lymphoma which gave rise
to only a single focus of transformed cells with a low
efficiency like that obtained with normal cell DNA. We were
able to clone the transforming sequence present in NIH
transformants by using hybridization with Alu repetitive
human DNA sequences. The transforming gene consisted of
approximately 40 kb of human DNA which was isolated in six
overlapping lambda clones. Blot hybridization using a

series of probes from this transforming gene to examine the organization of the sequences in transformed NIH cells, in normal human cells, and in the T-cell lymphoma which gave rise to the initial transformant indicated that all three types of DNAs were co-linear with the cloned transforming sequences at the left and right-hand ends of the cloned gene. However, when a fragment from the middle of the clone was used as a probe, we found that sequences in the transformed NIH cells were co-linear with the cloned sequences, but that this fragment hybridized to a more complex pattern of DNA sequences in human DNAs; either human DNAs of normal human cells or of the original T-cell lymphoma. Analysis of these human sequences further indicated that the ret gene in the NIH cells was formed by recombination of two segments of human DNA which were unlinked, that is separated by at least 30 kilobases, in either the genome of normal human cells or the T-cell lymphoma, suggesting that this recombination event occurred during the transfection assay. Different segments of the ret gene were co-transcribed into the same mRNAs in transformed NIH cells, indicating that the recombination event generated a new biologically active transcriptional unit.

To further analyze this recombination process, we have cloned cDNAs corresponding to the ret transcript (Takahashi and Cooper, manuscript in preparation). The smallest ret mRNA is 3 kb, most of which was isolated as two overlapping cDNAs clones spanning 2.6 kb. The site of recombination between the two unlinked segments of human DNA is approximately in the middle of this cDNA. The entire sequence of the 2.6 kb cDNA was determined and found to contain a single open reading frame extending from the beginning of the cloned sequence up until about 100 nucleotides before a poly A tail. Thus, the two human sequences which recombined to form the active ret gene did so by generating not only a recombinant transcript but also a new recombinant fusion protein which contains coding sequences from both halves. Computer homology analysis of this sequence indicated that the 5' half was not related to any known protein coding sequences, but the 3' half of the gene was homologous to the family of tyrosine kinase oncogenes. The sequence of ret is not identical to any of the other known tyrosine kinase oncogenes or surface receptors, such as epidermal growth factor or insulin receptor, but displays 40%-50% homology in regions which are common between members of this gene family. Ret then appears to represent a new tyrosine kinase activated by recombination which may have involved loss of its normal amino-terminal sequences, as was the case with the raf gene.

A variety of neoplasms thus contain active transforming genes of several types which can be either related or unrelated to known viral transforming genes. The examples that I have illustrated here include ras, which is a membrane guanine nucleotide binding protein believed to be involved in signal transduction; raf, which is a serine/threonine kinase; ret which appears to be a tyrosine kinase family member; and Blym, which is a nuclear protein. Thus, the number of genes in neoplasms and the diversity of biochemical mechanisms by which they may act is broad. Major challenges in the field include detailed analysis of the biochemical mechanisms by which these transforming proteins can influence cell growth and attempts to define the roles that transforming genes may play in the pathogenesis of the neoplasms from which they have been isolated.

REFERENCES

Albino, A.P., LeStrange, R., Oliff, A.I., Furth, M.E., and Old, L.J. Transforming ras genes from human melanoma: a manifestation of tumor heterogeneity? Nature 308, 69-72, 1984.

Bos, J.L., Toksoz, D., Marshall, C.J., Verlaan-de Vries, M., Veeneman, G.H., Van der Eb, A.J., Van Boom, J.H., Janssen, J.W.G., and Steenvoorden, A.C.M. Amino-acid substitutions at codon 13 of the N-ras oncogene in human acute myeloid leukemia. Nature 315, 726-730, 1985.

Chang, E.H., Furth, M.E., Scolnick, E.M., and Lowy, D.R. Tumorigenic transformation of mammalian cells induced by a normal human gene homologous to the oncogene of Harvey murine sarcoma virus. Nature 297, 479-483, 1982.

Cooper, G.M. and Lane, M.A. Cellular transforming genes and oncogenesis. Biochim. Biophys. Acta Rev. on Cancer 738, 9-20, 1984.

Cooper, G.M. and Neiman, P.E. Transforming genes of neoplasms induced by avian lymphoid leukosis viruses. Nature 287, 656-659, 1980.

Cooper, G.M., Okenquist, S., and Silverman, L. Transforming activity of DNA of chemically transformed and normal cells. Nature 284, 418-421, 1980.

Der, C., Finkel, T., and Cooper, G.M. Biological and

biochemical properties of human ras^H genes mutated at codon 61. Cell, 1986, in press.

Der, C.J., Krontiris, T.G., and Cooper, G.M. Transforming genes of human bladder and lung carcinoma cell lines are homologous to the ras genes of Harvey and Kirsten sarcoma viruses. Proc. Natl. Acad. Sci. USA 79, 3637-3640, 1982.

Diamond, A., Cooper, G.M., Ritz, J., and Lane, M.A. Identification and molecular cloning of the human Blym transforming gene activated in Burkitt's lymphomas. Nature 305, 112-116, 1983.

Diamond, A., Devine, J., and Cooper, G.M. Nucleotide sequence of human Blym transforming gene activated in a Burkitt's lymphoma. Science 225, 516-519, 1984.

Finkel, T., Der, C.J., and Cooper, G.M. Activation of ras genes in human tumors does not affect localization, modification, or nucleotide binding properties of p21. Cell 37, 151-158, 1984.

Fukui, M., Yamamoto, T., Kawai, S., Maruo, K., and Toyoshima, K. Detection of raf-related and two other transforming DNA sequences in human tumor maintained in nude mice. Proc. Natl. Acad. Sci. USA 83, 5954-5958, 1985.

Furth, M.E., Davis, L.J., Fleurdelys, B., and Scolnick, E.M. Monoclonal antibodies to the p21 products of the transforming gene of Harvey murine sarcoma virus and of the cellular ras gene family. J. Virol. 43, 294-304, 1982.

Gilman, A.G. G proteins and dual control of adenylate cyclase. Cell 36, 577-579, 1984.

Goubin, G., Goldman, D.S., Luce, J., Neiman, P.E., and Cooper, G.M. Molecular cloning and nucleotide sequence of a transforming gene detected by transfection of chicken B-cell lymphoma DNA. Nature 302, 114-119, 1983.

McGrath, J.P., Capon, D.J., Goeddel, D.V., and Levinson, A.D. Comparative biochemical properties of normal and activated human ras p21 protein. Nature 310, 644-649, 1984.

Molders, H., Defesche, D., Muller, T.I., Bonner, U.R., and Muller, R. Integration of transfected LTR sequences into the c-raf proto-oncogene: activation by promoter insertion. EMBO J. 4, 693-698, 1985.

Parada, L.F., Tabin, C.J., and Weinberg, R.A. Human EJ bladder carcinoma oncogene is homologue of Harvery sarcoma virus ras gene. Nature 297, 474-478, 1982.

Reddy, E.P., Reynolds, R.K., Santos, E., and Barbacid, M. A point mutation is responsible for the acquisition of transforming properties by the T24 human bladder carcinoma oncogene. Nature 300, 149-152, 1982.

Santos, E., Tronick, S.R., Aaronson, S.A., Pulciani, S., and Barbacid, M. T24 human bladder carcinoma oncogene is an activated form of the normal human homologue of BALB- and Harvey-MSV transforming genes. Nature 298, 343-347, 1982.

Schafer, R., Griefel, S., Dubbert, M.A., and Willecke, K. Unstable transformation of mouse 3T3 cells by transfection with DNA from normal human lymphocytes. EMBO J. 3, 659-663, 1984.

Scolnick, E.M., Papageorge, A.G., and Shih, T.Y. Guanine nucleotide-binding activity as an assay for src protein of rat-derived murine sarcoma viruses. Proc. Natl. Acad. Sci. USA 76, 5355-5359, 1979.

Seeburg, P.H., Colby, W.W., Hayflick, J.S., Capon, D.J., Goeddel, D.V., and Levinson, A.D. Nature 312, 71-75, 1984.

Sefton, B.M., Trowbridge, I.S., Cooper, J.A., and Scolnick, EM. The transforming proteins of Rous sarcoma virus, Harvey sarcoma virus, and Abelson virus contain tightly bound lipid. Cell 31, 464-474, 1982.

Shimizu, K., Goldfarb, M., Perucho, M., and Wigler, M. Isolation and preliminary characterization of the transforming gene of a human neuroblastoma cell line. Proc. Natl. Acad. Sci. USA 80, 383-387, 1983.

Shimizu, K., Yoshimichi, N., Sekiguchi, M., Hokamura, K., and Tanaka, K. Molecular cloning of an activated human oncogene, homologous to v-raf, from primary stomach cancer. Proc. Natl. Acad. Sci. USA 82, 5641-5645, 1985.

Tabin, C.J., Bradley, S.M., Bargmann, C.I., Weinberg, R.A., Papageorge, A.G., Scolnick, E.M., Dhar, R., Lowy, D.R., and Chang, E.H. Mechanism of activation of a human oncogene. Nature 300, 143-149, 1982.

Takahashi, M., Ritz, J., and Cooper, G.M. Activation of a novel human transforming gene, ret, by DNA rearrangement. Cell 42, 581-588, 1985.

Taparowsky, E., Suard, Y., Fasano, O., Shimizu, K., Goldfarb, M., and Wigler, M. Activation of the T24 bladder carcinoma transforming gene is linked to a single amino acid change. Nature 300, 762-765, 1982.

Yuasa, Y., Srivastava, S.K., Dunn, C.Y., Rhim, J.S., Reddy, E.P., and Aaronson, S.A. Acquisition of transforming properties by alternatieve point mutations within c-bas/has human proto-oncogene. Nature 303, 775-779, 1983.

HORMONE RECEPTORS

MONOCLONAL ANTIBODIES

CELLULAR RESPONSES MEDIATED BY ESTROGEN RECEPTORS - FUNDAMENTAL ASPECTS.

G. LECLERCQ

Laboratoire de Cancérologie Mammaire, Service de Médecine, Institut J. Bordet, 1000 Brussels, Belgium.

Estrogens are acting on their target tissues trough binding to a specific receptor (estrogen receptor; ER). According to a classical concept, estradiol (E2) binds to ER in the cytoplams. In a subsequent step, E2 promotes the transformation of the receptor in an "active" form which enters into the nucleus where it interacts with the chromatin at some specific acceptor sites. RNA and protein syntheses derive from the interaction. Recent observations cast some doubt on this model. ER would be, in fact, a nuclear protein which would only be "activated" by E2 to interact with specific acceptor sites; the cytosolic form of the receptor would only be a consequence of a nuclear protein release during the homogenization (Jensen and Desombre, 1972; King and Greene, 1984).

In both models, the activation process of ER is a key step for the appearance of specific responses. Studies are presently undertaken in several laboratories to further analyse the mechanism as well as consequences of this process. It is our purpose to review here our own investigations.

1. Measure of the activation potency of a compound

A whole cell assay for measuring ER in monolayer culture of human breast cancer cell lines has been recently developed in our laboratory (Olea-Serrano et al., 1985 a). It is based on the measurement of incorporated 3H-E2 during 50 min. of incubation. This assay has been modified for evaluating the binding affinity of compounds interacting with ER in cytosol preparations (Stoessel and Leclercq, submitted).

Growing MCF-7 were incubated with 3H-E2 and increasing amounts of unlabeled E2 (control) or test compounds. For both steroid and diethylstilbestrol-based estrogens, relative binding affinities were in the same order of magnitude than those previously established on cytosol using a classical dextran-coated charcoal (DCC) assay. These values were directly related to the estrogen potency of the compounds as established in conventional tests (i.e. Allen-Doisy). In contrast, in the case of triphenylethylene estrogens and antiestrogens, whole cell assays gave systematically low values which were shown to be directly related to the weak estrogenicity of the compounds. These data indicated that the whole cell test provided a measure of the ability of a compound to stabilize the "active" form of the receptor, i.e. the conformation which promotes transcription.

Whole cell assay in competitive binding studies appears, therefore, as a powerful additive test to the classical DCC test performed in the cytosol which is totally unable to discriminate between active and non-active complexes. Since the test would provide a measure of the activation potency of a compound it seems logic to denominate it as "relative activation potency" (RAP) test. In further studies, it would be extremely interesting to analyse whether the RAP value of a given compound correlates with its ability to favor the binding of the cytosolic receptor to chromatographic matrices recognizing the activated form of the latter (i.e. ATP-Sepharose) (Singh et al., 1984). Correlation studies between RAP values and estrogenic-induced differences in elution or sedimentation characteristics of the receptor (Eckert and Katzenellenbogen, 1982) would be other instructive investigations.

Introduction of a RAP test in drug screening for the selection of antineoplastic compounds acting through ER seems of prominent importance. In this regard, an "improved" antiestrogen devoid of agonistic activity would logically be characterized by a very high RBA value (cytosol assay) and a very weak RAP value (whole cell assay). Obviously, in some cases, this relationship would not hold since the whole cell assay is also influenced by physiological factors independent of the receptor activation such as the cell membrane permeability or metabolism.

2. Physiological responses resulting from the activation process of estrogen receptor

Studies are presently conducted to analyse the influence of ER activation on the ability of isolated nuclei to incorporate 3H-actinomycin D (3H-AMD). This ability, which is an index of genomic derepression was found to be highly increased by the activation process. Investigations are pursued in parallel to analyse the consequence of this derepression mechanism on the synthesis and secretion of proteins. The relevance of our observations in regard to the trophic action of estrogens is also analysed. An overview of our findings is given in the following sections.

2.1. Genomic derepression

Nuclear transfer of cytosolic E2-ER complexes produces an increase in RNA synthesis most probably by derepressing genomic sites. Some years ago, we investigated this phenomenon by the autoradiographic method of 3H-AMD labeling introduced by

---

RAP: Relative Activation Potency
RBA: Relative Binding Affinity

Brachet and Ficq (1985) for the identification of derepression
processes. Uterine nuclei were incubated with uterine cytosol
and subsequently smeared on histological slides for the 3H-AMD
labeling. Under these experimental conditions, we found that a
preincubation of the cytosol with E2 allowing the nuclear transfer of the receptor produced a significant increase of 3H-AMD
binding (Leclercq et al., 1973) (Fig. 1). The phenomenon did
not occur under conditions giving no increase in RNA synthesis
indicating the high specificity of the assay. Noteworthy, our
observations were biochemically confirmed by Mainwaring and
Jones (1975) on isolated chromatin from prostatic tissue.

Pursuing our investigations, we recently showed that uterine cytosol preincubated with the strong antiestrogen hydroxy-
tamoxifen did not produce any increase or decrease of 3H-AMD
binding (Verrijdt et al., 1985). On the contrary, the compound
counteracted the increase of binding induced by E2 which is consistent with its known antagonistic activity.

All these data led us to investigate mammary carcinomas
(Verrijdt et al., 1985). In a preliminary study, MCF-7 breast
cancer cells (ER+) were used. As previously found with uterine
cells, a significant increase of 3H-AMD binding occurred in
isolated MCF-7 cell nuclei exposed to cytosol preincubated with
E2. Again, the increase was not found under various experimental
conditions giving no nuclear transfer of the receptor (i.e.,
cytosol alone, estradiol alone, cytosol in which E2 was added
at the time of the exposure to the nuclei). The increase did
not occur in a control ER-cell line (Evsa-T) clearly confirming the involvement of the receptor for its observation.

MXT mouse mammary carcinomas (Watson et al., 1977) gave
similar results (Verrijdt et al., 1985) (Fig. 1). Moreover, in
this experimental tumor model, an ultrastructural study revealed that the receptor-induced increase of 3H-AMD was associated
with a marked modification of the chromatin structure. In the
control, clumps of condensed chromatin were located near the
nuclear envelope, while after E2 treatment, chromatin was dispersed in the whole of the nucleoplasm.

Further studies to establish the optimal conditions of
3H-AMD labeling revealed that the increase only occurred after
30 min. of fixation of the nuclei in ethanol-acetic. Moreover,
the basal (unstimulated) 3H-AMD binding appeared always higher
after fixation with this mixture than with neutral formol which
is consistent with the concept that neutral formol maintains
and reinforces the bonds between the basic nuclear proteins and
the DNA thereby masking site for AMD. On the other hand, that a
prolonged fixation of the nuclei in ethanol-CH_3COOH was required
for demonstrating a receptor-induced increase of 3H-AMD binding
indicated that the removal of the basic proteins from the DNA
is essential for the observation of the phenomenon. This observation also suggested that the receptor largely reduces the
interaction between the basic proteins and the DNA so that they

could be extracted during the fixation procedure.

2.2. Protein induction and secretion

Incubation of cells with a labeled aminoacid (i.e. ^{35}S-methionine) in absence or presence of a hormone is a common methodology for assessing its inductive effect on protein synthesis. Identification of such induced proteins are usually performed by analytical SDS-polyacrylamide gel ectrophoresis and subsequent fluorography. This classical approach was used for investigating the effect of E2 on mammary tumor synthesis.

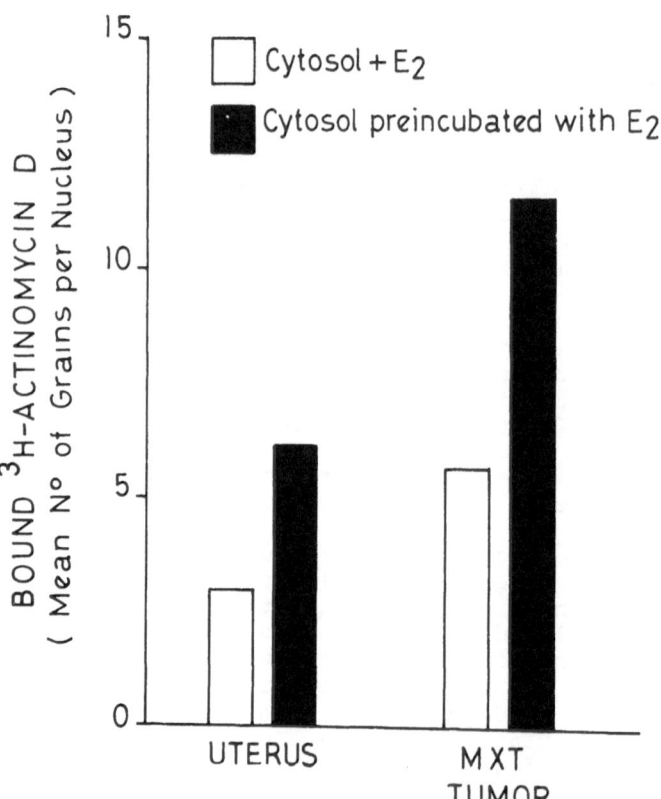

Fig. 1. Binding of ^{3}H-actinomycin D to purified nuclei exposed to cytosol + 10^{-8} M estradiol or cytosol preincubated with 10^{-8} M estradiol. Binding was assessed by autoradiography.

Preliminary investigations (Mairesse et al., 1980) revealed the constitutive synthesis of a cytosolic protein of Mr 46K in two breast cancer cell lines, respectively containing (MCF-7) and lacking (Evsa-T) ER. Estradiol at 10^{-8}M, a concentration producing a growth stimulatory effect (see below), stimulated the synthesis of this protein in the MCF-7 cells only (Fig. 2). Subsequent studies (Mairesse et al., 1985) indicated that this protein corresponds in fact to a group of 4 proteins of 46, 52, 54 and 60 K. All of them differ from a known uterine estrogen-induced protein (IP; Mr 48 K) by the absence of crea-

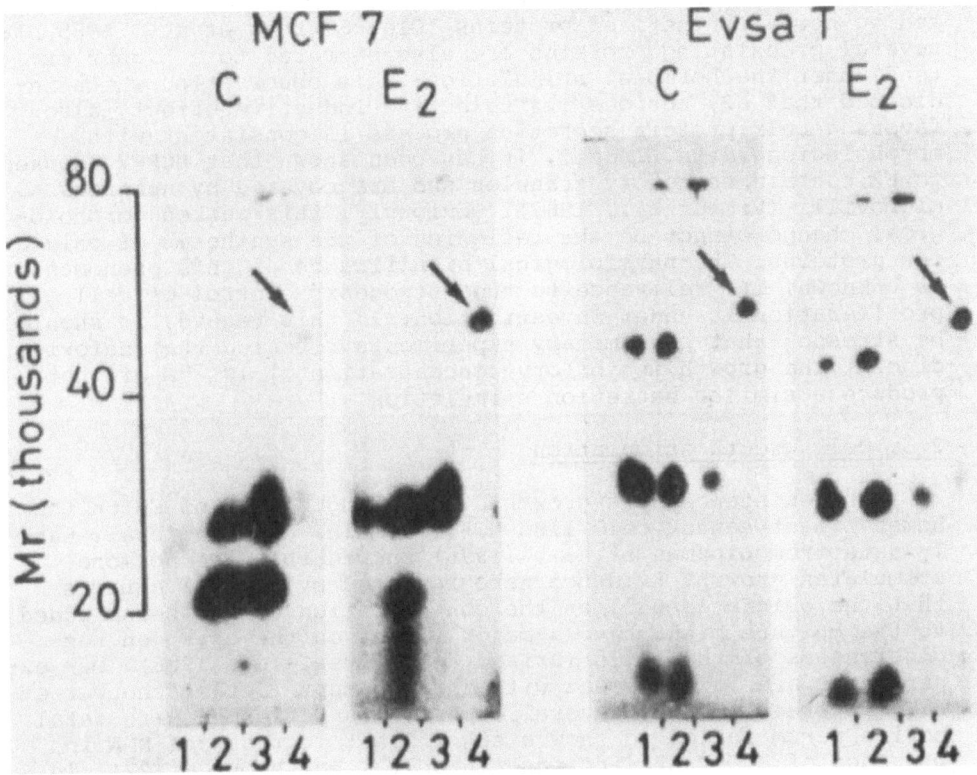

Fig. 2. Fluorogram of SDS polyacrylamide gel electrophoresis of MCF-7 (ER+) and Evsa-T (ER-) cytosols. Samples of [^{35}s]-labeled cytosol proteins from control and estradiol-treated cells were subjected to Cellogel electrophoresis. The Cellogel region corresponding to the uterine IP (Mr 48K) was excised and separated into 4 fractions that were submitted to polyacrylamide gel electrophoresis, The arrows indicate the constitutively synthetized proteins of Mr 48K. For further details, see Mairesse et al., ref. 12.

tine kinase activity as well as an increased acidity. Additional investigations showed that the antiestrogen nafoxidine does not stimulate the synthesis of any similar proteins at concentration ranging from 10^{-8} to $10^{-6}M$ (Mairesse et al., 1983). Moreover, at $10^{-6}M$, the drug totally suppressed the inductive effect of E2.

We also confirmed the observations of other investigators (Edwards and Mc Guire, 1982; Vignon et al., 1983) that E2 stimulates the secretion of some newly synthetized proteins. Moreover, we demonstrated that this secretion process is not limited to newly synthetized proteins (Olea-Serrano et al., 1985 b): several preexisting proteins are also secreted to a higher extend under the hormonal stimulation. This observation which indicated that E2, besides its selective inductive effect, also favors a bulk protein secretion process is consistent with morphological data. Indeed, it has been shown that MCF-7 exposed to E2 contain secretory granules and are covered by numerous microvilli (Vic et al., 1982). Obviously, this marked morphological change cannot be the reflexion of the synthesis of only a few proteins. The physiological significance of this phenomenon is unknown. Its relevance to the estrogenic control of cell proliferation is under investigation. In this regard, it should be stressed that preliminary experiments revealed that nafoxidine at the growth inhibitory concentration of $10^{-6}M$ did not produce a similar secretion stimulation.

2.3. Cell growth stimulation

The existence of a growth-stimulating effect of E2 on the human breast cancer cell line MCF-7 remains controversial. Early data from Lippman et al., (1976) showed that the hormone stimulates growth. Evidence were reported by several authors that the origin as well as the concentration of the serum added to the culture might have a major effect on the estrogen responsiveness of the cells (Briand and Lykkesfeldt, 1986). Our experiments are in agreement with this concept (Devleeschouwer et al., in press). Thus, several experiments performed with fetal bovine serum failed to show a significant increase of DNA in presence of $10^{-8}M$ E2 (increase in only 1 batch out of 22). In contrast, the hormone always produced a strong increase in a series of freshly prepared human serum (9 batches)(Fig. 3); this effect occurred at various serum concentration (1, 5, 10 and 20%) Reassessment of 2 batches of sera after prolonged storage at -20°C (6 and 8 months) did no more show this stimulatory effect, suggesting an alteration of (a) factor(s) mediating the effect of E2. Remarkably, several freshly prepared sera from various other origins (bovine, cat, dog) showed such a stimulatory effect, others from commercial origins were also effective in some cases.

Nature of these seric factors mediating the effect of E2 is unknown. Whether they are mitogens acting in synergy with E2 or growth inhibitors whom action is suppressed by the hormone is a controversial question (Briand and Lykkesfeldt, 1986; Sirbascu and Benson, 1979; Sato and Sonneschein, 1984). Experiments are carried in our laboratory to elucidate this problem. Such factors being most probably in very low amounts, we developed a microtechnique of cell culture to test a large spectrum of seric fractions under various experimental conditions (Maddedu et al., 1986). Cells cultures in 96-multiwell in presence or in absence of E2 and serum or fraction are fixed with ethanol and colored with hematoxylin. The intensity of the coloration is then measured with a multiscan spectrophotometer. This intensity which is related to the cell number, rapidly provides an accurate estimate of the effect of each experimental condition.

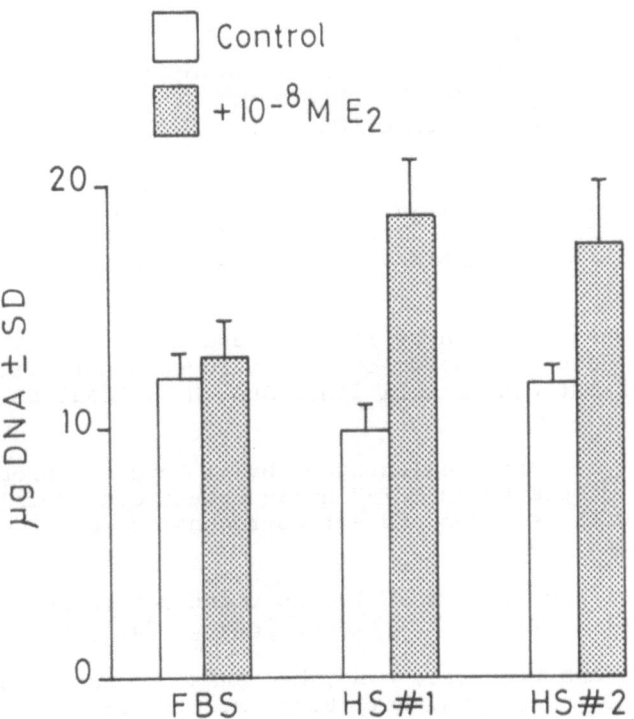

Fig. 3. Effect of 10^{-8}M estradiol on MCF-7 cell growth. Cells were cultured for 5 days in absence or presence of estradiol in either fetal (FBS) or human (HS; 2 batches) serum. For experimental details, see Leclercq et al., J. steroid Biochem. 19 : 75-85 (1983).

Implication of our studies in the clinical practice is not obvious. Nevertheless, the observation of a higher binding of 3H-AMD under E2 stimulation suggests that an estrogenic treatment may increase the vulnerability of the tumor cells to cytotoxic drugs. An attractive pursue of our investigations would be the development of an improved receptor assay for the detection of the hormone insensitive ER-positive tumors which contain an altered receptor activation mechanism. Finally, the search for new estrogen-inductible markers is another extension of our studies which should be extremely helpful for the management of the disease.

ACKNOWLEDGEMENTS

This work was supported by Belgian grants from the Fonds Cancérologique de la Caisse Générale d'Epargne et de Retraite and the Fonds National de la Recherche Scientifique.

REFERENCES

1. Brachet, J. and Ficq, A.: Binding sites of 14C-actinomycin in amphibian ovocytes and an autoradiography technique for the detection of cytoplasmic DNA. Expl. Cell Res. 38: 153-159, 1985.

2. Briand, P. and Lykkesfeldt, A.E.: Long-term cultivation of human breast cancer cell line, MCF-7, in a chemically defined medium. Effect of estradiol. Anticancer Res. 6: 85-90, 1986.

3. Devleeschouwer, N., Olea-Serrano, N. and Leclercq G.: Influence of the nature of serum on the estrogen-sensitivity of the MCF-7 breast cancer cell line. Ann. N.Y. Acad. Sci. (in press).

4. Eckert, R.L. and Katzenellenbogen, B.S.: Physical properties of estrogen complexes in MCF-7 human breast cancer cells: difference with estrogen and antiestrogens. J. Biol. Chem. 257: 8840-8846, 1982

5. Edwards, D.P. and McGuire, W.L.: Estrogen action in human breast cancer (review). Anticancer Res. 2: 297-308, 1982.

6. Jensen, E.V. and Desombre, E.R., Mechanism of action of the female sex hormones. Ann. Rev. Biochem. 41: 203-230, 1972.

7. King, W.J. and Greene, G.L.: Monoclonal antibodies localize estrogen receptor in the nuclei of target cells. Nature 307: 745-747, 1984.

8. Leclercq, G., Hulin, N. and Heuson, J.C.: Interaction of activated estradiol-receptor complex and chromatin in isolated uterine nuclei. Europ. J. Cancer Clin. Oncol. 9: 681-685, 1973.

9. Lippman, M., Bolan, G. and Huff, K.: The effect of estrogens and antiestrogens on hormone responsive human breast cancer in long-term tissue culture. Cancer Res. $\underline{36}$: 4595-4601, 1976.

10. Maddedu, L., Roy, E. and Leclercq, G.: A new method for evaluating the inhibitory potency of antiestrogens on breast cancer cell lines. Anticancer Res. $\underline{6}$: 11-16, 1986.

11. Mainwaring, W.I.P. and Jones, D.M.,Influence of receptor complexes on the properties of prostate chromatin, including its transcription by RNA polymerase. J. Steroid Biochem. $\underline{6}$: 475-481, 1975.

12. Mairesse, N., Devleeschouwer, N., Leclercq, G. and Galand, P.: Estrogen-induced protein in the human breast cancer cell line MCF-7. Biochem. Biophys. Res. Commun. $\underline{97}$: 1251-1257, 1980.

13. Mairesse, N., Devleeschouwer, N., Leclercq, G. and Galand, P.: Nafoxidine antagonism on estrogen "induced proteins" synthesis in the human breast cancer cell line MCF-7. IRCS Med. Sc. $\underline{11}$: 165, 1983.

14. Mairesse, N., Devleeschouwer, N., Leclercq, G. and Galand, P.: Estrogen-induced synthesis and secretion of proteins in the human breast cancer cell line MCF-7. J. Steroid Biochem. $\underline{15}$: 375-381, 1985.

15. Olea-Serrano, N., Devleeschouwer, N., Leclercq, G. and Heuson, J.C.: Assay for estrogen and progesterone receptors of breast cancer cell lines in monolayer culture. Eur. J. Cancer Clin. Oncol. $\underline{21}$: 965-973, 1985 a.

16. Olea-Serrano, N., Leclercq, G., Mairesse, N. and Heuson, J.C.: Bulk protein secretion induced by estradiol in MCF-7 cells. Eur. J. Cancer Clin. Oncol. $\underline{21}$: 1267-1271, 1985 b.

17. Sato, A.M. and Sonneschein, C.: Mechanism of estrogen action on cellular proliferation: evidence for indirect negative control on cloned breast tumor cells. Biochem. Biophys. Res. Commun. $\underline{122}$: 1097-1103, 1984.

18. Singh, R.K., Ruh, M.F. and Ruh, T.S.: Activation of 3H -estradiol- and 3H - H 1285-receptor complexes: effect of salt versus ATP on molybdate stabilized estrogen receptors. J. Steroid Biochem. $\underline{21}$: 205-208, 1984.

19. Sirbascu, D.A. and Benson, R.H.: Estrogen-inductible growth factors that may act as mediators (estromedins) of estrogen-promoted tumor cell growth. In: Hormones and cell culture, Book A (Sato G.H. and Ross R. eds). New York, Cold Spring Harbor Lab. $\underline{6}$: 477-497, 1979.

84

20. Stoessel, S. and Leclercq, G.: Competitive binding assay for estrogen receptor in monolayer culture: measure of receptor activation potency. Submitted for publication.

21. Verrijdt, A., Leclercq, G., Devleeschouwer, N. and Danguy, A.: Tritiated actinomycin D staining method: a valuable tool to study estrogen receptor-induced modifications of transcriptional activity in normal and neoplastic cells. Arch. Int. Physiol. Biochim. 93: 65-73, 1985.

22. Vic, P. Vignon, F., Derocq, D. and Rochefort, H.: Effect of estradiol on the ultrastructure of the MCF-7 human breast cancer cells in culture. Cancer Res. 42: 667-673, 1982.

23. Vignon, F., Capony, F., Chalbos, D., Garcia, M., Veith, F., Westley, B. and Rochefort, H.: Estrogen-regulated 52 K protein and control of cell proliferation in human breast cancer cells. Progress in Cancer Research and Therapy 31: 147-170, 1983.

24. Watson, C., Medina, D. and Clarck, J.H.: Estrogen receptor characterization in a transplantable mouse mammary tumor. Cancer Res. 37: 3344-3348, 1977.

MONOCLONAL HUMAN ANTITUMOR ANTIBODIES: SEARCH FOR SPECIFIC B-LYMPHOCYTES SUITABLE FOR FUSION

E. R. WAELTI, R. KRAFT, H. COTTIER

Department of Pathology, University of Bern,
Freiburgstrasse 30, CH-3010 Bern,
Switzerland

INTRODUCTION

Since the production of human monoclonal antibody has proved more difficult than the production of mouse monoclonal antibody, the obvious question must be asked: Is it worth the effort? The answer must be yes! Human monoclonal antibodies may obviate many of the difficulties that murine monoclonal antibodies used for therapy have encountered. The difficulties range from minor allergic reactions to anaphylaxis. Human monoclonal antibodies in this regard would also be safer and more useful in in vivo diagnostic and therapeutic applications. Moreover, murine monoclonal antibodies, being foreign proteins, are cleared by the reticuloendothelial system after several administrations due to their recognition by the human immune system. It should also be noted that murine monoclonal antibodies recognize a different range of antigens than do humans. The mouse immune system primarily recognizes xenogeneic antigens on human cells. A clinically relevant set of antigens on human tumor cell surfaces may generate a poor, if any, immune response in mice. Humans, on the other hand, may be better able to distinguish between normal and tumor cells.

The production of human monoclonal antibodies by the hybridoma technique is a time-consuming, often fruitless, and very expensive work. Despite great effort, the progress made to date has been very limited. The majority of laboratories engaged in this work have to make thousands of fusions using lymphocytes from patients with breast cancer, kidney cancer, lung cancer, and malignant melanoma to find a few clones secreting antibodies that react with tumor cell surface antigens. Moreover, human monoclonal antibodies, reacting to intracellular structures and to a variety of nontumor antigen specificities such as autoantigens, infectious disease antigens, and private antigens, occur at a significantly higher frequency than do antibodies to cell surface components. Therefore, the search for antibodies of the desired specificity may be likened to looking for a needle in a haystack.

Some data shall illustrate this point: In a screen for human antibodies to cellular antigens, Houghton et al. (1983) have found that 0.8% of clones secreted antibodies to cell surface components. Cote et al. (1983) at Memorial Sloan-Kettering Cancer Center, New York, tested the production of antibody reactive against cell surface or intracellular antigens in 422 Ig-secreting cultures; <1% of the cultures showed detectable antibody to cell-surface antigens, whereas 9% produced antibody to intracellular antigens.

It is against this background that we are looking for some new experimental strategies which would allow an increased yield of stable hybridomas producing human monoclonal antibodies to tumor cell surface antigens. We think that a preselection of tumor-specific lymphocytes may enhance the frequency of tumor-specific hybridomas. Cell affinity chromatography of lymphocytes which is currently being studied in our laboratory may provide the basis for the preselection. In this connection, our major effort is now involved in the generation of human monoclonal antibodies to breast cancer. The sources of B cells we have chosen are lymph nodes and, for the first time, malignant effusions, too.

It is well known that the draining lymph nodes of cancer patients are a source of sensitized lymphocytes. Schlom et al. (1980), Imam et al. (1982, 1985), and Cote et al. (1983) have demonstrated that B lymphocytes in the regional draining lymph nodes of breast cancer patients are primed to synthesize antibodies against tumor-associated antigens.

We suppose that in malignant effusions, tumor-specific B cells may also be found. However, the isolation of B cells from such fluids containing a mixture of cancer cells, mesothelial and endothelial cells, and inflammatory cells is not so easy to perform as from the lymph nodes. In addition, every effusion has a different composition, and the number of lymphocytes is usually low. Moreover, only 10% of the lymphocytes are B cells; the greatest part are T cells.

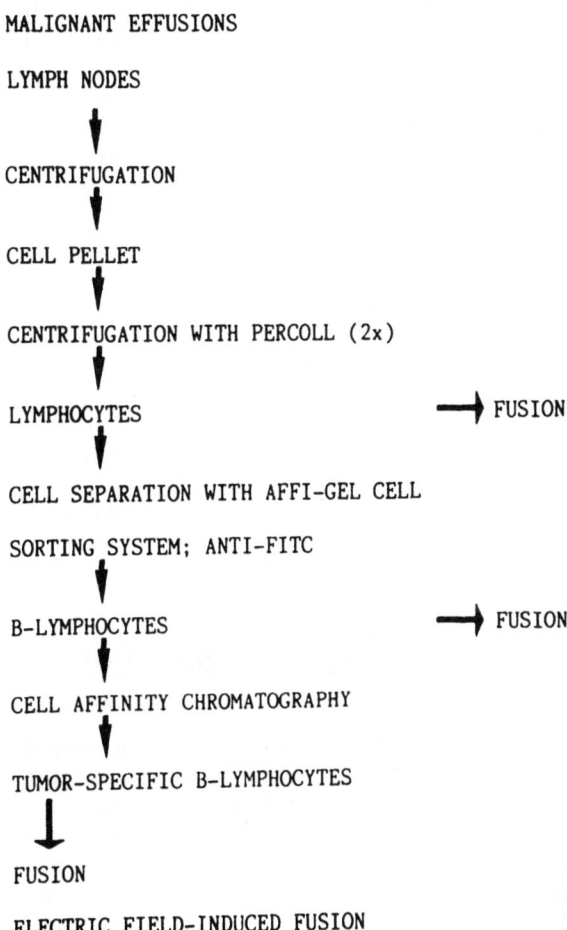

MALIGNANT EFFUSIONS

LYMPH NODES

CENTRIFUGATION

CELL PELLET

CENTRIFUGATION WITH PERCOLL (2x)

LYMPHOCYTES   → FUSION

CELL SEPARATION WITH AFFI-GEL CELL

SORTING SYSTEM; ANTI-FITC

B-LYMPHOCYTES   → FUSION

CELL AFFINITY CHROMATOGRAPHY

TUMOR-SPECIFIC B-LYMPHOCYTES

FUSION

ELECTRIC FIELD-INDUCED FUSION

Fig. 1.   Flow diagram illustrating the strategy for the isolation of tumor-specific B lymphocytes from malignant effusions and lymph nodes.

STRATEGY FOR THE ISOLATION OF TUMOR-SPECIFIC B LYMPHOCYTES

Figure 1 shows the flow diagram illustrating the sequence of events our laboratory uses in isolating the B cells from 1 to 2 litres of effusion.

After a first centrifugation of the fluid, the pelleted sediment of cells is resuspended and centrifuged two times over a Percoll density gradient. Sometimes, the resulting purification may not be sufficient for hybridization because of contamination with mammary carcinoma cells that outgrow the hybrid cells in the culture. Therefore, we have included as a second purification step an immunoselective cell separation that makes possible an enrichment of B cells by a factor of at least 30.

The Anti-FITC Cell Sorting System of Bio Rad which offers a rapid, sensitive, and easily reproducible means for obtaining purified cell populations was adapted and used to isolate human blastic B lymphocytes: Lymphocytes, preincubated with a commercially available FITC-conjugated antibody to surface Ig, are separated on a column of anti-FITC cell sorting beads. Before separation, cytophilic Ig is removed from the cells by an overnight $37^{\circ}C$ incubation. Bound lymphocytes can be released from the column by agitating the beads. A higher viability of released cells will be achieved by using appropriate non-specific FITC-Ig to compete with anti-FITC sites on the beads.

Cell affinity chromatography for preselection of tumor-specific lymphocytes

The next step we are planning is a preselection of tumor-specific lymphocytes. Membrane-bound antibodies on the B-cell surface serve as antigen receptors, while after stimulation by antigen, the same antibodies are produced in secreted form. Thus, if there are any tumor-specific B cells in malignant effusions of breast carcinoma patients, they should bind to mammary carcinoma cells by their appropriate antigen-binding Ig-receptors. They may also bind to cell-surface antigens of human breast cancer cell lines.

Table 1.

Cell Affinity Chromatography for Preselection of
B-Lymphocytes

Living cells	Culture on beads (Microcarriers)
Human breast car- cinoma cell lines:	Cytodex (Pharmacia)
MCF-7, BT-20, T-47D, etc.	
Cell membranes of human breast carcinoma cells	Polycationic beads Affi-Gel 731 (Bio Rad)

Our theoretical fractionation experiments aim at two possibilities summarized in Table 1. Firstly, the whole B-cell population is applied to an adsorbent column containing immobilized living mammary carcinoma cells on a solid matrix. A 20-min incubation at room temperature allows binding of B cells before commencing elution of unbound B cells. Specifically bound B cells are then recovered by competitive elution using human IgG.

Mai and Chung (1984) recently reported that MCF-7 cells rapidly attach on uncoated Cytodex 2 beads. A better possibility is to use extracellular matrix-coated beads. In this case, cells will proliferate and remain attached to these beads as monolayers even after 12 days of culture. The method is certainly applicable to other cell lines.

Instead of living cells on beads, plasma membranes of cancer cells may also be used for cell affinity chromatography. Plasma membranes are isolated on polycationic beads; for example, polyacrylamide beads coated with polyethylenimine are useful as a polycationic solid support (Affi-Gel 731, Bio-Rad) (Gruenberg and Sherman, 1983).

If we have succeeded in isolating a fraction of tumor-specific B lymphocytes, we are facing a new problem:

we have to develop a fusion technique suitable for low numbers of cells. A fascinating possibility may be the electric field-mediated fusion of cells. Zimmermann (1982) have tested this technique for the production of murine hybridoma cells.

It seems possible to fuse one B lymphocyte with one myeloma cell. The molecular processes which are thought to occur during electrically-induced fusion are an electrical breakdown leading to a disruption of the membrane structure and then, bridges between the lipid bilayers of the new cell membranes are formed during the reorganization of the lipid molecules.

Lo et al. (1984) reported an interesting modification of electrically induced cell fusion. The antigen, covalently conjugated to avidin, binds to the surface immunoglobulins on B cells. This B-cell-antigen-avidin complex binds to biotin covalently attached to the surface of myeloma cells. An intense electric field across a bulk cell suspension then produces selective fusion of cells with B cells which make the appropriate antibody.

FUSIONS WITH SPAZ-4 CELLS

A second major drawback for the production of human monoclonal antibodies is the lack of a suitable human myeloma fusion partner. Only a handful of human myeloma cells appears to be satisfactory for fusion. Beside the lymphoblastoid cell lines for fusion, only one myeloma cell line, SKO-007, a derivative of the U266 cell line, has been drug-marked and shown to produce hybridomas after fusion (Olsson and Kaplan, 1980; Cote et al., 1983; Houghton et al., 1983).

Because of availability of mouse myeloma cell lines, it is not surprising that from the beginning of the development of hybridoma technology, human B lymphocytes would be fused with murine fusion partners. Although mouse x human hybridomas are easy to produce and exhibit good in vitro growth characteristics, their genetic instability due to selective elimination of human chromosomes prevents a stable Ig-secretion. One of the first successful attempts to fuse human lymphocytes obtained from the tumor patient's draining lymph nodes with mouse myeloma cells was reported by Schlom et al. (1980). Some of the double cloned hybrid cell lines produced human monoclonal antibodies for at least 6 months

(Wunderlich et al., 1981). The mouse x human hybrids established by Sikora and Wright (1981) also lost the ability to secrete human Ig by the 10th week after fusion.

In our experiments, we successfully used the mouse x human myeloma SPAZ-4 as a fusion partner which was developed by Lars Oesterberg and Edith Pursch at the Sandoz Research Institute, Vienna (1983). This xenogeneic myeloma was produced by fusing the mouse SP2/0 myeloma to human peripheral blood lymphocytes obtained from a healthy nonimmunized donor. From five selected subclones resistant to 8-azaguanine and showing no antibody production, the best growing cell line was chosen and named SPAZ-4. The cells grow rapidly in the same semiadherent manner as mouse hybridomas and have doubling times of 18 to 23 hr. Hybridomas producing human anti-influenza antibodies have now been reported to be maintained for more than two years.

As a result of our experiences, we can confirm the SPAZ-4 is a rapidly growing, non-Ig-producing partner cell with good fusion properties. The cell line is optimal to use with respect to the number of Ig-secreting hybridomas generated and their stability over long-term culturing. It bears comparison with the human myeloma cell line SKO-007.

Cell cultures and cell fusions

SPAZ-4 cells were cultured at $37^{o}C$ in an atmosphere containing 5% CO_2 in Dulbecco's MEM (DMEM) supplemented with 10% FCS. After fusion, cells were maintained in cultures in DMEM with high glucose (4.5 g/L) supplemented with 20% FCS and 10% NCTC-109 medium (Microbiological Associates, Walkersville, MD, USA).

Human breast cancer cells (MCF-7, MDA, BT-20, SK-BR-3, T-47D, ZR-75-1) were maintained in continuous tissue culture in Richter's IMEM supplemented with 10% FCS and 10 g/ml insulin. Penicillin (100 IU/ml) and streptomycin (100 g/ml) were added to all cell cultures.

Single cell suspensions were prepared by straining the tissue of the lymph nodes through a fine stainless steel mesh. The resultant suspension was layered on Percoll (d = 1.072) and centrifuged at 400x g for 45 min. Effusions from breast cancer patients were centrifuged at 400x g for 10 min. The resultant cell pellets were resuspended in DMEM. The lymphocytes were separated from the carcinoma cells by repeated Percoll centrifugation. Before fusion, the isolated lymphocytes were cultured in DMEM for 24 hr in the incubator.

SPAZ-4 cells and lymphocytes were mixed at a ratio of 1 to 1, respectively, and fused using 50% (w/v) polyethylene glycol (PEG) 4000 (Merck, Darmstadt, FRG) containing 15% dimethylsulfoxide as described by Oi and Herzenberg (1980). One ml of cell suspensions was plated into each well of a 24-well tissue culture plate in a concentration of 1×10^5 to 5×10^5 cells/well. After incubation for 24 hr, the culture fluid was replaced with HAT medium. At 2-day intervals, 500 µl of spent medium were removed from each well and replaced by an equal volume of fresh made HAT medium. Instead of the commonly used feeder cells, the medium was supplemented with human endothelial culture supernatant (Costar Biologicals, Cambridge, MA, USA) as described by Astaldi et al. (1980). First growth was observed generally after 2 weeks. Feeding was continued with HT medium. Subsequent cell culture of the hybridomas was performed in vertical 75-ml flasks.

Ig detection and purification

Human Ig-secreting hybridomas were detected by an ELISA as described by Imam et al. (1985). IgG antibodies were purified by adsorption on Protein A-Sepharose (Pharmacia, Uppsala, Sweden) and elution with 0.05 M sodium acetate, 0.15 M NaCl, pH 4.3, and 0.1 M sodium citrate buffer, pH 3.0.

Determination of heavy chain isotypes

The heavy chain isotypes were determined using isotype-specific mouse antisera (Bio-Yeda, Rehovot, Israel) in a dot immunobinding assay on purified antibody preparations. One µl of antibody solution was applied on nitrocellulose paper squares. After incubation with the isotype-specific mouse antisera, the paper squares were incubated for 1 hr with biotinylated anti-mouse IgG. 0.05% (v/v) Tween 20 was present in all incubation and washing steps to prevent the nonspecific binding of the antibodies. Reactions were localized by the avidin-biotin-peroxidase technique (Vectastain ABC Kit). Color reactions were developed with 4-chloro-1-naphthol and hydrogen peroxide by the method of Hawkes et al. (1982).

TABLE 2.
FUSION FREQUENCIES OF SPAZ-4

Case	No. of wells seeded	No. of wells with hybrids	No. of wells with human Ig	IgG_1	Isotypes IgG_2	IgG_3	IgG_4
LYMPH NODES							
L2-85	48	6	6	x	x	x	
L4-85	48	4	4	x			
L5-85	48	6	4	x			
B.J.	48	6	0				
T.S.	48	4	3	x			
G.D.	48	5	5	x			
B.M.	48	2	0				
E.T.	48	15	7	x	x		
8	384	48	29 (60%)				
MALIGNANT EFFUSIONS							
M.H.	48	3	1	x			
G.M.	48	7	3	x			
V.E.	48	3	1	x			
3	144	13	5 (38%)				

Antibody reactivity to cell surface and intracellular antigens

Purified fractions of monoclonal antibodies were screened for reactivity to cellular antigens using a panel of human breast carcinoma cell lines. Breast carcinoma cells of malignant effusions were isolated by centrifugation on Percoll. Carcinoma cells were harvested from the upper layer. Lymphocytes were collected from the interphase. Target cells growing on polylysine-coated glass slides were fixed with 1:1 (v/v) methanol/acetone mixture for 5 min at room temperature. The cells were incubated with the antibody fractions for 1 hr at room temperature. The subsequent immunostaining was carried out by use of avidin-biotin-peroxidase complex (ABC) as detailed in the instructions of the Vectastain ABC Kit (Vector Laboratories, Burlingame, CA, USA). Purified human IgG fractions as a negative control were routinely negative for reactivity to carcinoma cells.

Results and discussion

The fusion frequencies of SPAZ-4 with human lymphocytes from lymph nodes and pleural malignant effusions are shown in Table 2. In 8 fusion experiments with lymphocytes of lymph nodes, 29 antibody-secreting hybrids were identified in a total of 16 24-well plates. Lymphocytes isolated from lymph nodes yielded higher fusion frequencies than those from malignant pleural effusions. The IgG_1 producers were more prevalent than IgG_2 or IgG_3. Levels of human Ig-synthesis ranged from 0.1 to 25 µg/ml of supernatant fluid. The cells have now been maintained for 6 months in culture, showing stable Ig production. Hybridomas have been cloned by limiting dilution without the use of feeder cells. The medium was supplemented with human endothelial culture supernatant that contains factor(s) that promote the growth and the stability of hybridoma cells and in these respects may be superior to the commonly used feeder cells (Astaldi et al., 1980).

Imam et al. (1985) fused lymphocytes of axillary lymph nodes from patients with metastatic breast carcinoma with M5, a non-secreting variant of the mouse myeloma cell subline of SP2/0. Wells exhibiting colonies of hybrid cells ranged from 4% to 73% of the wells seeded, but only 5% of these hybrid cells produced human immunoglobulin. In comparison to it, we obtained a much higher percentage of Ig-producer.

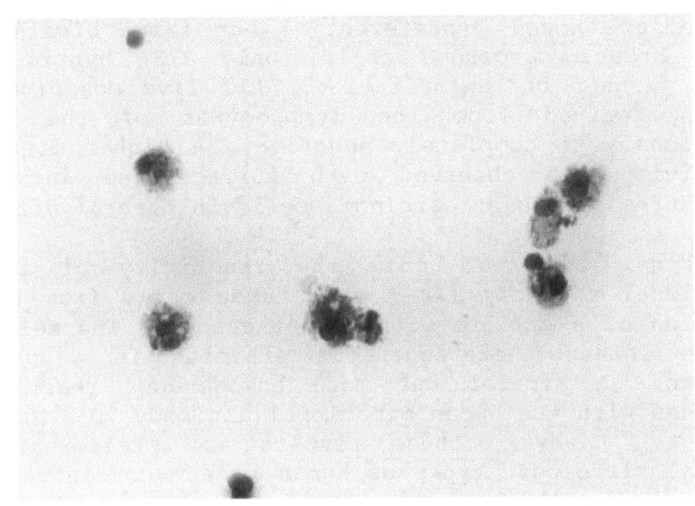

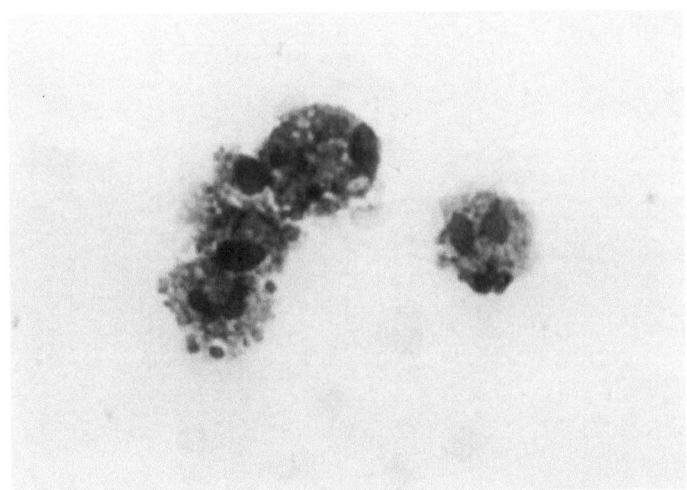

Figs. 2 and 3. Immunoperoxidase staining of human breast carcinoma cells from pleural effusion with human monoclonal antibody 12H-3. Cells were counterstained with hematoxylin (original magnification x 320). Note the marked heterogeneous cytoplasmic staining of the tumor cells.

To screen the Ig-producing hybridomas, we examined the binding of our monoclonal antibodies to a panel of human breast carcinoma cell lines (MCF-7, MDA, BT-20, SK-BR-3, T-47D, ZR-75-1) with a biotin-conjugated goat antihuman IgG antibody. The reaction was amplified with an avidin-biotin-peroxidase complex. Although a part of the antibodies showed a preferential but faint binding to the human breast carcinoma cells, only 3/34 hybridomas were worth further characterization. All five monoclonal antibodies derived from the lymphocytes of the malignant effusions were completely negative. A higher frequency of reactivity was observed with surface and intracellular structures of breast carcinoma cells in pleural effusions.

Figs. 2 and 3 show the reactivity of the human monoclonal antibody 12H-3 with tumor cells from a pleural effusion of a patient with breast cancer. The cells demonstrate intense hetereogeneous staining in a cytoplasmic pattern. A similar but more homogeneous reactivity was observed with the human monoclonal antibody 7D-3 as shown in Fig. 4. However, these results are preliminary, since several histologic types of human breast carcinomas have to be examined with the produced monoclonal antibodies.

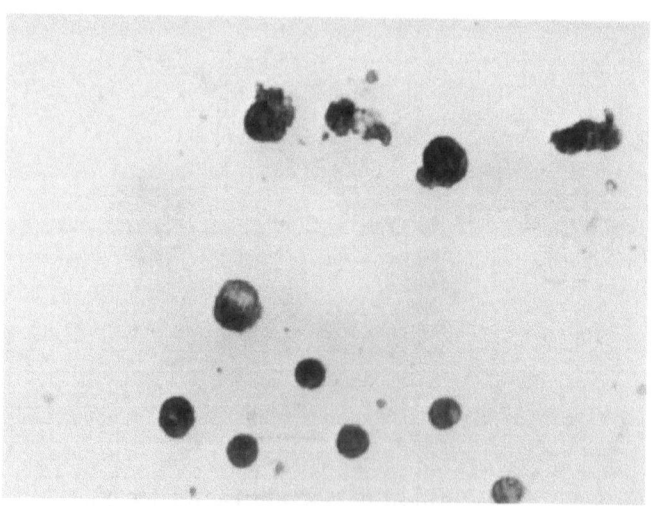

Fig. 4.   Immunoperoxidase staining of human breast carcinoma cells from pleural effusion with human monoclonal antibody 7D-3. Cells were counterstained with hematoxylin (original magnification x 320). Note the more homogeneous staining of the tumor cells.

REFERENCES

Astaldi, G.C.B., Janssen, M.C., Lamsdorp, P., Willems, Ch.,
    Zeijlemacher, W.P., and Oosterhof, F. Human
    endothelial culture supernatant (HECS): A growth
    factor for hybridomas. J. Immunol. 125:1411-1414,
    1980.
Cote, R.J., Morrissey, D.M., Houghton, A.N., Beattie, Jr.,
    E.J., Oettgen, H.F., and Old, L.J. Generation of human
    monoclonal antibodies reactive with cellular antigens.
    Proc. Natl. Acad. Sci. USA, 80:2026-2030.
Gruenberg, J. and Sherman, W. Isolation and
    characterization of the plasma membrane of human
    erythrocytes infected with the malarial parasite
    Plasmodium falciparum. Proc. Natl. Acad. Sci. USA
    80:1087-1091, 1983.
Hawkes, R., Niday, E., and Gordon, J. A dot-immunobinding
    assay for monoclonal and other antibodies. Anal.
    Biochem. 119:142-147, 1982.
Houghton, A.N., Brooks, H., Cote, R.J., Taormina, M.C.,
    Oettgen, H.F., and Old, L.J. Detection of cell surface
    and intracellular antigens by human monoclonal
    antibodies. J. Exp. Med. 158:53-65, 1983.
Imam, A., Taylor, C.R., and Tokes, Z.A. Use of human
    monoclonal antibodies for the detection of antigenic
    heterogeneity in the population of breast carcinoma
    cells. J. Histochem. Cytochem. 30:573 (abstract),
    1982.
Imam, A., Drushella, M.M., and Tokes, Z.A. Generation and
    immunohistological characterization of human monoclonal
    antibodies to mammary carcinoma cells. Cancer Res.
    45:263-271, 1985.
Lo, M.M.S., Tsong, T.Y., Conrad, M.K., Srittmatter, S.M.,
    Hester, L.D., and Snyder, S.H. Monoclonal antibody
    production by receptor-mediated electrically induced
    cell fusion. Nature 310:792-793, 1984.
Mai, S. and Chung, A.E. Cell attachment and spreading on
    extracelluar matrix-coated beads. Exp. Cell. Res.
    152:500-509, 1984.
Oesterberg, L. and Pursch, E. Human x (mouse x human)
    hybridomas stably producing human antibodies.
    Hybridoma 2:361-367, 1983.
Oi, V.T. and Herzenberg, L.A. Immunoglobulin producing
    hybrid cell lines. In: Selected Methods in Cellular
    Immunology. W.H. Freeman, San Francisco, 1970, pp
    351-372.
Olsson, L. and Kaplan, H.S. Human-human hybridomas
    producing monoclonal antibodies of predefined antigenic

specificity. <u>Proc</u>. <u>Natl</u>. <u>Acad</u>. <u>Sci</u>. <u>USA</u> <u>77</u>:5429-5431, 1980.

Schlom, J., Wunderlich, D., and Teramoto, Y.A. Generation of human monoclonal antibodies reactive with human mammary carcinoma cells. <u>Proc</u>. <u>Natl</u>./<u>Sci</u>. <u>USA</u> <u>77</u>:6841-6845, 1980.

Sikora, K. and Wright, R. Human monoclonal antibodies to lung-cancer antigens. <u>Br</u>. <u>J</u>. <u>Cancer</u> <u>43</u>:696-700, 1981.

Wunderlich, D., Teramoto, Y.A., and Schlom, J. The use of lymphocytes from axillary lymph nodes of mastectomy patients to generate human monoclonal antibodies. <u>Eur</u>. <u>J</u>. <u>Cancer</u> <u>Clin</u>. <u>Oncol</u>. <u>17</u>:719-730, 1981.

Zimmermann, U. Electric field-mediated fusion and related electrical phenomena. <u>Biochim</u>. <u>Biophys</u>. Acta <u>694</u>:227-277, 1982.

ANTIESTROPHILIN MONOCLONAL ANTIBODIES AS IMMUNOCYTOCHEMICAL PROBES OF ESTROGEN RECEPTOR IN TISSUE SECTIONS OF BREAST CARCINOMAS

L. OZZELLO, C. DE ROSA, D.V. HABIF, AND R. LIPTON

Arthur Purdy Stout Laboratory of Surgical Pathology and Department of Surgery, Columbia University, College of Physicians and Surgeons, New York, N.Y. 10032, U.S.A.

INTRODUCTION

In recent years, it has become apparent that a reliable histochemical technique for the demonstration of estrogen receptor (ER) in tissue sections would be very useful for the evaluation of breast cancer patients. Indeed, the biochemical assays for ER currently used in clinical laboratories, although of proven value, suffer from several limitations (Poulsen, 1981), a very important one being that of sampling. This is especially true for tumors with abundant or unevenly distributed stroma in which the specimen given to the biochemist may not be representative of the tumor as a whole, and for small lesions in which the amount of tissue available is not sufficient for biochemical analysis. The histochemical visualization of ER could obviate some of these limitations and offer the advantage of providing a better appreciation of the topographic distribution of ER in any given tumor and of the percentage of ER-positive carcinoma cells.

Several histochemical techniques utilizing the uptake of estradiol by sections of neoplastic tissue have been proposed in the past. These techniques, each with its own merits and flaws, provide an assessment of the estrogen-binding capabilities of a tumor, but not a direct evaluation of the receptor proper (Chamness et al., 1980). In this report, we shall review our experience on the immunostaining of ER using antiestrophilin monoclonal antibodies. These antibodies are highly specific and bind selectively to both free and occupied ER, thus fully visualizing the receptor itself.

ANTIESTROPHILIN MONOCLONAL ANTIBODIES

Three antibodies were used in these studies: D75P3γ and D547Spγ prepared and kindly provided by Dr. G.L. Greene and H222Spγ developed by Dr. L.S. Miller and supplied by Abbott Laboratories. These antibodies were prepared by immunizing Lewis rats with purified estrophilin isolated from the cytosolic fraction of MCF-7 cells, and subsequently fusing the immunized rat spleen cells with mouse myeloma cells to make hybridomas (Greene and Jensen, 1982; Greene et al., 1980; Miller et al., 1982). They were characterized and found to be ER-specific by several criteria (Greene et al., 1984). They were shown not to cross-react with other steroid receptors or other cellular proteins and to recognize different antigenic determinants on the ER molecule (Greene et al., 1984).

IMMUNOCYTOCHEMICAL ASSAY ON FROZEN SECTIONS

Most of the investigative work on the immunocytochemistry of ER using antiestrophilin monoclonal antibodies has been done on frozen sections of target tissues both human and animal (King and Greene, 1984; King et al., 1985; Ozzello et al., 1986; Pertschuk et al., 1985; Press and Greene, 1984). In this laboratory, the antibody H222Spγ was used on frozen sections of human breast carcinomas. Some of this work was carried out in collaboration with the Diagnostic Division of Abbott Laboratories as part of the evaluation of a kit (ER-ICA Monoclonal) subsequently commercialized by the Abbott Company. Part of the results were presented at a symposium on "Estrogen Receptor Determination with Monoclonal Antibodies" (Monte Carlo, December 14, 1984) and reported in the symposium proceedings (Ozzello et al., 1986).

Thirty-six breast carcinomas were obtained at the time of biopsy in the operating rooms of Columbia-Presbyterian Medical Center. Without delay, tissue samples were collected in cold phosphate buffered saline, 0.01M, pH 7.2-7.4 (PBS) and delivered to the laboratory where they were placed in freezing vials and frozen at -80°C. Some of the specimens were quick-frozen in liquid nitrogen or at -28°C and stored as soon as possible at -80°C. These different

freezing modalities proved to be equally satisfactory provided the freezing was done without delay and the tissue was
not allowed to dry at any time.

The staining technique was that proposed by the manu-
facturer. Briefly, cryostat sections 4-6 µm thick were
placed on glass slides previously coated with a tissue
adhesive (poly-L-lysine). Two adjacent sections from each
specimen were fixed in 3.7% formaldehyde in PBS at room
temperature and then passed through cold methanol and cold
acetone. All subsequent incubations were carried out at
room temperature in a humidified chamber. Following incubation with blocking reagent (normal goat serum), one section
from each pair was incubated with H222Spγ monoclonal antibody for 30 minutes, while the other section was exposed to
control antibody (normal rat IgG). All sections were then
incubated with bridging antibody (goat anti-rat antibody)
and with peroxidase-anti-peroxidase (PAP) complex (rat anti-
PAP in Tris buffer). Diaminobenzidine tetrachloride was
used as chromogen and Harris hematoxylin as nuclear counterstain. MXF-7 cells attached to glass slides served as ER-
positive controls and were processed simultaneously with the
diagnostic sections.

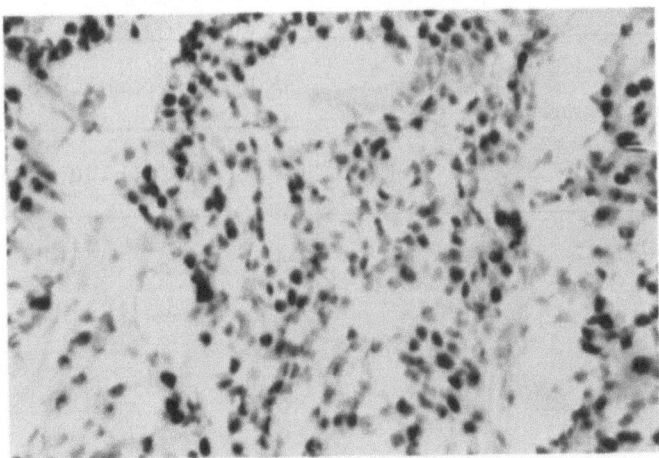

Fig. 1   Infiltrating ductal carcinoma of the breast in an
          86-year-old woman (DCC: 1228 fmol/mg cytosol
          protein). Most, but not all, nuclei of the
          carcinoma cells are ER-positive, the intensity of
          the immunoreactivity ranging from weak to strong.
          ER-ICA, X200.

A quantitative assay for ER [Dextran-Coated Charcoal (DCC) analysis] was performed on every tumor in another laboratory.

The sections were evaluated by two observers (L. Ozzello and C. De Rosa), who had no knowledge of the DCC results. Tumors were regarded as being ER-positive when showing brown staining in the nuclei of the neoplastic cells, and were scored as to intensity of staining (weak, moderate, strong) and as to number of stained nuclei (less than 1/3, between 1/3 and 2/3, and over 2/3). All positive tumors displayed variable proportions of negative and positive nuclei of different staining intensities (Fig. 1). Such heterogeneous pattern was presumably due to functional heterogeneity of the carcinoma cells. No staining was seen in the cytoplasm of the tumor cells nor in the stromal cells, although light, nonspecific background staining was present in some sections.

Table 1

COMPARISON OF IMMUNOSTAINING WITH DCC ASSAY VALUES
FOR 36 BREAST CARCINOMAS*

Nuclear staining	fmol/mg cytosol protein		
	<3	10-100	>100
Negative	4	0	0
Borderline	3	2	0
Positive			
<1/3 cells	0	8	0
>1/3 cells	0	6	13

*ER-ICA, frozen sections

The preferential immunostaining of ER in the nuclei as observed by us and by others (King and Greene, 1984; King et al., 1985; Ozzello et al., 1985; Poulsen et al., 1985; Press and Greene, 1986) raises questions as to the localization of ER in target cells. According to the original theory, free ER are present in the cytoplasm and are translocated to the nucleus after binding with estrogen (Jensen et al., 1968). The immunocytochemical findings, however, together with recent biochemical and autoradiographic evidence, suggest that occupied as well as free ER are located predominantly in the nucleus, although small amounts may be present in the cytoplasm (Jensen, 1984; King and Greene, 1984; King et al., 1985; Martin and Sheridan, 1982; Ozzello et al., 1985; Welshons et al., 1984).

Table 1 summarizes the comparison of the immunostaining with the DCC results. It can be seen that no ER staining was detected in tumors with negative DCC values (<3 fmol/mg cytosol protein), and that the nuclei of all specimens with positive DCC values (>10 fmol/mg cytosol protein) were stained. Statistically, this correlation was found to be highly significant (p<0.001). Furthermore, the number of positively stained nuclei tended to be greater in tumors with DCC values above 100 fmol/mg (p<0.01). Five additional cases were classified as "borderline" because it was difficult to be sure that any ER staining was present. Of these 5 cases, 3 were DCC negative and 2 had low DCC values (22 and 30 fmol/mg).

In this material, no statistically significant correlation was found between staining intensity and DCC values.

These findings indicate that ER-ICA is a reliable technique and can be used to provide valuable information when the conventional biochemical assays cannot be done. It appears that, although a quantitative evaluation of the ER content of a tumor is not yet possible by this technique, breast carcinomas with nuclear immunostaining are likely to be ER-positive and to be ER-rich when over 1/3 of their nuclei are stained.

IMMUNOSTAINING OF ER IN PARAFFIN EMBEDDED TISSUE

Often it becomes necessary to assess the ER status of a breast cancer patient after the biopsy material has been processed for routine histological examination. Under these circumstances, it would be very desirable to be able to visualize ER in paraffin sections. In this laboratory, a first attempt to stain paraffin sections of breast carcinomas using antiestrophilin monoclonal antibodies was made in collaboration with Dr. H.S. Poulsen of the University of Aarhus and Drs. G.L. Green and W.J. King of the University of Chicago (Poulsen et al., 1985).

This study was carried out on 68 breast carcinomas from the files of our surgical pathology laboratory. Most of these tumors had been fixed in Bouin's solution and embedded in paraffin at 60°C. The length of fixation was not known, but according to the routine of this laboratory, it could range from 4 to 24 hours or longer; nor was the delay between excision and fixation known. The ER status of all these tumors had been assessed at the time of surgical excision by the DCC assay.

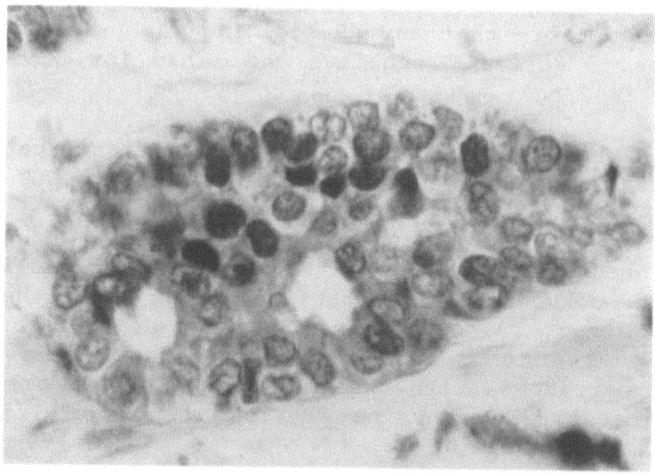

Fig. 2   Infiltrating ductal carcinoma of the breast in a 61-year-old woman (DCC: 252 fmol/mg cytosol protein). Finely granular immunoreactivity of variable intensity in several nuclei of carcinoma cells. This type of reaction was seen in paraffin sections stained with either the PAP or the avidin-biotin techniques. X480.

Staining was done with the PAP technique according to a schedule worked out by Poulsen et al. (1985). Following deparaffinization and pre-incubation with normal goat serum (50% in PBS) for 40 minutes at room temperature, the sections were incubated with primary antibody at 4°C overnight in a humidified chamber, taking care that the sections did not dry. As primary antibody, we used the D75P3γ and D547Spγ of Dr. G.L. Greene, combined in equal amounts to final concentrations of 10 µg or 25 µg. This was done on the assumption that these two monoclonal antibodies might react additively and enhance immunoreactivity since they recognize different antigenic sites on the ER molecule (Greene and Jensen, 1982). The bridging antibody (goat anti-rat IgG diluted in 50% goat serum) was used at a concentration of 500 µg/ml incubating the sections for 60 minutes at room temperature. The sections were then incubated with rat PAP at a 1:40 dilution in 50% goat serum for 30 minutes followed by diaminobenzidine (1.7 mM with 0.03% hydrogen peroxide in PBS) for 10 minutes, and counterstained with methylene blue.

We accepted as positive immunoreactivity a brown granular staining which we found localized predominantly in the nuclei (Fig. 2). All positive tumors displayed hetereogeneous staining with variations in the number and in the intensity of stained nuclei. The slides were read independently by H.S. Poulsen and L. Ozzello, who agreed in all cases on whether or not the tumors contained positive cells, but only in 80% of the cases as to the number of positive cells and in 2/3 of the cases as to the intensity of the immunoreactivity. To further check reproducibility of results, 19 paraffin blocks were sent to Dr. Greene's laboratory where Dr. King repeated the staining and obtained the same results in 18 of the 19 specimens.

The correspondence between immunostaining and ER status by DCC assay is outlined in Table 2. Of the tumors that were DCC-negative, the majority (21/25) had no nuclear staining, but 4 of them did, whereas 9 of 11 with DCC values above 50 fmol/mg were positive by immunostaining and 2 were not. Among the tumors with borderline or low DCC values (3-50 fmol/mg), 18 were negative and 14 were positive by immunocytochemical assay. Conversely, of the 41 tumors with no ER staining, 21 were negative and 20 were positive by DCC assay, but among the latter, only 2 had values above 50 fmol/mg. Among the tumors with positive nuclear staining, 23 were also positive by DCC assay while 4 were negative. These findings indicate that the correspondence between ER immunostaining on paraffin sections and DCC values is not as

Table 2

COMPARISON OF IMMUNOSTAINING WITH DCC ASSAY VALUES
FOR 68 BREAST CARCINOMAS*

Nuclear staining	fmol/mg cytosol protein		
	<3	3-50	>50
Negative	21	18	2
Positive			
<10% cells	3	6	0
>10% cells	1	8	9

*D75P3 γ + D547SPγ, paraffin sections, PAP

good as that for frozen sections. Nevertheless, a positive
stain would appear to indicate that the tumor is most likely
DCC-positive, especially when more than 10% of the cells are
stained, while a lack of immunoreactivity is of lesser value
as an indicator and could only suggest that a negatively
stained tumor is either DCC-negative or is in the borderline
ER-poor group.

Discrepancies between immunostaining and DCC assays are
probably due to flaws in either techniques. It is possible
that various parameters in tissue processing including
delays in fixation, type of fixative and duration of fixation may modify or mask antigenic determinants. In our
experiments on paraffin embedded material, immunoreactivity
is seen in tissues fixed in Bouin's solution but not in
those fixed in formalin. This is a crucial technical point
which is currently under investigation. It is also possible
that the methodology used here is not sensitive enough to
reveal some of the tumors with low ER content. On the other
hand, limitations in the biochemical assays may be responsible for some false results. For instance, a tumor with
extensive fibrosis may give a borderline or negative biochemical result, but show a positive immunoreactivity in the
tumor cells buried in the dense stroma (Ozzello et al.,
1985).

In a separate study, we attempted to determine whether ER immunoreactivity correlated with response to antiestrogen therapy (Ozzello et al., 1985). This was done on a group of 28 patients, all of whom were treated with Tamoxifen citrate (Nolvadex, Stuart) in addition to other forms of therapy. All of them had surgery, ranging from excisional biopsy to modified radical mastectomy, and some received chemotherapy and/or radiotherapy. In several of these patients, multiple specimens of recurrences and metastases were available in addition to the primary tumors.

The immunostaining was done using monoclonal antibody D75P3γ (kindly provided by Dr. G.L. Greene) at a concentration of 25 µg/ml, visualized with the avidin-biotin technique (Vectastain Kit, Vector Laboratories). The slides were read by L. Ozzello and C. De Rosa without knowledge of the DCC results. As previously, we accepted as positive reactivity a brown granular staining which we found predominantly in the nuclei of carcinoma cells (Fig. 2), although cytoplasmic staining was also observed in some cases. Heterogeneous staining was seen in all positive cases. Variations in immunoreactivity were also seen among different samples from any one specimen and between different specimens from any one patient. Table 3 shows the correlation between immunostaining and the DCC assay values; and in agreement with the previous group of tumors, it shows that the largest number of specimens with positive ER staining and the largest proportions of stained nuclei were found in tumors with high DCC values. But also in this group of patients, among DCC positive tumors we found a few with no immunoreactivity and vice versa.

The correlation between ER staining and response to antiestrogen therapy is outlined in Table 4. The overall evaluation of the clinical outcome in this group of patients is difficult because many of them had advanced disease and received other forms of therapy in the course of their disease in addition to antiestrogens. Therefore, the clinical evaluation was limited to the response to endocrine therapy: patients were regarded as failures if their local disease persisted or if metastases or recurrences became clinically manifest during or following Nolvadex administration. Table 4 shows that about one-half of the patients with positive ER status by immunocytochemistry and by DCC assay (>50 fmol/mg) responded favorably to therapy, whereas the majority of the patients with negative ER immunostaining and with negative or low DCC values failed to respond. Although the number of cases is small, it appears

Table 3

COMPARISON OF IMMUNOSTAINING WITH DCC ASSAY VALUES
FOR 44 BREAST CARCINOMAS*

Nuclear staining	fmol/mg cytosol protein		
	<3	3-50	>50
Negative	1	8	5
Positive			
<1/3 cells	1	3	4
>1/3 cells	0	6	16

*D75P3γ, paraffin sections, avidin-biotin

Table 4

ER STATUS AND RESPONSE TO ANTI-ESTROGEN THERAPY

ER status	Remissions	Failures
Immunocytochemistry		
negative	1	7
positive	11	9
DCC assay		
<3 fmol/mg	1	0
3-50 fmol/mg	2	6
>50 fmol/mg	9	10

that there is concordance between immunocytochemical and DCC assays with respect to antiestrogen therapy, and that ER-immunoreactivity might be a somewhat better predictor. They suggest that patients with negative ER staining are poor candidates for this type of hormonal manipulation, while those with positive ER-immunoreactivity have about 50% chance of responding. Similar findings have been reported by others (Pertschuk et al., 1985).

In conclusion, we are of the opinion that immunohisto-chemistry for the detection of ER using antiestrophilin monoclonal antibodies both on frozen sections and on paraffin sections has a definite place in the evaluation of the ER status of breast cancer patients. The results on paraffin sections are not as good as we would like them to be since the technique has not yet been adequately standardized. Nevertheless, we believe that these techniques are valid and can be regarded as valuable adjuncts to conventional biochemical assays, not only as a substitute when the latter cannot be performed, but also by providing additional and more detailed information on the distribution of ER within any one tumor or in multiple lesions of any one patient.

ACKNOWLEDGMENTS

This work was supported in part by the Ambrose Monell Foundation, the Milstein Medical Research Foundation, Columbia University Research in Surgery Gift, Mr. and Mrs. G.M. Shapiro, and Abbott Laboratories.

REFERENCES

Chamness, G.C., Mercer, W.D., and McGuire, W.L. Are histological methods for estrogen receptor valid? J. Histochem. Cytochem. 28, 792-798, 1980.
Greene, G.L. and Jensen, E.V. Monoclonal antibodies as probes for estrogen receptor detection and characterization. J. Steroid Biochem. 16, 353-359, 1982.
Greene, G.L., Nolan, C., Engler, J.P., and Jensen, E.V. Monoclonal antibodies to human estrogen receptor. Proc. Natl. Acad. Sci. (USA) 77, 5115-5119, 1980.
Greene, G.L., Sobel, N.B., King, W.J., and Jensen, E.V. Immunochemical studies of estrogen receptors. J. Steroid Biochem. 20, 51-56, 1984.

Jensen, E.V. Intracellular localization of estrogen
    receptors: implication for interaction mechanism.
    Lab. Invest. 51, 487-488, 1984.
Jensen, E.V., Suzuki, T., Kasashima, T., Stumpf, W.E.,
    Jungblut, P.W., and DeSombre, E.R. A two-step
    mechanism for the interaction of estradiol with rat
    uterus. Proc. Natl. Acad. Sci. (USA) 459, 632-638,
    1968.
King, W.J. and Greene, G.L. Monoclonal antibodies localize
    estrogen receptor in the nuclei of target cells.
    Nature (Lond.) 307, 745-747, 1984.
King, W.J., DeSombre, E.R., Jensen, E.V., and Greene, G.L.
    Comparison of immunocytochemical and steroid-binding
    assays for estrogen receptors in human breast tumors.
    Cancer Res. 45, 293-304, 1985.
Martin, P.M. and Sheridan, P.J. Toward a new model for the
    mechanism of action of steroids. J. Steroid Biochem.
    16, 215-229, 1982.
Miller, L.S., Tribby, H.E., Miles, M.R., Tomita, J.T., and
    Nolan, C. Hybridomas producing monoclonal antibodies
    to human estrogen receptor. Abstract 1459. Fed. Proc.
    41, 520, 1982.
Ozzello, L., De Rosa, C., Habif, D.V., and Lipton, R.
    Immunostaining of estrogen receptors in paraffin
    sections of breast cancers using antiestrophilin
    monoclonal antibodies. In: Monoconal Antibodies and
    Breast Cancer, R.L. Ceriani ed., Martinus Nijhoff
    Publish., Dordrecht-Boston-Lancaster, 1985, pp. 3-12.
Ozzello, L., De Rosa, C.M., Konrath, J.G., Yeager, J.L., and
    Miller, L.S. Detection of estrophilin in frozen
    sections of breast cancers using an estrogen receptor
    immunocytochemical assay. Cancer Res., 1986, in press.
Pertschuk, L.P., Eisenberg, K.B., Carter, A.C., and Feldman,
    J.G. Immunohistologic localization of estrogen
    receptors in breast cancer with monoclonal antibodies.
    Correlation with biochemistry and clinical endocrine
    response. Cancer 55, 1513-1518, 1985.
Poulsen, H.S. Oestrogen receptor assays. Limitation of the
    method. Eur. J. Cancer 17, 495-501, 1981.
Poulsen, H.S., Ozzello, L., King, W.J., and Greene, G.L.
    The use of monoclonal antibodies to estrogen receptors
    for immunoperoxidase detection of ER in paraffin
    sections of human breast cancer tissue. J. Histochem.
    Cytochem. 33, 87-92, 1985.
Press, M.F. and Greene, G.L. An immunocytochemical method
    for demonstrating estrogen receptor in human uterus
    using monoclonal antibodies to human estrophilin. Lab.
    Invest. 50, 480-486, 1984.

Welshons, W.V., Lieberman, M.E., and Gorski, J. Nuclear
    localization of unoccupied oestrogen receptors. Nature
    (Lond.) <u>307</u>, 747-749, 1984.

HISTOCHEMICAL DEMONSTRATION OF ENDOGENOUS ESTROGEN

IN BREAST CARCINOMAS; METHOD AND CLINICAL SIGNIFICANCE

I. KATAYAMA, S. WAKATSUKI, I. IINO, AND M. IZUO

Department of Pathology, Saitama Medical School, Saitama 350.04, Japan, and Department of Surgery, Gunma University School of Medicine, Gunma, Japan

INTRODUCTION

Because of the proved capability of predicting the response to endocrine therapy, biochemical assays of estrogen receptors have been used as an essential test in the management of patients with breast carcinomas although these tests require fresh tissue and elaborate equipment. In contrast, morphological methods have several fundamental methodological flaws and are considered unacceptable for clinical application although they have multiple potential advantages over the biochemical methods such as applicability to routine paraffin sections.

There are two kinds of morphological methods for demonstrating estrogen receptors: indirect and direct. The indirect method tries to visualize estrogen presumably taken up by the receptors rather than visualizing estrogen receptors per se. The direct method tries to visualize estrogen receptors with the use of monoclonal antibodies developed against the receptor proteins. The subject of the present study pertains to the indirect method.

One major pitfall of the indirect morphologic method is the high concentrations of exogenous estrogen used for binding with the estrogen receptors in breast carcinomas. The concentrations of the exogenously administered estrogen are so high that they are likely to bind nonspecifically with the types II and III binders (Chamness and McGuire, 1982). In our preceding study (Shimizu et al., 1983), we circumvented this particular pitfall by trying to demonstrate endogenous estrogen without prior exposure of tissues to exogenous estrogen. At that time, our experiments using DMBA/treated rats proved that the intravenously administered estrogen was taken up and became demonstrable in the rat breast tumors biochemically with scintillation counting and morphologically with microautoradiography. The results served as evidence that the endogenous estrogen remains in formalin-fixed paraffin-embedded human breast carcinomas in amounts detectable by the morphological methods. Accordingly, we applied the method to breast carcinomas from 277 patients in the foregoing study (Katayama et al., 1984) and found a good correlation between results of the morphological method and those of the biochemical assays and clinical features. Similarly using the same method, Okazaki et al. (1985) obtained results which correlated even better with biochemical assays and clinical features of 122 patients with breast carcinomas. The present study was undertaken in order to test reproducibility and clinical utility of the method through its application to a different group of 225 patients with breast carcinomas.

MATERIALS AND METHODS

Patients

    Two hundred twenty-five patients with breast carcinomas were selected for this study on accounts of complete follow-up from the pool of patients seen at the University Hospital of the Gunma University Medical School during the period of 1965 to 1980. All 225 patients were women; 149 were premenopausal and 76 postmenopausal. Stages at the diagnosis were stage I for 76 patients, stage II for 88, stage III for 45, and stage IV for 16. Response to adjuvant therapies for the first relapse after radical mastectomy was recorded for 27 patients according to the criteria of UICC (Hayward et al., 1977). Each patient received a single or combined form of endocrine therapy (oophorectomy, adrenalectomy, or anti-steroid hormone chemotherapy) and/or in addition, radiation, chemotherapy, and local excision. Single mode of therapy was given to 13 patients, combination of two modes to eight patients, and three modes to five, to a total of 47 modes of therapy to 27 patients. When listing the response to more than one mode of therapy for one patient, the response was listed repeatedly for individual modes of therapy; for example, for a patient who had a partial response to a combination of three modes of therapy, the partial response was listed for each of the three different modes of therapy (Fig. 1).

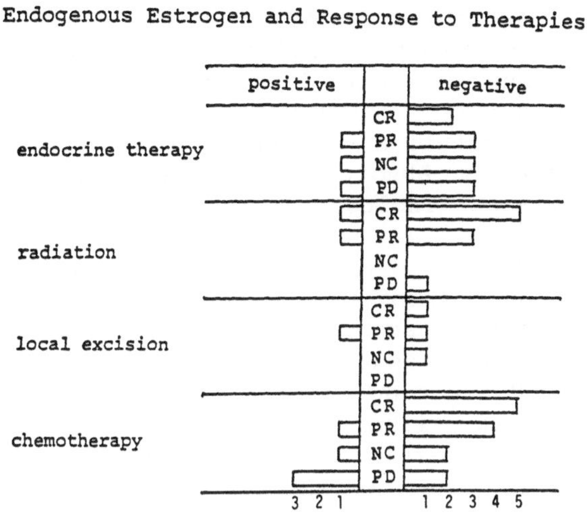

Endogenous Estrogen and Response to Therapies

Figure 1. Endogenous estrogen and effects of adjuvant
therapies. On the abscissa, 3 - 1 and 1 - 5
indicate numbers of patients. Abbreviations are
CR for complete reponse, PR for partial response,
NC for no change, and PD for progressive disease.

Sixty patients died, of whom 54 died of breast carcinomas
and the remaining six of other causes. Five-year survival
rate was calculated with the number of survivors as the
numerator and the number of dead patients plus that of
survivors at the end of five years as the denominator.
Ten-year survival rate was calculated likewise.

Histopathology

The histologic subtyping of breast carcinomas was made
according to the classification of WHO. There were five
cases of noninvasive carcinomas and 220 cases of invasive
carcinomas. Of the latter, there were 21 cases of special
histologic subtypes and 199 cases of common type ductal
carcinomas.

Immunocytochemical method

New sections were cut from the permanently stored
paraffin blocks of mastectomy specimens and were stained

according to the previously reported method with minor modifications (Shimizu et al., 1983). Following pretreatment with swine serum, sections were incubated with rabbit anti-17β-estradiol-6-bovine serum albumin (Ortho) diluted to 1:2, followed by swine anti-rabbit serum, PAP complex, diaminobenzidine and finally by counterstain with hematoxylin. Controls included omission of the primary antiserum and substitution of the primary antiserum with normal rabbit serum. Absorption of the primary antiserum with estradiol was not included in the present study.

The results were read positive when more than one-third of the cancer tissue demonstrated reactions intense enough and distinct from the background, reaction-positive cancer cells prevailing over scattered reaction-negative cancer cells, and nuclear staining discrimination whereby positive cancer cells showed either clearly positive or clearly negative nuclear staining in addition to positive cytoplasmic staining (Fig. 2A and B).

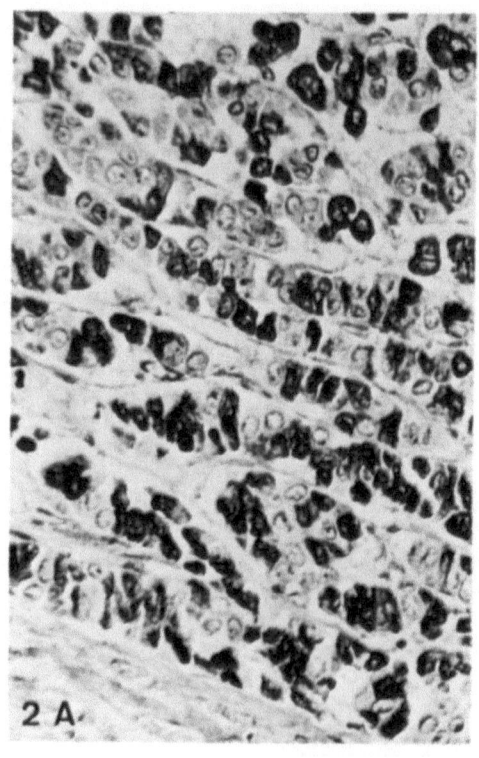

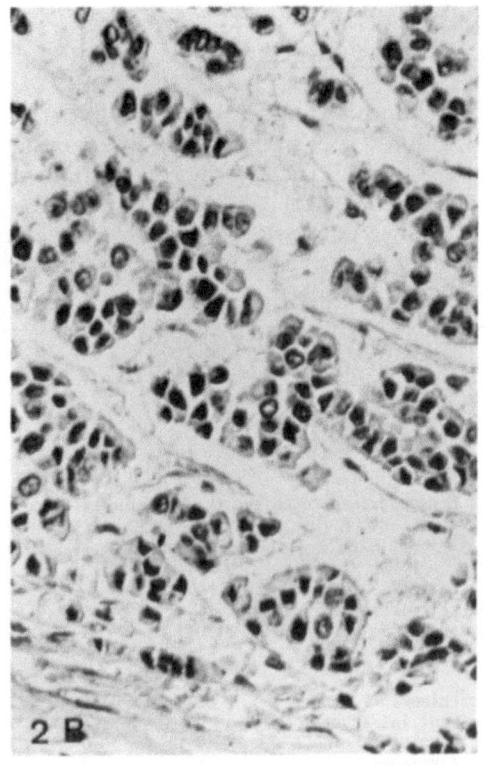

Figure 2A and B.: Breast carcinoma positively stained for endogenous estrogen (A) and negative control with omission of anti-estradiol serum (B).

Biochemical assay of estrogen receptors

Sucrose density gradient (SDG) assay of estrogen receptors was performed on fresh cancer tissues from 44 patients according to the method of Kato et al. (1976), while the immunocytochemical staining was made on paraffin sections prepared from the same specimen. The results of SDG assays were read positive when the values were over 10 fmol/mg cytosol protein.

RESULTS

Positive rate and staining patterns

Endogenous estrogen was positive in 93 of 225 patients as a whole (41.3%). When positive for endogenous estrogen, the sections of breast carcinomas demonstrated brown reaction products in the cytoplasm of some cancer cells and in the nucleus as well as cytoplasm of other cells in variable proportions. The reaction-positive cancer cells comprised the majority of cancer cells in most cell nests with the remaining cells free of reaction products (Fig. 2A and B).

Table 1. Endogenous estrogen and the histological type

	Positive	Negative	Total
1. Non-invasive			
a) intraductal carcinoma	1	3	4
b) lobular carcinoma in situ	0	1	1
2. Invasive			
a) ductal carcinoma	86	113	199
b) c̄ predominant intraductal comp	0	4	4
c) invasive lobular carcinoma	0	0	0
d) mucinous carcinoma	1	3	4
e) medullary carcinoma	3	5	8
f) papillary carcinoma	1	0	1
g) tubular carcinoma	1	2	3
h) adenoid cystic carcinoma	0	1	1
Total	93	132	225

Histologic classification (Table 1)

Endogenous estrogen was positive in one of five patients with noninvasive carcinomas and in 92 of 220 invasive carcinomas. There were 21 patients with special histologic subtypes, of whom six were positive for endogenous estrogen. These results disagreed with those of the preceding study in which nearly all noninvasive carcinomas and most of special histologic subtype invasive carcinomas were positive for endogenous estrogen (Katayama et al., 1984).

Table 2. Endogenous estrogen in relation to menopause and clinical stage

	Positive	Negative	Total
Premenopuase	66	83	149
Postmenopuase	27	49	76
Total	93	132	225
Stage I	32	44	76
Stage II	43	45	88
Stage III	14	31	45
Stage IV	4	12	16
Total	93	132	225

Menopause and clinical stage (Table 2)

Endogenous estrogen was positive in 66 of 149 premenopausal patients (44.2%) and 27 of 76 postmenopausal patients (35.5%). As for the clinical stages at diagnosis, the largest number of patients were diagnosed at stage II followed by stages I, III, and IV in the descending order of frequency of both groups of patients with positive and negative endogenous estrogen. The number of patients at stage IV was significantly fewer in the positive group, four as opposed to 12 in the negative group.

Modes of adjuvant therapy and their effects (Figure 1)

First relapse after radical mastectomy was often treated by a combination of two or three modes of therapy as described before, and, as a result, 27 patients received a total of 47 modes of therapy. In the 14 patients who received endocrine therapy solely or in combination with other modes of therapy, there was no apparent correlation between endogenous estrogen and responses to the endocrine therapy. Partly because the number of patients was limited, it was difficult to make any correlation between endogenous estrogen and responses to radiation for 11 patients and those to local excision for four patients. As for chemotherapy on 18 patients, responses of five patients with positive endogenous estrogen were CR in none, PR in one, NC in one, and PD in three, and responses of 13 patients with negative endogenous estrogen were CR in five, PR in four, NC in two, and PD in two. These results suggested a higher rate of response to chemotherapy for patients with negative endogenous estrogen.

Table 3. Endogenous estrogen and 5 & 10 year survivals

		Positive	Negative	Total
	Stage I	21/24(87.5%)	34/38(89.5%)	55/62(88.7%)
	Stage II	28/31(90.3%)	34/40(85.0%)	62/71(87.3%)
5 year	Stage III	5/10(50.0%)	15/33(45.5%)	20/43(46.5%)
	Stage IV	2/4 (50.0%)	6/11(54.5%)	8/15(53.3%)
	Total	56/69(81.2%)	89/122(73.0%)	145/191(75.9%)
	Stage I	9/9 (100.0%)	21/26(80.7%)	30/35(85.7%)
	Stage II	8/10(80.0%)	8/12(66.7%)	16/22(72.7%)
10 year	Stage III	2/6 (33.3%)	2/16(12.5%)	4/22(18.2%)
	Stage IV	0/1 (0 %)	1/4 (25.0%)	1/5 (20.0%)
	Total	19/26(73.1%)	32/58(55.2%)	51/84(60.7%)

Five-year and ten-year survival rates (Table 3)

As a whole, five-year survival rate was 81.2% (56/69) for positive patients and 73.0% (89/122) for negative patients. The ten-year survival rate was 73.1% (19/26) for positive patients and 55.2% (32/58) for negative patients. Table 3 gives further subdivisions of the survival rates according to the clinical stages of the patients.

Table 4. Endogenous estrogen and length of survival in months
(number of patients / mean / range)

	Positive	Negative	Total
Stage I	3/36.0/25-48	7/47.4/31-77	10/44.0/25-77
Stage II	4/45.8/19-71	8/58.3/13-141	12/54.1/13-141
Stage III	6/38.0/16-71	18/59.2/25-123	24/57.5/16-123
Stage IV	4/20.0/ 9-34	4/34.0/ 4-61	8/27.0/ 4-61
Total	17/32.8/ 9-71	37/52.4/ 4-141	54/46.3/ 4-141

Average length of survival in months (Table 4)

Table 4 lists the length of survival in months for 54
dead patients according to the clinical stage. As a whole,
17 patients with positive endogenous estrogen survived a
mean of 32.8 months (range 9 - 71 months), and 37 patients
with negative endogenous estrogen a mean of 52.4 months
(range 4 - 141 months). There was a trend for patients with
negative endogenous estrogen to survive longer than those
with positive endogenous estrogen.

Table 5. Endogenous estrogen by PAP method
and estrogen receptor by SDG method

PAP(+), SDG(+)	12
PAP(+), SDG(−)	7
PAP(−), SDG(+)	7
PAP(−), SDG(−)	18
Total	44

Biochemical assay of estrogen receptors (Table 5)

For 44 patients studied both by SDG assays and by the
present method, the concordance rate was 68.2% (30/44), 12
patients being positive for both tests and 18 patients
negative for both tests.

DISCUSSION

Results of the present immunocytochemical study for demonstrating endogenous estrogen on 225 patients with breast carcinomas seemed to correlate on one hand with those of SDG assays of estrogen receptors (concordance in 68.2%) and with ten-year survival rates of 73.1 and 55.2% respectively for patients with positive and negative endogenous estrogen. On the other hand, an inverse correlation, if any, was observed in the average length of survival in months for patients who died of breast carcinomas; viz., 32.8 and 52.4 months respectively for patients with positive and negative endogenous estrogen. Furthermore, there was no apparent correlation between results of the present immunocytochemical study and effects of endocrine and other adjuvant therapies. Below, we shall consider the reasons why the present study failed to reproduce the good correlation seen in the foregoing study.

In addition to the high concentrations of estrogen that are likely to produce nonspecific staining, the immunocytochemical method has the problem inherent with the use of anti-estradiol antibodies; viz., mixture of unknown and unwanted antibodies in the anti-estradiol serum and the tight clathrate-type binding of estrogen with the receptors which makes the bound estrogen hardly accessible to anti-estradiol (Chamness and McGuire, 1982; Underwood et al., 1982). These problems of anti-estradiol sera remain just the same for the present immunocytochemical method despite elimination of problems associated with exogenous estrogen pretreatment in high doses.

We ran controls for checking the specificity of the primary antiserum; its omission, its substitution with normal rabbit serum, and its absorption with estradiol, as did Walker et al. (1980) and Taylor et al. (1981). All these controls were negative, as expected. However, these controls turned out insufficient for excluding the cross-reactivity of the primary antiserum. Since the anti-estradiol antibodies used in the present method were produced by rabbits immunized with a conjugate consisting of estradiol as haptene and BSA as protein carrier, the sera may contain anti-BSA and other antibodies as well as anti-estradiol antibodies. For this reason, Mercer et al. (1980) ran a control using the primary antiserum preabsorbed by BSA, and Pertschuk et al. (1978) ran labelled rabbit antiserum as conjugate control and unlabelled anti-sheep serum prior to labelled serum as blocking control.

To our surprise, when we substituted the primary
antiserum with anti-BSA antibody, we obtained the same
staining pattern as seen with the primary antiserum. We,
therefore, concluded that what we saw as positive staining
in the present study had much to do with cross-reactivity
related to the anti-BSA antibodies. The primary antiserum
used in the present study was that of Immunoperoxidase
Staining Kit (Histoset, Ortho). According to the broch_ure
enclosed in the commercial package, the anti-estradiol serum
had a quality-control for the specificity by radioimmuno-
assay, and its cross-reactivity had been reduced by liquid
or solid phase absorption. The brochure recommends omission
of the primary antiserum and its substitution with nonimmune
serum for negative controls but offers no further precaution
for checking the anti-BSA antibodies. The brochure does not
include cross-reactivity due to anti-BSA antibodies among
the lists for trouble-shooting items, either. The lesson is
that the quality control of pharmaceutical laboratories
cannot always be taken for granted.

According to Pertschuk et al. (1980), each new batch of
anti-steroid serum may vary considerably in its specific
antibody titers and may frequently contain unknown and
unwanted antibodies against tissue components such as nuclei
and mitochondria. Therefore, it is necessary to readjust
the entire steps in the procedure each time one batch of the
anti-seroid serum is to be changed to the next. The procedure is so painstakingly complex that he concluded the
immunocytochemical method to be unsuitable for routine
clinical application. Accordingly, Pertschuk et al. (1980)
turned from the immunocytochemical method to a histochemical
method and then most recently to direct morphologic method;
viz., the novel technique of demonstrating estrogen receptors by means of monoclonal antibodies (Pertschuk et al.,
1985).

In summary, the indirect morphological methods, either
histochemical or immunocytochemical, have several methodo-
logical pitfalls which keep them unsuitable for clinical
utilization. In contrast, the direct morphologic methods
using monoclonal antibodies are now receiving the limelight.
The direct methods are theoretically superior to the indirect methods because of precise correlation with the
biochemical assays since the direct methods measure the
receptors per se as do the biochemical assays, while the
indirect methods measure estrogen and not estrogen receptors. The direct methods are now being tested not only on
frozen sections (Pertschuk et al., 1985; McCarty et al.,

1985; Shimada et al., 1985) but also on sections from paraffin embedded tissues after fixation in Bouin's solution (Poulsen et al., 1985), buffered cold formalin (Shimada et al., 1985), or formalin at room temperature (Garanis et al., 1983). In the context of these new developments, the need appears declining for further efforts toward standardizing the immunocytochemical methods for demonstrating endogenous estrogen.

SUMMARY

In order to evaluate reproducibility and clinical utility of a morphological method for demonstrating endogenous estrogen (Shimizu et al., 1983) which produced a good correlation with the biochemical assays and clinical features in a preceding study (Katayama et al., 1984), the same method was applied to 225 patients with breast carcinomas. Positive results were obtained in 93 of 225 patients as a whole (41.3%) and in 66.2% (66/149) for premenopausal and in 33.8% (27/76) for postmenopausal women. Five-year survival rate for patients with positive and negative results were 81.2% (56/69) and 73.0% (89/122) respectively, and ten-year survival rate 73.1% (19/26) and 55.2% (32/58) respectively. For 54 dead patients, the mean survival in months was 32.8 (range 9 - 71) for 17 patients with positive results and 52.4 (range 4 - 141) for 37 patients with negative results. Of 44 patients who had both the histological study and SDG assays of estrogen receptors on the same specimen, results of the two studies agreed in 30 patients (68.2%). There was no apparent correlation between results of the endogenous estrogen staining and those of endocrine and other adjuvant therapies. In summary, the present study failed to reproduce the good correlation seen in the preceding study. The problem was traced to cross-reacting antibodies in the batch of the primary antiserum in the Immunoperoxidase Staining Kit (Ortho), the quality control of which it was our mistake to have taken for granted. The antiserum may vary considerably in its specific antibody titers and may frequently contain unknown and unwanted antibodies.

REFERENCES

Chamness, G.C., McGuire, W.L. Questions about histochemical methods for steroid receptors. Arch. Pathol. Lab. Med. 106, 53-54, 1982.

Garanis, J.C., Miller, L.S., Tomita, J.T., Tieu, T.M., Clowry, L.J., Jr. Immunoperoxidase localization of estrogen receptors in human breast carcinoma. Cancer Detection and Prevention 6, 235-239, 1983.

Hayward, J.L., Carbone, P.P., Heuson, J.C., Kumaoka, S., Segaloff, A., Robens, R.D. Assessment of response to therapy in advanced breast cancer: a project of the Programme on Clinical Oncology of the International Union Against Cancer, Geneva, Switzerland. Cancer 39, 1289-1294, 1977.

Katayama, I., Shimizu, M., Miura, M., Maruyama, M., Kobayashi, M., Iino, Y., Izuo, M., Wakatsuki, S. Histochemical demonstration of endogenous estrogen in breast carcinomas: Biochemical and clinical correlation. Virchows Arch (Pathol. Anat.) 402, 353-359, 1984.

Kato, J., Nomura, Y., Matsumoto, K., Onouchi, T. Radioreceptor assay of estrogen. Nippon Rinsho 34, 510-517, 1976 (in Japanese)

McCarty, K.S., Jr., Miller, L.S., Cox, E.B., Konrath, J., McCarty, K.S., Sr. Estrogen receptor analyses. Correlation of biochemical and immunohistochemical methods using monoclonal antireceptor antibodies. Arch. Pathol. Lab. Med. 109, 716-721, 1985.

Mercer, M.D., Lippman, M.E., Wahl, T.M., Carlson, C.A., Wahl, D.A., Lezotte, D., Teague, P.O. The use of immunocytochemical techniques for the detection of steroid hormones in breast cancer cells. Cancer 46, 2859-2868, 1980.

Okazaki, U., Asaischi, K., Okazaki, C., Mikami, T., Toda, K., Okazaki, M., Totsuka, M., Hayasaka, A., Narimatsu, H. Estradiol staining of breast carcinoma cells and its significance. Proceedings of Japan Mammary Cancer Society 42, 75, 1985 (in Japanese).

Pertschuk, L.P., Eisenberg, K.B., Carter, A.C., Feldman, J.G. Immunohistologic localization of estrogen receptors in breast cancer with monoclonal antibodies. Correlation with biochemistry and clinical endocrine response. Cancer 55, 1513-1518, 1985.

Pertschuk, L.P., Tobin, E.H., Gaetjens, E., Carter, A.C., Degenschein, G.A., Bloom, N.D., Brigati, D.J. Histochemical assay of estrogen and progesterone receptors in breast cancer: Correlation with biochemical assay and patients' response to endocrine therapies. Cancer 46, 2896-2901, 1980.

Pertschuk, L.P., Tobin, E.H., Brigati, D.J., Kim, D.S., Bloom, N.D., Gaetjens, E., Berman, P.J., Carter, A.C., Degenschein, G.A. Immunofluorescent detection of estrogen receptors in breast cancer: Comparison with dextran-coated charcoal and sucrose gradient assays. Cancer 41, 907-911, 1978.

Poulsen, H.S., Ozzello, L., King, W.J., Greene, G.L. The use of monoclonal antibodies to estrogen receptors (ER) for immunoperoxidase detection of ER in paraffin sections of human breast cancer tissue. J. Histochem. Cytochem. 33, 87-92, 1985.

Shimada, A., Kimura, S., Abe, K., Nagasaki, K., Adachi, I., Yamaguchi, K., Suzuki, M., Nakajima, T., Miller, L.S. Immunocytochemical staining of estrogen receptor in paraffin sections of human breast cancer by use of monoclonal antibody: Comparison with that in frozen sections. Proc. Natl. Acad. Sci. USA 82, 4803-4807, 1985.

Shimizu, M., Wajima, O., Miura, M., Katayama, I. PAP immunoperoxidase method demonstrating endogenous estrogen in breast carcinomas. Cancer 52, 486-492, 1983.

Taylor, C.R., Cooper, C.L., Kurman, R.J., Goeblesmann, U., Markland, F.S. Detection of estrogen receptor in breast and endometrial carcinoma by immunoperoxidase technique. Cancer 47, 2634-2640, 1981.

Underwood, J.C., Sher, E., Reed, M., Eisman, J.A., Martin, T.J. Biochemical assessment of histochemical methods for oestrogen receptor localisation. J. Clin. Pathol. 35, 401-406, 1982.

Walker, R.A., Cove, D.H., Howell, A. Histological detection of oestrogen receptor in human breast carcinomas. Lancet 1, 171-173, 1980.

World Health Organization. Histological Typing of Breast
    Tumors. 2nd ed., International Histological Classi-
    fication of Tumors, No. 2, WHO, Geneva, 1981.

IMMUNOCYTOCHEMISTRY OF PUTATIVE ESTROGEN RECEPTORS:

A REAPPRAISAL

VINCENZO EUSEBI[1], FLORIANA C.M. FRATAMICO[1], AND STEFANO MIGNANI[2]

1.   Istituto di Anatomia e Istologia Patologica,
     Universita di Bologna, 40138 Bologna, Italy
2.   Istituto di Radiologia, Universita di Bologna

An immunocytochemical method for estrogen receptor (ER) analysis of breast carcinomas was reported by one of us in 1981 (Eusebi et al., 1981). This technique was compared with the dextran-coated charcoal assay and a cytochemical method. We felt at the time that an improvement in existing techniques for assaying estrogen receptors was needed in view of conflicting evidence in the literature concerning correlation between the morphological and functional parameters of breast tumours. While some authors found a correlation between high ER content and a low histologic grade of malignancy (Fisher et al., 1980; Maynard et al., 1978), others did not (Johansson et al., 1970; Paszko et al., 1978; Rosen et al., 1978). Several groups of workers detected a positive correlation between ER positivity and the lobular type of invasive carcinoma (Antoniades and Spector, 1979; Eusebi et al., 1977; Rosen et al., 1975), but this was not corroborated by other investigators (Fisher et al., 1980; Maynard et al., 1978; Poulson et al., 1982).

Furthermore, while Rosen et al. (1978) reported that five tubular carcinomas were all ER-negative, Lagios et al. (1980) observed that four out of six tubular carcinomas were ER-positive. Lastly, while a direct relationship between the degree of tumour elastosis and the presence of ER has been reported (Masters et al., 1979), Fisher et al. (1980) have suggested, on the basis of a multivariate analysis, that tumour elastosis is more closely related to the patient's age than to ER status per se.

Such discrepancies became more patent when data from a single group were analyzed. In 1975, Rosen et al. (1975)

reported that 92 per cent of lobular carcinomas of the breast were ER-positive. Subsequently, the same authors reported 89 per cent positivity for the same type of carcinoma (Rosen et al., 1978), and later, 49 per cent positivity (Lesser et al., 1981).

For a direct demonstration of estrogen receptors on isolated breast carcinoma cells or on fresh tissue sections, several techniques have been described. Basically, the signal given by the single estrogen binding site is magnified by means of a large fluorescent complex or enzyme reactions.

Lee (1978) developed a cytochemical fluorescent method to visualize ER-positive cells with E-BSA-FITC complexes. Nenci et al. (1976) and Pertschuk et al. (1978) described immunofluorescent methods with anti-estrogen sera, and Walker et al. (1980) used anti-estrogen antibodies bound to horseradish peroxidase. These authors employed sections previously fixed in acetone, an estrogen solvent, and as a result, the method was highly criticized by Eusebi et al. (1981).

It became clear that the advantages of all these procedures could be enhanced by means of a two-stage method consisting of a fluorescent cytochemical procedure followed by an immunohistochemical method employing anti-estrogen sera (Eusebi et al., 1981) (Fig. 1). In a second phase, E-BSA complexes were visualized by means of anti-estradiol serum and an immunoperoxidase procedure with peroxidase anti-peroxidase complexes. An original immuno-galactosidase procedure was proposed as an additional improvement to the method (Bondi et al., 1982, 1984; Eusebi and Bussolati, 1985), (Fig. 2).

More recently, the traditional model of steroid hormone receptor function (Schrader, 1984) as well as the reliability of histochemical methods (Chamne et al., 1980; Underwood et al., 1982) have been questioned. In addition to technical errors, there has been some debate as to whether the added estrogens used in the various published methods bind to receptors only.

As a result, the introduction of anti-receptor antibodies seemed to provide a solution to these various problems. Unfortunately, these antibodies appear to give different results. The polyclonal anti-receptor antibody used by Raam et al. (1982) located the receptor in the

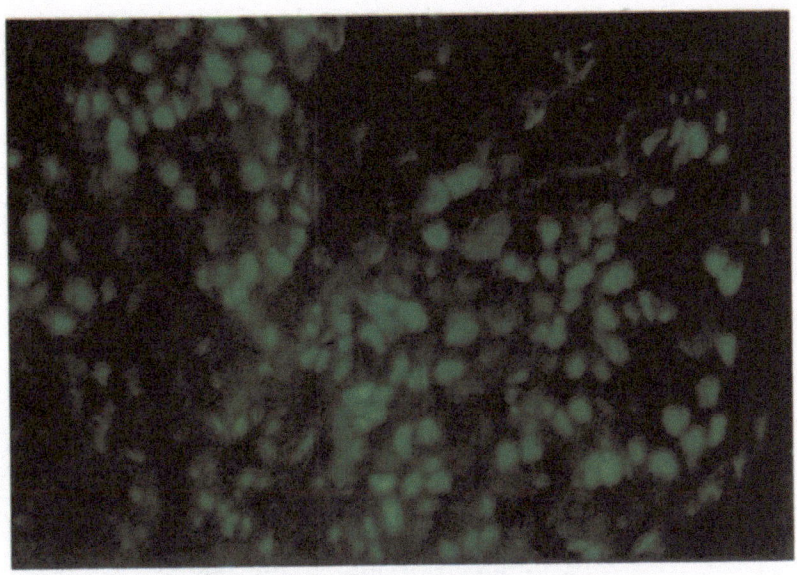

Fig. 1.   Breast carcinoma. Numerous neoplastic cells
display positive fluorescent nuclei (E-BSA-FITC).
X 180.

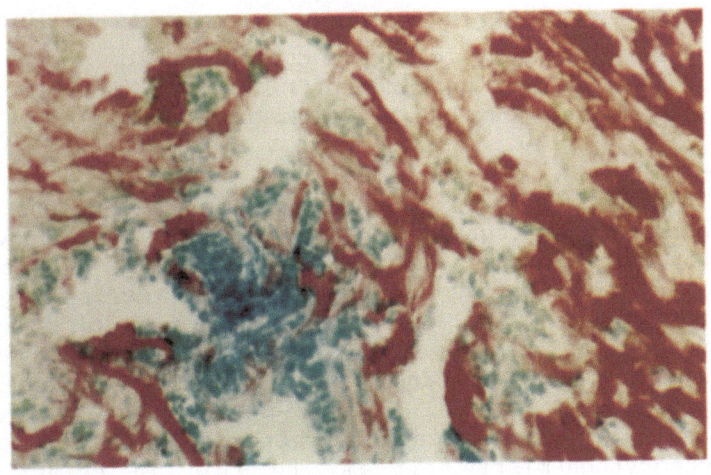

Fig. 2.   Same case as Fig. 1. Positive cells with blue
nuclei. The stroma is counterstained with van
Gieson's solution
(Anti-estradiol-beta-galactosidase). X 140.

cytoplasm, whereas the monoclonal anti-receptor antibody tested by Jensen et al. (1982) stained the cytoplasm only. In another study (King and Green, 1982), the same antibody located the receptor in the nucleus only (Fig. 3). On the basis of the results produced by this antibody, the classical theory according to which estrogen receptors are present in the cytoplasm and translocate to the nucleus has been dismissed in favor of the presence of the receptors in the nucleus only.

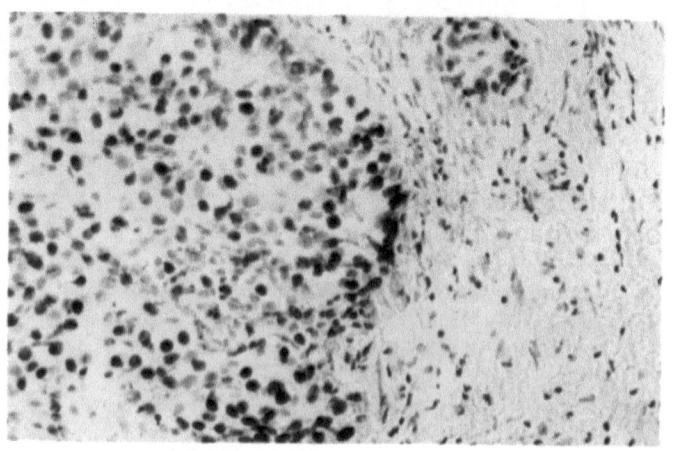

Fig. 3.   Breast carcinoma. Most of nuclei appear stained by this anti-receptor antibody (ABC-peroxidase) (by courtesy of Professor G. Bussolati, Torino). X 140.

More recently, a human-specific monoclonal antibody against an estrogen receptor component of the cytosol has been described by Coffer et al. (1985). This antibody stains the cytoplasm of breast cancer cells (Fig. 4), but unfortunately, it also stains cells from squamous cell carcinoma of the lung (G. Bussolati, personal communication) (Fig. 5). This finding is not surprising since it is well known that monoclonal antibodies, although very selective, often bind to the most unexpected sites. In addition, in immunocytochemistry, it is the rule in establishing the specificity of a reaction to preadsorb an antiserum with its respective antigen. This cannot be done with the available anti-ER monoclonal antibodies which have been produced against the "estrogen receptor machinery" since the actual structure of the estrogen receptors has not been elucidated

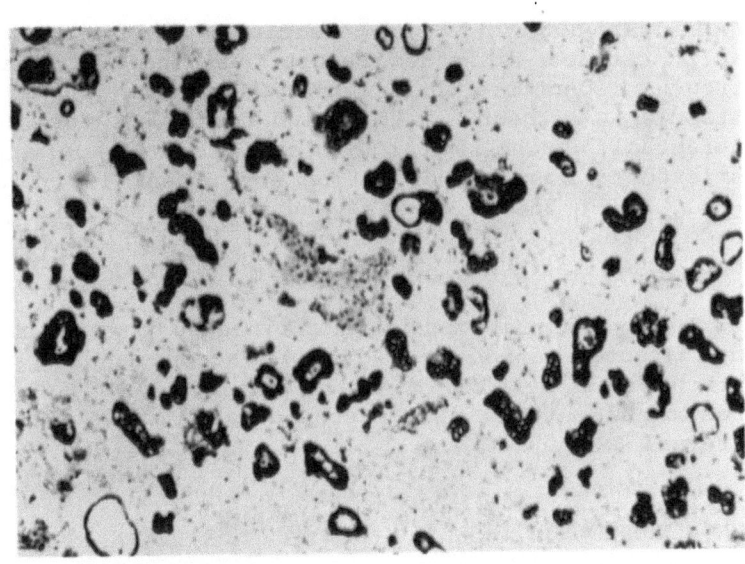

Fig. 4.   Pleural effusion from breast carcinoma. Most of
the cells display positive cytoplasm using this
monoclonal antibody anti-estrogen receptor
(ABC-peroxidase) (by courtesy of Professor G.
Bussolati). X 80.

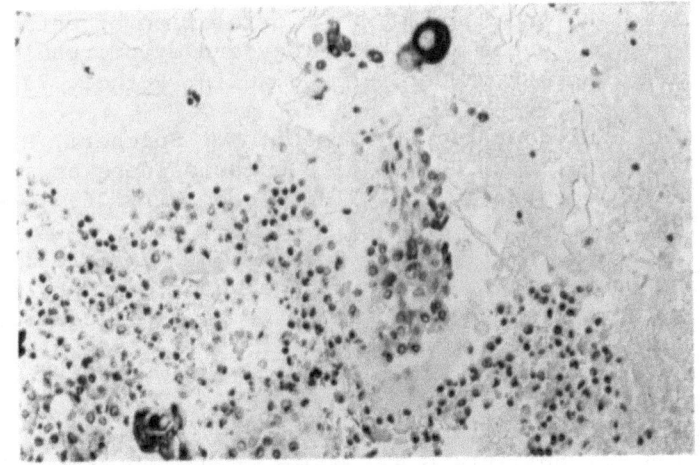

Fig. 5.   Pleural effusion from a bronchial squamous cell
carcinoma. Using the same antibody
(ABC-peroxidase) as in Fig. 4, several cells
appear immunologically positive (by courtesy of
Professor G. Bussolati). X 80.

and it has not yet been possible to purify them. As a result, caution is needed before assuming the presence of estrogen receptors solely on the basis of monoclonal antibodies. A theory of this kind could well turn out to be non-factual, much like the classical one now apparently dismissed by most authors (King and Green, 1984; Pertschuk et al., 1985) but which was very much in favour for over a decade (Jensen and Jacobson, 1962; McGuire et al., 1977; Nenci, 1981).

In conclusion, more work is needed on the physiology and characterization of ER before accepting the published histochemical methods as reliable for routine practice, since these methods differ considerably while all claiming to reveal ER.

ACKNOWLEDGMENTS

Work supported by Grants of MPI and CNR, project "Oncologia" no. 85.02158.44.

REFERENCES

Antoniades, K. and Spector, H. Correlation of estrogen receptor levels with histology and cytomorphology in human mammary cancer. Am. J. Clin. Pathol. 71, 497-503, 1979.
Bondi, A., Chieregatti, G., Eusebi, V., Fulcheri, E., and Bussolati, G. The use of B-galactosidase as a tracer in immunocytochemistry. Histochemistry 26, 153-158, 1982.
Bondi, A., Morichelli, M.P., Ghidoni, D., Bertarelli, C., and Eusebi, V.E. Immunobetagalactosidasi nella evidenziazione dei recettori ormonali in carcinomi mammari. Istocitopatologia 6, 29-31, 1984.
Chamne, G.C. Marcer, W.D., and McGuire, W.L. Are histochemical methods for estrogen receptors valid? J. Histochem. Cytochem. 28, 792-798, 1980.
Coffer, A.I., Spiller, G.H., Lewis, K.M., and King, R.J.B. Immunoradiometric studies with monoclonal antibody against a component related to human estrogen receptor. Cancer Research 45, 3694-3698, 1985.
Eusebi, V. and Bussolati, G. A two-stage immunocytochemical method for putative estrogen receptor analysis. In: Morphologic localization of putative steroid receptors. Techniques and Applications, Vol. I. Lee, S.H. and Pertschuk, L.P., eds. CRC Press, Boca Raton, FL, 1985.

Eusebi, V., Pich, A., Macchiorlatti, E., and Bussolati, G. Morpho-functional differentiation in lobular carcinoma of the breast. Histopathology 1, 304-314, 1977.

Eusebi, V., Cerasoli, P.T., Guidelli-Guidi, S., Grilli, S., Bussolati, G., and Azzopardi, J.G. A two-stage immunocytochemical method for oestrogen receptor analysis: correlation with morphological parameters of breast carcinomas. Tumori 6, 315-323, 1981.

Fisher, E.R., Redmond, C.K., Liu, H., Rochette, H., Fisher, B., and collaborating NSAPS investigators. Correlation of estrogen receptor and pathological characteristics of invasive breast cancer. Cancer 45, 349-353, 1980.

Jensen, E.V. and Jacobson, H.I. Basic guides to the mechanism of estrogen action. Recent Prog. Horm. Res. 18, 387, 1962.

Jensen, E.V., Greene, G.L., Closs, L.E., De Sombre, E.R., and Nadji, M. Receptors reconsidered: a 20-year perspective. Rec. Prog. Horm. Res. 38, 1-39, 1982.

Johansson, H., Terenius, I., and Thoren, I. The binding of estradiol-17 to human breast cancers and other tissues in vitro. Cancer Res. 30, 692-698, 1970.

King, W.L. and Greene, G.L. Monoclonal antibodies localize oestrogen receptro in the nuclei of target cells. Nature 307, 745-747, 1984.

Lagios, M.D., Rose, M.R., and Margolin, F.R. Tubular carcinoma of the breast. Am. J. Clin. Pathol. 73, 25-30, 1980.

Lee, S.H. Cytochemical study of estrogen receptor in human mammary cancer. Am. J. Clin. Pathol. 70, 197-203, 1978.

Lesser, M.L., Rosen, P.P., Senie, R.T., Duthie, K., Menendez-Botet, L., and Schwartz, M. Estrogen and progesterone receptors in breast carcinoma: correlations with epidemiology and pathology. Cancer 48, 299-309, 1981.

Masters, J.R.W., Millis, R.R., King, R.J.B., and Rubens, R.D. Elastosis and response to endocrine therapy in human breast cancer. Br. J. Cancer 39, 536-639, 1979.

McGuire, W.L., Horwitz, K.B., Pearson, O.H., and Segaloff, A. Current status of estrogen and progesterone receptors in breast cancer. Cancer 39, 2934-2947, 1977.

Maynard, P.V., Davies, C.J., Blamey, R.W., Elston, C.W., Johnson, J., and Griffiths, K. Relationship between oestrogen-receptor content and histological grade in human primary breast tumours. Br. J. Cancer 38, 745-748, 1978.

Nenci, I. Estrogen receptor cytochemistry in human breast cancer: status and prospects. Cancer 48, 2674-2686, 1981.

136

Nenci, I., Beccati, M.D., Piffanelli, A., and Lanza, G. Detection and dynamic localization of estradiol receptor complexes in intact target cells by immunofluorescence technique. J. Steroid. Biochem. $\underline{7}$, 505-510, 1976.

Paszko, Z., Padzik, H., Dabska, M., and Pienkowska, F. Estrogen receptor in human breast cancer in relation to tumor morphology and endocrine therapy. Tumori $\underline{64}$, 495-506, 1978.

Pertschuk, L.P., Eisenberg, K.B., Carter, A.C., and Feldman, J.G. Immunohistologic localization of estrogen receptors in breast cancer with monoclonal antibodies. Cancer $\underline{55}$, 1513-1518, 1985.

Pertschuk, L.P., Tobin, E.H., Brigati, D.J., Kim, D.S., Blom, N.D., Gaetjens, E., Berman, P.J., Carter, A.C., and Degenshein, G.A. Immunofluorescent detection of estrogen receptors in breast cancer. Cancer $\underline{41}$, 907-911, 1978.

Poulsen, H.S., Ozzello, L., and Andersen, J. Oestrogen receptors in human breast cancer. Virchows Arch. (Anat. Pathol.) $\underline{397}$, 103-108, 1982.

Raam, S., Nemeth, H., Tamura, D.S., O'Brian, D.S., and Cohen, J.L. Immunohistochemical localization of estrogen receptors in human mammary carcinoma using antibodies to the receptor protein. Eur. Cancer Clin. Oncol. $\underline{18}$, 1-12, 1982.

Rosen, P.P., Menendez-Botet, C.J., Nisselbaum, J.S., Urban, J.A., Mike, V., Fracchia, A., and Schwartz, M.K. Pathological review of breast lesions analysed for estrogen protein. Cancer Res. $\underline{35}$, 3187-3194, 1975.

Rosen, P.P., Menendez-Botet, C.J., Senie, R.T., Schwartz, M.K., Schottenfeld, D., and Farr, G.H. Estrogen receptor protein (ERP) and histopathology of human mammary carcinoma. In: Hormones, Receptors and Breast Cancer, McGuire, W.L., ed., Raven Press, New York, 1978.

Schrader, W.T. New model for steroid hormone receptors? Nature $\underline{308}$, 17-18, 1984.

Underwood, J.C.E., Sher, E., Reed, H., Eisman, J.R., and Martin, T.J. Biochemical assessment of histochemical methods for oestrogen receptor localization. J. Clin. Pathol. $\underline{35}$, 401-406, 1982.

Walker, R.A., Cove, D.H., and Howell, A. Histological detection of estrogen receptor in human breast carcinomas. Lancet $\underline{1}$, 171, 1980.

MONOCLONAL ANTIBODIES IN THE MANAGEMENT OF BREAST CANCER

F. MORNEX[1], D. COLCHER[2], M.O. WEEKS[2], and J. SCHLOM[2]

1. Centre Léon Bérard, 28, rue Laennec, 69000 Lyon, France
2. Laboratory of Tumor Immunology and Biology, National Cancer Institute, Bethesda, Md 20205, U.S.A.

For many years antibodies have had a major role in the diagnosis, investigation and treatment of a wide variety of diseases. At the same time, immunologists have continued to develop methods of immunization that would produce large amounts of homogeneous antibodies (Krause, 1970; Haber, 1970). These approaches have not been generally applicable to the routine production of serologic reagents against many antigens. The identification of human tumor associated antigens (TAAs) and the development of specific immunologic reagents directed against these targets have long been sought (Pressmann and Korngold, 1953). In past decades, the classical method of generating antibodies to TAAs has been the hyperimmunization of an animal with an extract of a human tumor and the absorption of the resultant sera with a variety of normal tissues. For example, if an extract of human breast carcinoma was used as immunogen, then the serum has to be absorbed with extracts of normal breast, benign breast tumor, as well as extracts of normal human red blood cells, liver, etc. This absorbed hyperimmune serum has then to be tested for its ability to react with the immunogen (in this case breast carcinoma). All too often, only weak reactivity was observed and only enough sera were obtained to complete a finite number of tests; thus, the entire process has to begin over again. Furthermore, since hyperimmune sera are estimated to contain some tens of thousands of different types of immunoglobulins which differ in isotype, affinity and specifity, reproductibility of results from laboratory to laboratory was difficult if not impossible to achieve.

The advent of hybridoma technology in 1975 represented a quantum leap in the field of tumor immunology (Kohler and Milstein, 1975, Kohler et al., 1976). For the first time, single cell populations of B-lymphocytes from immunized hosts could be immortalized via fusion with drug selected non-immunoglobulin secretor murine myeloma cells. The fused cell product could now be cloned and propagated indefinitely. The supernatant fluids of cultures from literally thousands of different cloned cell populations (termed hybridoma) could now be assayed to select for homogeneous populations of immunoglobulins with the desired reactivity. As a direct result of this technology, numerous monoclonal antibodies (MAbs) have been generated that have led to the identification of novel TAAs from various human carcinomas, melanomas, leukemias and lymphomas (Boven and Pinedo, 1986). To date, at least a dozen monoclonal antibodies against human mammary carcinomas have been reported in the literature (Arklie et al., 1982; Colcher et al., 1983 a; Menard et al., 1983; Nuti et al., 1982; Schlom et al., 1984 a, 1984 b, Sloane and Omerod, 1981); each one has been characterized with respect to range of reactivity and reactive antigen. In general, these MAbs can be classified into four groups based on the immunogen used to generate the monoclonal antibody. These include antibodies generated using (a) breast tumor cell lines, (b) milk fat globule membrane (c) membrane enriched extracts of breast carcinoma metastases, or (d) lymph nodes from mastectomy patients. Each of the MAbs thus far described, including those prepared by several different groups from milk fat globule membrane (Arklie et al., 1982; Foster et al., 1982; Rasmussen et al., 1982; Taylor-Papadimitriou et al., 1981) appears to be unique with respect to percent of reactive mammary tumors, percent of reactive cells within tumors, location of reactive antigen within the tumor cell, or degree of reactivity with non-mammary tumors as well as normal tissues.

An analysis of the monoclonal antibody literature as it relates to breast cancer (Arklie et al., 1982; Colcher et al., 1981, 1983 a; Epenetos et al., 1982 a, 1982 b; Foster et al., 1982; Hand et al., 1983; Menard et al., 1983; Nuti et al., 1982; Rasmussen et al., 1982; Schlom et al., 1984 a; Sloane and Omerod, 1981; Taylor-Papadimitriou et al., 1981) reveals several important concepts: (a) most breast cancer associated determinants (as defined by MAbs) are also found on other carcinoma cells, i.e., a large number of "pancarcinoma" antigens have recently been elucidated, (b) a great deal of antigenic heterogeneity exists in the expression of a given tumor antigenic determinant, both among cells of a given tumor and between different tumors of different patients, (c) established breast cancer cell lines may not reflect the phenotype or even genotype of breast cancer biopsy material. The latter findings most likely reflect the enormous selective pressure exerted on cell populations in attempts to establish appropriate culture conditions and subsequent immortal cell lines. The MAbs thus far characterized and future generations of MAbs, may ultimately find use in virtually all arms of patients management. The progress being made in several of these areas as well as the problems that have been encountered will be discussed.

Serum assays

MAbs to detect tumor associated antigens in serum can eventually be used in early detection of carcinoma lesions, monitoring for recurrence and monitoring the efficacy of specific therapeutic regimens. Whereas no monoclonal antibody has yet been reported that can be used to detect tumor in asymptomatic individuals as an early diagnostic test, several MAbs have been reported that may be used to monitor tumor burden in breast cancer patients. Thus, a recent study describes the use of a monoclonal antibody (DF3) (Kufe et al., 1984) in a radioimmuno-assay (RIA) to monitor the appearance of a 300,000 dalton reactive antigen in serum. The results (Hayes et al., 1985) indicate that 76% (33 of 43) of patients with metastatic breast cancer had elevated antigen levels as compared to 3 of 36 normal controls ($p < 0.001$). Further studies with this and other MAbs, either used alone or as a part of a MAb cocktail, are being evaluated to monitor the clinical course of patients.

Immunohistochemical and Immunocytochemical Methods to Detect and Phenotype carcinoma.

Perhaps the most immediate applications of monoclonal antibodies in the management of human breast cancer will be their use to detect occult tumor cells and to phenotype carcinoma cell populations. Recently, Johnston et al., (1985) have shown that a particular MAb (B 72.3) can be used as an adjunct in the detection of breast carcinoma cells in pleural effusions.

B 72.3 was generated using a membrane-enriched fraction from a mammary carcinoma metastasis (Colcher et al., 1981; Nuti et al., 1982). Immunoperoxidase studies have demonstrated that B 72.3 reacts with approximately 50% of breast carcinomas, with more than 80% of colon carcinomas, and also with other adenocarcinomas, but shows no significant reactivity with a large variety of normal tissues (Johnson et al., 1986; Johnston et al., 1985). The reactive antigen (TAG-72 = Tumor Associated Glycoprotein), which is a $> 10^6$ dalton mucin-like molecule,was found on carcinoma cells of 22/23 samples from all 21 patients tested with metastatic breast cancer. Conversely, monoclonal antibody B 72.3 failed to react with effusions from 41 patients without cancer (Johnston et al., 1985). Since these studies were conducted retrospectively with formalin fixed blocks of effusion material, the accuracy of diagnosis and the clinical outcome of each patient was already known. Most cytopathologists will admit difficulties in the definitive diagnosis of carcinoma in approximately 10% of effusion samples, due to the presence of often atypical single cells or scattered tumor cells among clusters of reactive mesothelial cells.

The use of monoclonal antibody appeared to complement standard cytologic procedures in those particular situations (Johnston et al., 1985).

Figures 1-4 show different pleural effusions which presented diagnostic problems at the time of routine diagnostic interpretation, in patients with widely metastatic breast carcinoma. The diagnostic interpretation was aided by the use of MAb B 72.3 allowing discrimination of tumors cells with bland cytological features from reactive mesothelial cells (Fig. 1, 2) and identification of isolated clusters of malignant cells in an extre-

mely cellular sample (Fig 3,4). These studies are being ex-
panded by several groups to use various MAbs as an adjunct to
the diagnosis of mammary carcinoma with fine-needle aspiration
biopsy, and for the detection of occult cancer cells in bone
marrow.

Monoclonal antibodies are more and more used in immunohis-
topathology to phenotype carcinomatous lesions. Thus, various
monoclonal antibodies to estrogen receptor are currently being
evaluated in comparison to immunoassays of tumor extracts
(Lundy et al., 1985; Rasmussen et al., 1982). Immunohistochemical assays have the advantage of defining reactivity to specific cell types and overcome the criticism that values obtained

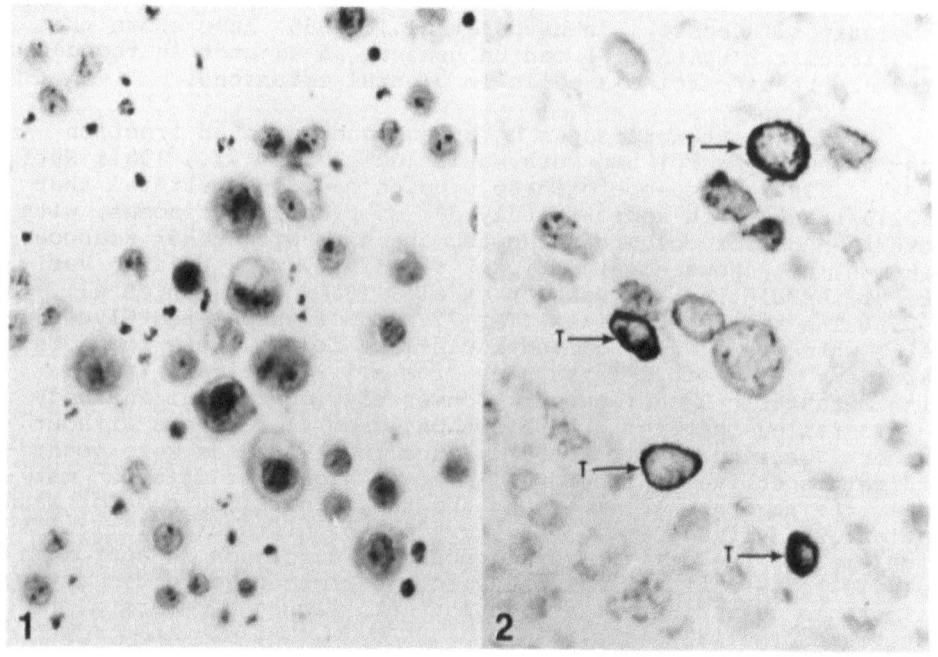

Fig. 1: Membrane filter preparation of a malignant effusion
        from a patient with infiltrating lobular carcinoma of
        the breast. Papanicolaou stain. x 480.

Fig. 2: Reactivity of the same specimen as in Fig. 1 with
        MAb B 72.3 showing staining of single tumor cells (T)
        against a background of inflammatory cells. The dark
        cytoplasmic staining of carcinoma cells reflects the
        reaction of the diaminobenzidine substrate and thus
        MAb B 72.3 binding. x 550.

from biochemical assays may be more indicative of the percent of tumor cells present in the sample than the actual amount of estrogen receptor per tumor cell.

Monoclonal antibodies are presently studied in immunopathology and immunocytopathology for differential diagnosis. Monoclonal antibody B 72.3 is reactive with breast carcinoma but is nonreactive with lymphoma. Lesions in regional lymph nodes in the absence of a primary breast lesion will thus be assayed for the presence of B 72.3 reactive antigen. It can be envisioned that several MAbs used in concert will help the pathologist in the future in a variety of differential diagnoses.

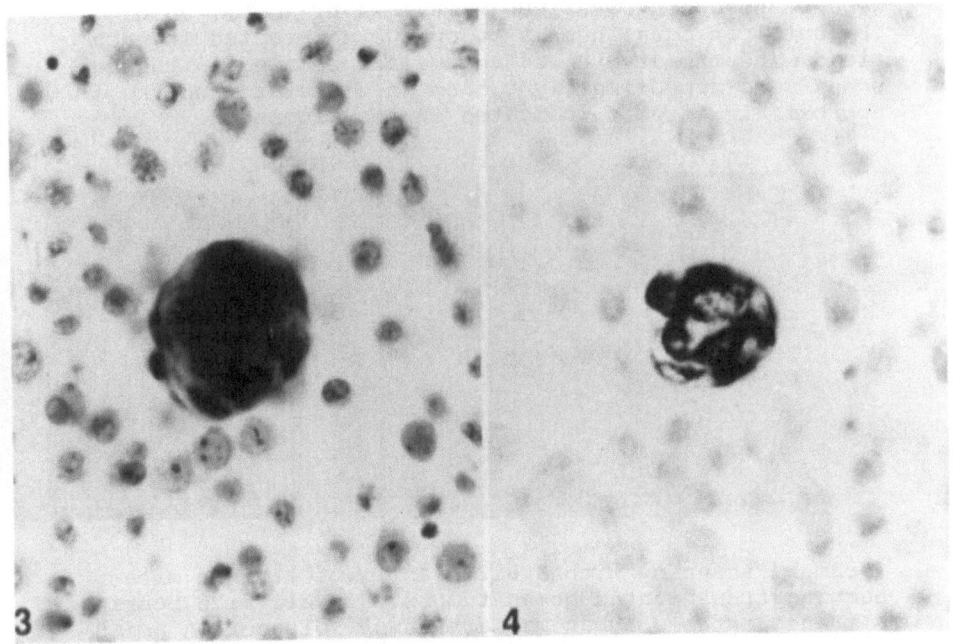

Fig. 3: Member filter preparation of a malignant effusion from Patient B with infiltrating ductal carcinoma of the breast. Papanicolaou stain. x 380.

Fig. 4: Cell block preparation of the same specimen as Fig. 3 reacted with MAb B 72.3. A single cluster of malignant cells (center) is present against a background of non-staining inflammatory and mesothelial cells. x 550.

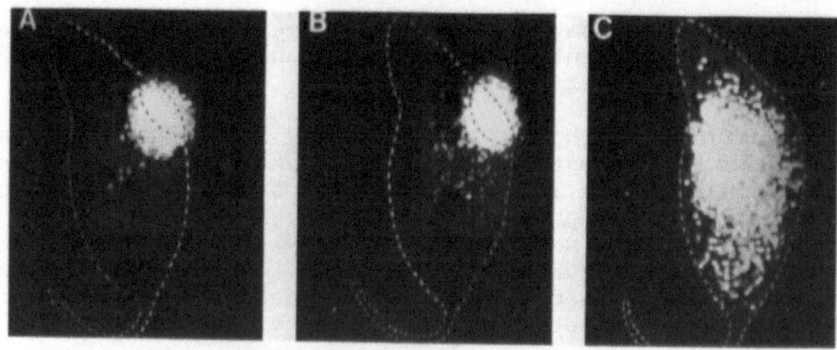

Fig. 5 γ-camera scanning with B 6.2 IgG of athymic mice bearing
        transplanted human tumors. Athymic mice bearing a trans-
        plantable human mammary tumor (Clouser) (A and B) or a
        human melanoma (A375) (C) were inoculated with approxi-
        mately 30 μCi of ^{125}I - B 6.2 IgG (53 μCi/μg). The mice
        were scanned after various times   24 hr (A,C), 96 hr
        (B) until an equal number of cpm were detected in each
        field. The mammary tumors and melanomas used in these
        scans were approximately 0.5 cm in diameter, and the
        approximate size is indicated in the figure.

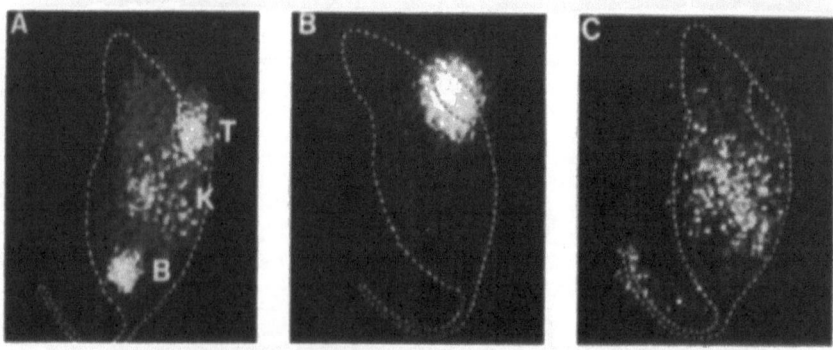

Fig. 6: γ-camera scanning with B 6.2 F(ab')$_2$ of athymic mice
         bearing transplanted human tumors. Athymic mice bearing
         a transplantable human mammary tumor Clouser (A and B)
         or a human melanoma   A375 (C)   were inoculated with
         approximately 30 μCi of ^{125}I - B 6.2 F(ab')$_2$ (19 μCi/μg).
         The mice were scanned after various times   (24 hr (A);
         96 hr (B and C) until an equal number of cpm were de-
         tected in each field. The mammary tumors and melanomas
         used in these scans were approximately 0.5 cm in diame-
         ter and the approximate size is indicated in the figure.
         In A, the tumor (T), kidneys (K) and bladder (B) are
         indicated.

RADIOLOCALIZATION OF HUMAN COLON CANCER
WITH I-131-B72.3 MONOCLONAL ANTIBODY

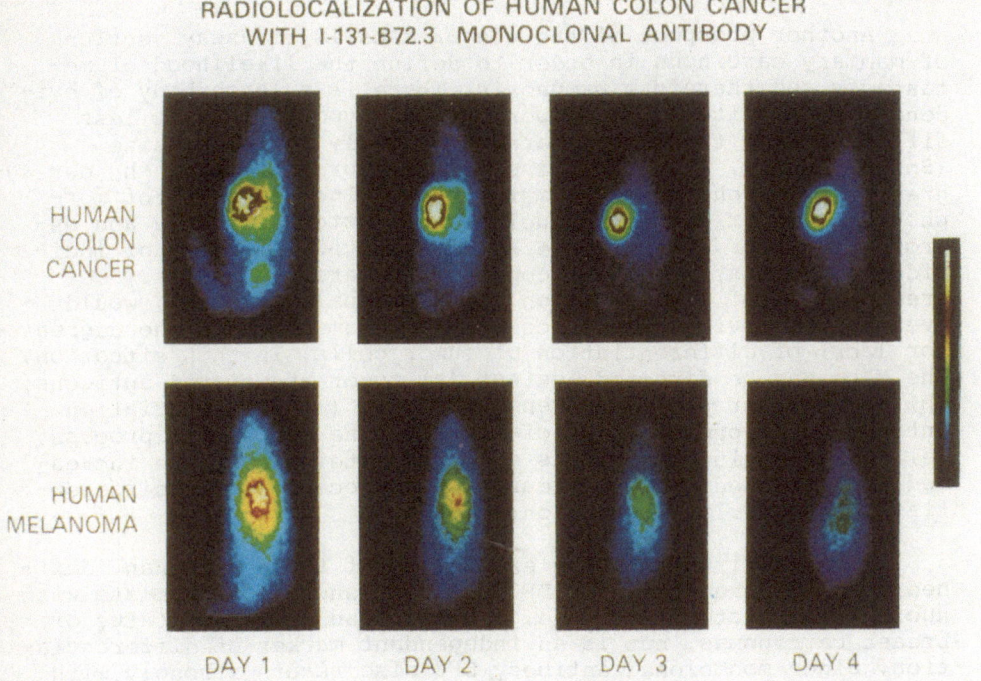

Fig. 7: Dorsal scintiphotos of athymic mice after i.v. injection
with 62 μCi of I-131 B 72.3. A through D: mouse bearing
0.8 cm human colon tumor on left flank is shown on Days
1, 2, 3 and 4. E through H: similar series for human
melanoma of comparable size and location.

Colon tumor becomes increasingly distinct as non specific background activity decreases, but no accumulation
is detected in melanoma. Bladder activity near base of
tail is visible on Day 1 (A and E) but not thereafter.
Body background was comparable in two animals but appears higher in melanoma-bearing mouse due to longer
counting times.

Each image consists of 50.000 counts acquired into 64-
by 64-pixel matrix, interpolated to a 256 X 256 matrix
without background subtraction or computer smoothing.
Color bar at right shows common scale used for all images, with highest value at top representing maximum
pixel value in image sequence.

Prognostic studies

Another prospect of the use of MAbs is to assay sections of mammary carcinoma in order to define the likelihood of metastasis and therefore prognosis. There is a large body of evidence in the literature supporting the hypothesis that less differentiated tumor cells are more likely to metastasize (Schlom et al., 1984 a, 1984 b). At the present time, the degree of differentiation is mainly determined on basis of morphologic criteria such as nuclear and histologic grade and estrogen receptor status. More subtle changes in levels of individual proteins, or the glycoprotein determinants (i.e., degree or type of glycosylation of individual proteins), would eventually provide a more accurate assessment as to the degree (or lack) of differentiation of tumor cells. In this situation, the MAbs may be directed against (a) tumor associated antigens, (b) oncogene or proto-oncogene products, (c) differentiation antigens, (d) proteins associated with the metastatic process, (e) normal cellular proteins or glycoproteins that are increased or decreased in levels during the processes of dedifferentiation and early progression.

In this direction, the expression of the determinant defined by monoclonal antibody DF3 has been shown to correlate with nuclear and histologic grade, and estrogen receptor status of breast carcinomas, but is an independant marker of differentiation. Since monoclonal antibody DF3 also reacts strongly with lactating mammary epithelial cells, it can be hypothesized to reveal a novel differentiation antigen (Lundy et al., 1985).

Other hypotheses involve the mechanism of attachment and invasion in the metastatic process i.e., (a) tumor cells that express high levels of exposed laminin receptor are more likely to bind to laminin in basement membranes, and (b) tumor cells expressing high levels of type IV collagenase are more likely to invade through basement membrane via the dissolution of type IV collagen. Thus, one could envision a panel of monoclonal antibodies such as DF3, anti-laminin receptor, anti-type IV collagenase, anti-oncogene products and growth factors as a means of better defining the probability of metastasis for a given carcinoma cell population.

Radionuclide - Conjugated Monoclonal Antibodies to Localize Tumor Lesions In Situ

A major concern in the evaluation of the primary breast cancer patient is the presence or absence of tumor in regional lymph nodes. Presently, the removal of the regional axillary nodes at time of lympectomy or mastectomy, and subsequent histopathologic evaluation of individual nodes, is the standard procedure. The absence of tumor in nodes is a favorable prognostic indicator and, in the vast majority of cases, no subsequent therapy is called for. Approximately 25% of "node negative patients, however, will eventually develop metastatic breast cancer. One reason for this situation may be that blood-borne cancer cells have already invaded distal organs at the time of mastectomy. Another, not necessary non-exclusive, possibility is that tumor cells have spread via lymphatics to the internal mammary, interpectoral, or supraclavicular lymph nodes. Since the removal of these nodes would require surgery, their tumor involvement is not always monitored.

It is clear that direct visualization of nodes for the presence of tumor cells is optimal. However, in view of (a) the lack of accessibility to many lymph nodes, and (b) the trend toward less agressive breast cancer surgery (questioning of whether axillary nodes need to be removed in all cases), a modality of monitoring the presence of tumor in both axillary and other lymph nodes would be advantageous. Thus, a monoclonal antibody or a mixture of monoclonal antibodies to tumor associated antigens, coupled with diagnostic radionuclides such as Iodine ^{131}, Technetium ^{99}m, or Indium ^{111}, could be used for this purpose in lymphoscintigraphy. In this procedure, radiolabeled monoclonal antibody is administered regionally (either subcutaneously or directly into lymphatics) and thus migrates through regional lymphatic nodes. At appropriate intervals, the patients will be scanned with a gamma camera for localization of radionuclide-coupled monoclonal antibody in tumor bearing lymph nodes. To evaluate this method, studies should be conducted on patients prior to mastectomy or lumpectomy, with axillary node resection. The nodes will then be weighed, counted for radioactivity in a gamma counter and sections studied by autoradiography to determine if the radionuclide-MAb conjugate is efficiently localized in the tumor spread.

A major issue in the management of the breast cancer patient is defining the appearance and location of metastatic lesions. Regardless of the nodal status of the patient at the time of mastectomy or lumpectomy, the patient and physician must in reality wait at least 10 years before ruling out metastatic spread. I.v. administration, at regular intervals, of a radionuclide-MAb-conjugate to a breast tumor associated antigen would potentially be useful. At this time, several monoclonal antibodies are being studied for optimal labeling conditions, and for immunoglobulin fragmentation in order to obtain a more rapid blood clearance. But it will most likely take several years to obtain definite results. Parameters to be investigated in the use of each monoclonal antibody include: (a) dose and specific activity of the radiolabeled MAb, (b) affinity of the MAb for the tumor antigen and the stability of the radionuclide monoclonal antibody complex, (c) route of antibody administration, (d) whether intact IgG, Fab'$_2$ or Fab fragments are used, (e) choice of radionuclide varying in energy and half life, (f) metabolism (i.e., clearance) of the radiolabeled MAb or fragment from the blood and/or lymphatics, (g) location of the tumor, i.e., depth within the body, (h) size of the tumor,

(i) degree of vascularity and other histologic properties of
the tumor, (j) the degree of expression of the specific tumor
associated antigen in the tumor mass, (k) the presence or appearance of human anti-murine Ig antibodies and (l) the presence of circulating tumor antigen (Boven and Pinedo, 1986;
Schlom et al., 1984 b). All these parameters are part of a network and must be evaluated as such. Thus, if one choses to use
a monoclonal antibody fragment which will clear from the blood
faster, the MAb dose, specific activity, and choice of radionuclide may have to be altered.

Development of Animal Models for Tumor Localization and Therapy

The first step in testing the efficacy of monoclonal antibodies as radiopharmaceutical agents is the development of an
appropriate animal model. The athymic mouse has been shown to
be an excellent recipient for human tumor xenografts (Rygaard
and Polvsen, 1969). Previous studies have used either cells
grown in culture or tumor pieces introduced subcutaneously
into the athymic mouse and this method has proven useful in
examining the potential of MAbs as radioimmunodetection agents.
However, the utility of this model may be limited for radiothe-
rapeutic studies because of differences between the subcutaneous tumor site in the mouse and metastases in visceral organs
in the human. Therefore, it will be necessary to establish
representative models of metastatic lesions in athymic mice.

In order to examine the use of MAbs as radiopharmaceuti-
cals for tumor localization it is initially necessary to determine what form of the antibody will best serve the specificity
and clearance needs in a given system and then to determine
how best to label that antibody or fragment. The intact immunoglobulin molecule is the easiest to use, but because of its
high molecular weight and potential for binding to F_C receptors, it may not be the ideal radiopharmaceutical. Immunoglobulin fragments may therefore be better agents to use because
elimination of the F_C region through fragmentation eliminates
binding to cellular F_C receptors which can alter antibody
biodistribution. The use of an antibody minus the F_C portion
may also reduce its immunogenicity in patients and thus minimize an immune response. The smaller fragment size also facilitates an antibody clearance from the body resulting in a
lower radiation dose to the patient. Studies were therefore
undertaken to radiolabel immunoglobulin and MAb fragments
reactive with human mammary and colon tumor antigens without
loss of immunoreactivity and to study their ability to localize human tumors grown in athymic mice (Colcher et al., 1983 b,
1984). The antibodies used were B 6.2 and B 72.3 which have
been shown to bind over 50% of human breast carcinoma and over
80% of human colon carcinoma.

Iodination of IgG and fragments

MAb B 6.2 (Colcher et al., 1983 b, Schlom et al., 1984 a,
1984 b) was purified by salt precipitation and ion exchange

chromatography. Purified IgG was then used to generate purified F(ab')$_2$ and Fab' fragments by pepsin digestion followed by molecular sieving; the fragments retained all immunoreactivity when compared on a molar basis to intact IgG. The IgG and fragments were labeled with iodine ^{125} via iodigen technique and examined for reactivity by binding to extracts of human breast cancer metastasis. Indeed they bound to extracts of breast tumor metastasis, but not to extracts of normal human liver, lymphoid cells, or rhabdomyosarcoma. The labeled antibody was shown to bind to the surface of MCF-7 breast cancer cells and was as specific as unlabeled antibody. More than 70% of the antibody remained immunoreactive after labeling. B 6.2 IgG and fragments have also been radiolabeled with isotopes such as iodine ^{123} and iodine ^{131} which have more clinical applications.

Based on the information obtained from the B 6.2 system, radiolabeling and localization studies were undertaken using MAb B 72.3. B 72.3 binds to a tumor associated glycoprotein, TAG-72, exhibiting some properties of a mucin of M_r 10^6 daltons (Johnson et al., 1986). B 72.3 exhibits a high degree of tumor specificity. Labeling studies using the method established for B 6.2 indicated that B 72.3 labeled efficiently under these conditions, but that its immunoreactivity was greatly reduced. It therefore became necessary to examine other techniques for radiolabeling (chloramine-T, lactoperoxidase, Bolton-Hunter). In each case, MAb B 72.3 was efficiently radiolabeled, but again, its immunoreactivity was greatly reduced. The iodogen technique was therefore re-examined and adjustments were made in the three major parameters affecting it: the ratios of immunoglobulin, iodine and iodogen. A final protocol was achieved (40 μg IgG, 0,5mCi Na ^{125}I, 20 μg iodogen) (Colcher et al., 1984), that yielded an iodinated antibody which bound over 80% of its radioactivity to tumor extracts as measured in sequential solid phase radioimmunoassay. The iodinated B 72.3 bound as well to the breast tumor metastasis as the original immunogen while showing no reactivity to a second breast tumor metastasis previously shown to lack TAG-72. No binding was observed to apparently normal liver or to a normal human lymphoid cell line. It was then tested for reactivity with a number of human tumor cell lines to assess its potential as an agent for radioimmunodetection. ^{125}I - B 72.3 exhibits substantial reactivity with a colon tumor (LS-174T) grown in athymic mice, but fails to bind to extracts of the A375 melanoma grown as a xenograft which was previously shown to lack TAG-72.

Tumor distribution studies using B 6.2

Athymic mice were trocared with pieces of Clouser transplantable human mammary tumor and analyzed for the ability of MAb B 6.2 to selectively bind tumor tissue. After approximately 10-20 days, the tumors grew to detectable nodules; the growth rate of these tumors varied as did the final size obtained

(0.5 to 2.5 cm in diameter). Athymic mice were also injected with A 375 human melanoma cells as a control for B 6.2 reactivity.

Athymic mice bearing the Clouser human mammary tumor were given injections of 0.1 µg ^{125}I-labeled B 6.2 IgG. MAb B 6.2, as already mentioned, is known to be reactive with human breast carcinomas (Colcher et al., 1983 b). Ratios of the counts in the tumor to those in various tissues were examined. Tumor to tissue ratios of cpm rose over a four days period and then fell at day seven. At day 4, tumor to tissue ratios were 10/1 or higher in the liver, spleen, and kidney (Chart 1, A to E), and in the brain and muscle greater than 50/1 and as high as 110/1. Lower tumor to tissue ratios were observed in the blood and the lungs. The absolute amount of ^{125}I-labeled IgG found in the tumor ranged from 2 to 15% of the injected dose, depending on tumor size.

When the Clouser mammary tumor-bearing mice were given injections of ^{125}I-F(ab')$_2$ fragments of B 6.2, higher tumor to tissues ratios were obtained. The tumor to tissue ratios in the liver and spleen were 15/1 to 20/1 at 96 hours (Chart 1, F to J). The tumor to tissue ratios were somewhat lower in the blood and lungs, but were still higher than those obtained using intact IgG. This is probably due to the faster clearance of the F(ab')$_2$ fragments over the intact IgG. The tumor to kidney ratios were relatively low and were probably a result of the more rapid fragment clearance. The absolute amount of ^{125}I-F(ab')$_2$ fragments in the tumor ranged from 1 to 12% of the injected dose, depending on tumor size, with a decrease in radioactivity/mg tumor over the 4-days period.

Athymic mice bearing the human melanoma (A375), a tumor without surface reactivity to B 6.2 in live cell RIA, were used as controls for non specific binding of the labeled antibody or fragments to tumor tissue. No preferential localization of the monoclonal antibody was observed in the tumor. In fact, the radioactivity (cpm/mg) in the tumor was lower than that found in many organs, resulting in ratios of less than 1 (Chart 1, A to J). Similarly, no localization was observed when either normal murine IgG or MOPC-21 IgG (the same isotype as B 6.2) from a murine myeloma, or their fragments were inoculated into athymic mice bearing Clouser mammary tumors or melanomas.

Athymic mice bearing Clouser mammary tumors were also given injections of ^{125}I-labeled B 6.2 Fab' (Colcher et al., 1983 b). The clearance rate of the Fab' fragments was considerably faster than that of the larger F(ab')$_2$ fragment or the intact IgG. Acceptable tumor to tissue ratios were obtained, but the fast clearance rate resulted in a large amount of the

---

cpm = counts per minute

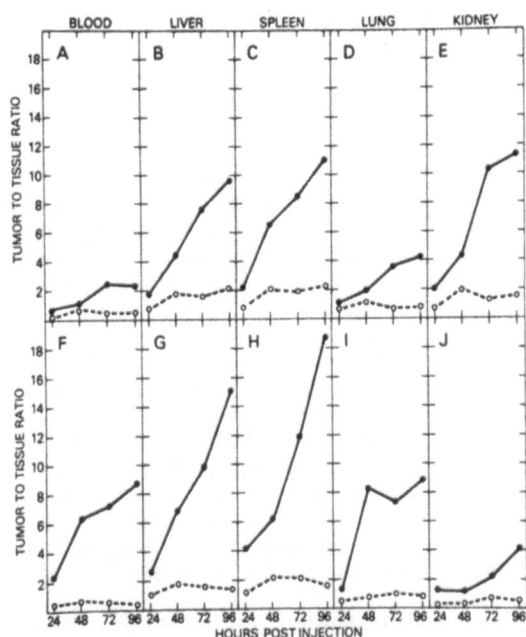

Chart 1. Tissue distribution of ^{125}I-B 6.2 IgG and F(ab')$_2$ in athymic mice bearing human tumor transplants. Athymic mice bearing a transplantable human mammary tumor (Clouser) (●) or a human melanoma (A375) (O) were inoculated with ^{125}I-B 6.2. Approximately 1.5 μCi of IgG (A to E) or F(ab')$_2$ (F to J) were injected i.v. and the mice were sacrificed at daily intervals. The radioactivity per mg of tumor was determined and compared to that of various tissues, the averages of 2 to 20 mice per group are shown.

labeled Fab' being found in the kidney and bladder, resulting in low tumor to kidney ratios. These studies therefore indicate that F(ab')$_2$ fragments were superior to Fab' or intact IgG in the radioimmunolocalization studies with MAb B 6.2. As expected the smaller Fab' fragment cleared more rapidly than the F(ab')$_2$ fragments, which in turn cleared more rapidly than intact IgG in these studies. While the molecular size probably accounts for this behavior, it is also possible that the smaller Fab' fragments are dehalogenated more rapidly, which could also accelerate the clearance of ^{125}I activity from the blood pool. The slow components for the blood clearance of B 6.2 IgG, F(ab')$_2$ and Fab' are 41 hr, 14 hr and 4 hr, respectively. Another way of expressing blood clearance, perhaps more relevant to a potential imaging application, is the calculation of the time when the activity in the blood pool has decreased to 10% of its initial value: this occurs at 69 hr, 32 hr and 4 hr for

^{125}I-labeled B 6.2 IgG, F(ab')$_2$ and Fab', respectively (Colcher
etet al., 1983 b).

Imaging of Xenografts in Athymic Mice with B 6.2

Studies were undertaken to determine whether the localization of the ^{125}I-labeled antibody and fragments in the tumors
was sufficient to be detected with a gamma camera. Athymic mice
bearing the Clouser mammary tumor or the A375 melanoma were
given i.v. injections of approximately 30 μCi of ^{125}I-B 6.2 IgG.
The mice were imaged and then sacrificed at 24 hr intervals.
The Clouser tumors were easily detected at 24 hr using radiolabeled B 6.2 IgG with a small amount of activity detectable in
the blood pool. The tumor remained strongly positive over the
4-day period, with the background activity decreasing to the
point where it was barely detectable at 96 hr (Fig. 5). No tumor localization was observed using radiolabeled B 6.2 IgG in
the mice bearing the control human melanoma transplants of similar size. Mice bearing Clouser mammary tumors or melanomas were
also given injections of normal murine IgG radiolabeled with
^{125}I. The scanning demonstrated no specific localization and
were consistent with the tissue distribution data given above.

Mice were also given injections of ^{125}I-B 6.2 F(ab')$_2$
fragments (Fig. 6). The mice cleared the fragments faster than
the intact IgG and a significant amount of activity was observed in the two kidneys and bladder at 24 hr but tumors were
clearly positive for localization of the ^{125}I-B 6.2 F(ab')$_2$
fragments. The activity was cleared from the kidneys and bladder by 48 hr, and the tumor to background ratio increased over
the 4-day period of scanning, with little background, and good
tumor localization observed at 96 hr. No localization of activity was observed with the radiolabeled B 6.2 F(ab')$_2$ fragments
in the athymic mice bearing the A375 melanoma nor was localization observed using normal murine F(ab')$_2$ in mammary tumor bearing mice. While B 6.2 F(ab')$_2$ fragments appeared to be best
for radioimmunodetection, a smaller percentage of the injected
dose was retained in the tumor as compared to the IgG. Thus,
for therapeutic studies the intact IgG may be better because it
will deliver a greater dose to the tumor.

Tumor Distribution Studies with B 72.3

Radiolocalization studies were also performed with B 72.3
using athymic mice bearing human colon carcinomas (LS-174T) in
comparison with a human melanoma xenograft (A375) as an antigen negative control for nonspecific uptake of immunoglobulin
(Colcher et al., 1984). Athymic mice were given s.c. injections
of 4 x 10^5 cells. Tumor growth was rapid with a doubling time
of approximately 2 to 3 days for the LS-174T cells. After 7 to
10 days when the tumors were approximately 0.3 to 0.5 cm in
diameter, the mice were given i.v. injections of approximately
1.5 μCi of ^{125}I-B 72.3 IgG or ^{125}I-MOPC-21 IgG (control antibody of the same isotype). The ratio of cpm radioactivity per mg

of tissue in the LS-174T tumor in comparison with that of various tissues was examined over a 7-day period. The tumor to tissue ratio rose over this period with tumor to liver, tumor to spleen or tumor to kidney ratios of approximately 18:1 at Day 7. Tumor to blood ratios also rose during this time, resulting in ratios of 5:1 at Day 7. There was no specific uptake of ^{125}I-B 72.3 IgG in any of the normal organs examined (Chart 2). Approximately 10% of the injected dose per g reached the tumor at Day 2 after injection of the radiolabeled antibody.

A major difference between the B 6.2 system and the B 72.3 system is that the amount of the B 72.3 radiolabel at the tumor stayed constant over a longer period of time. Then, the activity on a per g basis began to drop as the tumor progressed in size. The increased tumor to tissue ratios result primarily from the clearance of labeled IgG from the blood pool.

The absolute amount of radioactivity in the tumor rose over the first 2 days and then remained constant through Day 7.

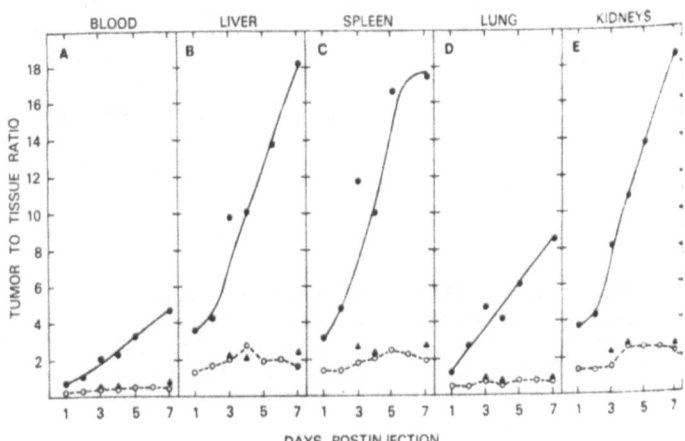

Chart 2. Tissue distribution of ^{125}I-B 72.3 IGg in athymic mice bearing human tumors. Athymic mice bearing LS-174T colon carcinomas (●) or A375 melanomas (O) were inoculated with approximately 1.5 μCi of ^{125}I-B 72.3 IgG. The mice were sacrificed over a 7-day period and radioactivity per mg of tissue was determined. The ratio of the activity in the tumor as compared to other organs was plotted. Mice bearing LS-174T colon carcinomas were also given injections of the control antibody MOPC-21. (▲).

Athymic mice bearing melanomas (A375, a melanoma tumor line that shows no reactivity with B 72.3 in live cell RIAs) were used as controls. No specific uptake of ^{125}I-B 72.3 was observed in the tumors of these control animals (Chart 2). Similarly no localization was observed in athymic mice bearing the colon carcinoma cell line when using ^{125}I-MOPC-21 IgG as a control antibody (Chart 2).

Imaging of Athymic Mice Bearing Human Tumors

Studies were then undertaken to determine whether localization of the ^{125}I-labeled B 72.3 was sufficient to be detected by gamma scanning. Athymic mice bearing colon carcinomas or melanomas were given injections of approximately 70 μCi (approximately 5 μg) of ^{125}I-B 72.3 IgG; the higher dose was necessary to minimize imaging time. The mice bearing the human colon carcinomas demonstrated significant uptake at early time points with most of the activity in the area of the tumor. The remaining activity in the mice was detected primarily in the area of the heart and lungs. No significant activity was seen in the liver, kidneys, bladder or stomach. The lack of activity in these organs indicates that there is no significant breakdown of the radiolabeled antibody, nor is there a large amount of iodine due to the deiodination of the antibody. At 48 hr, the activity was still seen primarily in the tumor, with the activity in the area of the heart and lungs significantly decreased. A similar pattern was seen at 72 hr with a continuing decrease in the activity in the vital organs. The proportion of the activity found in the tumor continued to increase (Keenan et al., 1984). Several mice bearing the control tumor, the A375 melanoma transplanted at the same site as the LS-174T tumors, were imaged at similar times. No significant activity of the ^{125}I-B 72.3 was detected in the area of the melanomas. The activity was primarily seen in the area of the heart and lungs (Fig. 7).

Therapy

Tumor therapy using MAbs can theoretically be mediated via (a) effector cell mechanisms, (b) complement, (c) conjugation with toxins or drugs and (d) conjugation with radionuclides (Boven and Pinedo, 1986, Schlom et al., 1984 b). There are two major reasons why the radionuclide-conjugate approach should be pursued. The first is the large antigenic heterogeneity that has been observed in most tumors using numerous monoclonal antibodies. When concerning drug conjugate or effector cell mediated mechanisms, the monoclonal antibody must bind to all cells of the tumor for efficient killing. Thus, tumor cells not expressing cell surface tumor antigen would be unaffected. Since killer isotopes (alpha or beta emitters) can kill several (up to 5 or more) cell diameters, the monoclonal antibody-radionuclide conjugate need not bind every tumor cell to kill the entire cell population. Secondly, many carcinoma associated antigens have been shown to be stable components of the cell membrane (Kufe et al., 1983 a); thus, monoclonal antibody-carcinoma antigen complexes on the cell surface have been shown not to internalize as do many monoclonal antibody-lymphocyte antigen cell surface complexes. Since monoclonal antibody-drug conjugates must internalize to mediate cell killing, they may be ineffectual in these cases. Radionuclide-monoclonal antibody complexes, however need not internalize for cell killing. Studies using therapeutic doses of radionuclide conjugated monoclonal antibody B 72.3 in the athymic mouse model have been initiated recently, but it is still too early to evaluate the results (Boven and Pinedo, 1986).

CONCLUSIONS

The diagnostic potential of monoclonal antibodies, especially MAb B 72.3 is shown by selective recognition of adenocarcinoma over most other cancers and reactive mesothelium in effusions, as well as efficiency for the detection, staging and management of human breast cancer. Furthermore, due to its in vivo characteristics, MAb B 72.3 is a potential therapeutic agent in the treatment of breast cancer. The future directions will involve the use of biologic response modifiers, such as recombinant interferon (Greiner et al., 1984), use of fragments, use of "Killer" isotopes, cocktails of MAbs, and production of genetically engineered human MAbs. Finally, monoclonal antibodies should permit a better understanding of some of the mechanisms underlying tumor cell initiation and progression (Schlom et al., 1984 a and 1984 b). Thus, MAbs research involving human carcinomas is proceeding in two directions simultaneously: one toward the mechanisms of oncogenesis and basic tumor cell biology, and the other toward more immediate clinical applications.

REFERENCES

1. Arklie, J., Taylor-Papadimitriou, J., Bodmer, W., Egan, M., and Millis, R., Differentiation antigens expressed by epithelial cells in the lactating breast are also detectable in breast cancers. Int. J. Cancer. 28: 23-29, 1982.

2. Boven, E. and Pinedo, H.M., Monoclonal antibodies in cancer treatment: where do we stand after 10 years? Radiother. Oncol. 5: 109-117, 1986.

3. Colcher, D., Horan-Hand, P., Nuti, M. and Schlom, J. A spectrum of monoclonal antibodies reactive with human mammary tumor cells. Proc. Natl. Acad. Sci. U.S.A., 78: 3199-3203, 1981.

4. Colcher, D., Horan-Hand, P., Nuti, M. and Schlom, J. Differential binding to human mammary and nonmammary tumors of monoclonal antibody reactive with carcinoembryonic antigen. Cancer investig., 1: 127-138, 1983 a.

5. Colcher, D., Zalutsky, M., Kaplan, W., Austin, F. and Schlom, J. Radiolocalization of human mammary tumors in athymic mice by a monoclonal antibody. Cancer Res., 43: 736-742, 1983 b.

6. Colcher, D., Keenan, A., Larson, S. and Schlom, J.; Prolonged binding of a radiolabeled monoclonal antibody (B 72.3) used for the in situ radioimmunodetection of human colon cancer xenografts. Cancer Res., 44: 5744-5751, 1984.

7. Epenetos, A.A., Britton, K.E., Mather, J., Shepherd, J., Granowska, M., Taylor-Papadimitriou, J., Nimnon, C.C., Durbin, H., Hawkins, L.R., Malpas, J.S. and Bodmer, W.F., Targeting of iodine-123-labelled tumor associated monoclonal antibodies to ovarian, breast and gastrointestinal tumours. Lancet, 2: 1000-1004, 1982 a.

8. Epenetos, A.A., Canti, G., Taylor-Papadimitriou, J., Curling, M. and Bodmer, W. Use of two epithelium specific monoclonal antibodies for diagnosis of malignancies in serous effusions. Lancet, 2: 1004-1006, 1982 b.

9. Foster, C.S., Dinsdale, E.A., Edwards, P.A.W. and Neville, A.M., Monoclonal antibodies to the human mammary gland, II, Distribution of determinants in breast carcinomas. Virchows Arch. (Path. Anat.), 394: 295-305, 1982.

10. Greiner, J.W., Horan-Hand, P., Noguchi, P., Fisher, P.B., Petska, S. and Schlom, J., Enhanced expression of surface tumor-associated antigens on human breast and colon tumor cells after recombinant leukocyte alpha-interferon treatment. Cancer Res., 44: 3208-3214, 1984.

11. Hand, P., Nuti, M., Colcher, D. and Schlom, J. Definition of antigenic heterogeneity and modulation among human mammary carcinoma cell populations using monoclonal antibodies to tumor-associated antigens. Cancer Res. 43: 728-735, 1983.

12. Haber, E., Antibodies of restricted heterogeneity for structural study, Fed. Proc., 29: 66-71, 1970.

13. Hayes, D.F., Sekine, H., Ohno, T., Abe, M., Keese, K. and Kufe, D.W. Use of a murine monoclonal antibody for detection of circulating plasma DF3 antigen levels in breast cancer patients. J. Clin. Invest., 75: 1671-1678, 1985.

14. Johnson, V., Schlom, J., Paterson, A.J., Bennett, J., Magnani, J. and Colcher, D., Analysis of a human tumor-associated glycoprotein (TAG-72) identified by monoclonal antibody B72.3. Cancer Res., 45: 850-857, 1986.

15. Johnston, W.W., Szpak, C.A., Lottich, S.A., Thor, A. and Schlom, J. Use of a monoclonal antibody (B72.3) as an immunocytochemical adjunct to diagnosis of adenocarcinoma in human effusions. Cancer Res., 45: 1894-1900, 1985.

16. Keenan, A.M., Colcher, D., Larson, S.M. and Schlom, J. Radioimmunoscintigraphy of human colon cancer xenografts in mice with radioiodinated monoclonal antibody B72.3. J. Nucl. Med. 25: 1197-1203, 1984.

17. Kohler, M. and Milstein, C., Continuous cultures of fused cells secreting antibody of predefined specifity. Nature, 256: 495-497, 1975.

18. Kohler, M., Howe, S.C. and Milstein, C., Fusion between immunoglobulin-secreting and nonsecreting myeloma cell lines Eur. J. Immunol., 6: 292-295, 1976.

19. Krause, R.M., The search for antibodies with molecular uniformity. Adv. Immunol., 12: 1-56, 1970.

20. Kufe, D.W., Nadler, L. and Sargent, L., Biological behavior of human breast carcinoma-associated antigens expressed during cellular proliferation. Cancer Res., 43: 851-857, 1983.

21. Kufe, D., Inghirami, G., Abe, M., Hayes, D., Justi-Wheeler, H. and Schlom, J., Differential reactivity of a novel monoclonal antibody (DF3) with human malignant versus benign breast tumors. Hybridoma, 3: 223-232, 1984.

22. Lundy, J., Thor, A., Maenza, R., Schlom, J., Forouhar, F., Testa, M. and Kufe, D., Monoclonal antibody DF3 correlates with tumor differentiation and hormone receptor status in breast cancer patients. Breast Cancer Res. Treat., 5: 269-276, 1985.

23. Menard, S., Tagliabue, E., Canevari, S., Fossati, G. and Colnaghi, M.I. Generation of monoclonal antibodies reacting with normal and cancer cells of human breast. Cancer Res., 43: 1295-1300, 1983.

24. Nuti, M., Teramoto, Y.A., Mariani-Constantini, R., Horan-Hand, P., Colcher, D. and Schlom, J., A monoclonal antibody (B 72.3) defines patterns of distribution of a novel tumor associated antigen in human mammary carcinoma cell population. Int. J. Cancer, 29: 539-545, 1982.

25. Pressmann, D. and Korngold, L., The in vivo localization of anti-Wagner-osteogenic-sarcoma antibodies. Cancer, 6: 619-623, 1953.

26. Rasmussen, B.B., Hilkens, J., Hilgers, J., Nielsen, H.H., Thorpe, S.M. and Rose, C., Monoclonal antibodies applied to human breast carcinoma: relationship to menopausal status, lymph node status and steroid hormone receptor content. Breast Cancer Res. Treat. 2: 401-405, 1982.

27. Rygaard, T. and Polvsen, C.O., Heterotransplantation of a human malignant tumor in nude mice. Acta Pathol. Microbiol. Scand., 77: 758-760, 1969.

28. Schlom, J., Greiner, J., Horan-Hand, P., Colcher, D., Inghirami, G., Weeks, M., Pestka, S., Fisher, P.B., Noguchi, P. and Kufe, D., Monoclonal antibodies to breast cancer-associated antigens as potential reagents in the management of breast cancer. Cancer, 54: 2777-2794, 1984 a.

29. Schlom, J. and Weeks, M.O.: Potential clinical utility of monoclonal antibodies in the management of human carcinomas. In: Important advances in oncology, V. De Vita, S. Hellman and S. Rosenberg, eds, J.B. Lippincott Co., Philadelphia, P.A., vol. 1, 1984 b, p.p. 170-192.

30. Sloane, J.P. and Omerod, M.J., Distribution of epithelial membrane antigen in normal and neoplastic tissues and its value in diagnostic tumor pathology. Cancer, 47: 1786-1795, 1981.

31. Taylor-Papadimitriou, J., Peterson, J.A., Arklie, J., Burchell, J., Ceriani, R.L. and Bodmer, W.F., Monoclonal antibodies to epithelium-specific components of the human milk fat globule membrane; Production and reaction with cells in culture. Int. J. Cancer, 28: 17-21, 1981.

ESTROGEN RECEPTORS IN BENIGN AND MALIGNANT BREAST DISEASES

PINOTTI, J.A.[1], PISANI, R.C.B. de [1], TEIXEIRA, L.C.[1], and BASTOS, S.[2].

1. Department of Obstetrics and Gynecology, School of Medical Sciences. State University of Campinas, 13.100 Campinas, Brazil.
2. Center of Gynecological Cancer Control, State University of Campinas.

INTRODUCTION

Nearly twenty years ago, JENSEN et al. (1967), using radioactive substances, detected a greater hormone concentration in target organs than in other tissues and began to isolate hormone receptor proteins. They probably did not realize the impact of these findings upon the prognosis and the treatment of breast cancer. The knowledge of hormonal receptors, particularly estrogen receptors, is of obvious importance in the choice of adjuvant treatment and for appropriate therapeutic decisions in cases of breast cancer metastases and local recurrence.

The role of hormonal receptors in the prognosis of breast cancer has been the focus of several controversial publications (Williams et al., 1985; Campbell et al., 1981). Today, the widespread belief that estrogen-receptor-negative tumors have a worse prognosis must be revised and rediscussed (Blamey et al., 1980).

The role of estrogen receptors in benign breast diseases and in non-cancerous contralateral breasts is another problem that is not yet well understood.

The present study is based on a number of reports concerning hormonal receptors in benign breast diseases, breast cancers and contralateral breasts. The findings were collected between 1977 and 1984 at the Department of Gynecology and Obstetrics of the School of Medical Sciences, State University of Campinas, and at the Clinic of Prof. J.A. Pinotti (CLAP).

MATERIALS AND METHOD

Between 1977 and 1984, estrogen receptors were determined in 288 cases of benign breast disease, 180 biopsies from contralateral breasts and 501 cases of breast cancer.

POSITIVE ESTROGEN RECEPTORS IN BENIGN BREAST DISEASES

Histologic lesions	Predominant lesions	Accompanying lesions
FIBROADENOMA	35/100 (35%)	
CYSTIC DISEASE	5/20 (25%)	
INFLAMMATORY PROCESS	2/9 (22%)	
DUCTAL ECTASIA	1/8 (12.5%)	
DYSPLASTIC LESIONS:	38/138 (28%)	
Microcystic disease	14/61 (23%)	6/8 (75%)
Macrocystic disease	4/8 (50%)	
Focal fibrosis	10/22 (45%)	5/40 (12.5%)
Diffuse fibrosis	3/18 (17%)	
Apocrine metaplasia	2/7 (29%)	7/32 (22%)
Sclerosing adenosis	2/7	7/25 (28%)
Typical ductal hyperplasia	2/3	10/29 (35%)
Atypical ductal hyperplasia	1/2	
TOTAL	86/288 (30%)	35/134 (26%)

TABLE 1

Estrogen receptor assays were carried out using a dextran-coated charcoal (DCC) technique based on the measurement of the capacity of cytosol to bind tritiated estradiol. The results were expressed as femtomoles (fm) per mg of cytosol protein.

The excised tissues were separated from normal tissue components and either rapidly frozen in liquid nitrogen or assayed immediately. The tissue samples were homogenized in a buffer and the homogenates centrifuged at 50,000 g for 30 min. at 4° C to obtain the cytosol fraction. The protein concentration in the cytosol was first estimated by a spectrophotometric absorption technique (Layne 1957) and later quantified by the method of Lowry et al., (1951). The estimated protein value served to indicate the appropriate dilution for each cytosol (1-2 mg/ml) for the DDC saturation method. The cytosol was then incubated at 4° C with increasing quantites of tritiated estradiol (Amersham, England), for I8 hours. At the same time, in a further set of cytosol samples, a 200-fold excess of estradiol was added prior to the incubation of tritiated estradiol in order to determine non-specific binding.

The binding data were analyzed by the method of Scatchard (Scatchard, 1949; Chamness and McGuire, 1975) and samples with concentrations greater than 5 fm of E/mg of cytosol protein were considered estrogen receptor positive.

RESULTS

Benign breast disease

The distribution of hormone receptors in different types of benign breast diseases is shown in Table 1. Fibroadenomas presented a higher incidence rate of positive estrogen receptors (35%) than dysplasia (28%) or cystic disease (25%), but without significant statistical difference between the first two pathological conditions ($x_1^2 = 1.519$, $0.2 < p < 0.3$). Among dysplastic lesions, i.e., micro or macrocystic disease, diffuse or focal fibrosis, apocrine metaplasia, sclerosing adenosis and ductal hyperplasia, there was no significant difference in the ER content ($X_4^2 = 5.3236$, $0.2 < p < 0.3$). Ductal hyperplasias, however, yielded a higher incidence rate of ER+ tissues (35%) than other dysplasias when they were non-predominant, accompanying lesions (statistically significant difference, $X_4^2 = 13.4810$, $0.001 < p < 0.1$).

These observations suggest a possible relationship between epithelial cellularity and the amount of ER protein (Rosen et al., 1975; May-Levin et al., 1977; Allegra et al., 1979; Martin et al., 1978), a correlation that might be expected since estrogen-receptors are situated in epithelial and not in stroma cells. This hypothesis correlates also with the higher ER content of neoplastic tissues, which have greater cellularity than

PLASMA LEVELS OF ESTRADIOL IN PATIENTS WITH MAMMARY DYSPLASIA
BEFORE, DURING AND AFTER TREATMENT WITH TAMOXIFEN

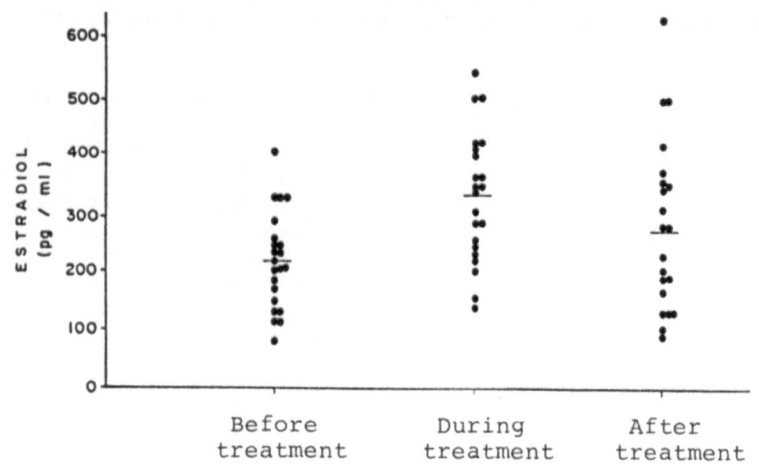

FIGURE 1

PLASMA LEVELS OF LH IN PATIENTS WITH MAMMARY DYSPLASIA
BEFORE, DURING AND AFTER TREATMENT WITH TAMOXIFEN

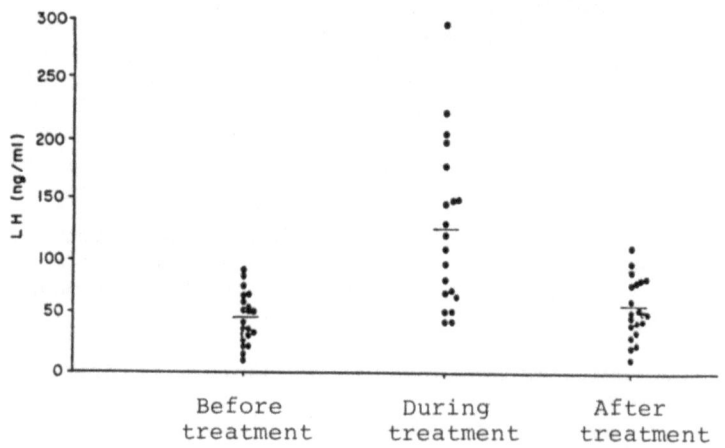

FIGURE 2

benign breast lesions (Hahnell et al., 1971; Hahnell and Twaddle, 1973).

Although our data are in agreement with those in the literature (Hahnell et al., 1971; Hahnell and Twaddle, 1973; Rosen et al., 1975; May-Levin et al., 1977), we must point out that the DCC technique assays only estrogen-free receptors and that in a young population in which the receptors are partially occupied by endogeneous hormone, false negative readings may occur. In these young women, however, the mammary epithelium is abundant, possibly explaining why there is good symptomatic response to hormonal treatment with tamoxifen in spite of the low incidence rate of ER-positive samples (Pinotti et al., 1979).

Tamoxifen, furthermore, blocks estrogenic action but induces submaximal increases in progesterone receptor levels (Katzenellenbogen et al., 1984; Martin et al., 1979 a and b; Mortel et al., 1981). This means that, besides its antiestrogenic effect, tamoxifen may increase, at least initially, the endogeneous action of progesterone at the level of mammary cells and increase plasma levels of LH/FSH and estradiol (Pinheiro, 1985), (Fig. 1 and 2).

The age distribution of patients with dysplasia showed a slight and gradual decrease in the incidence of estrogen-receptor-positive tissues up to the age of 50 and an increase just after this age, reflecting the interaction of hormonal status and changes in tumor cellularity in aging women (Table 2). In patients with fibroadenomas, a sharper decrease in the incidence of ER positiveness was observed with the increase in age (Table 3). The decrease in the incidence of ER+ tissues occurs as a result of fibrosis in the course of the disease (Allegra et al., 1979; Martin et al., 1978, 1979 a).

There is growing evidence in the literature that an imbalance between estrogen and progesterone exists in favour of estrogen (Mauvais-Jarvis et al., 1977; Melis et al., 1982). Other factors such as proteases, e.g., plasminogen activators, are involved in the permanent remodelling process of the breast and these enzymes are apparently under hormonal control (Ossowski et al., 1979; Mira-y-Lopez et al., 1983). Thus, we are currently investigating the presence of plasminogen activators in cytosols, since the increase in this enzyme has also been associated with malignant transformation (Christman et al., 1975).

Contralateral breast

The contralateral breast deserves special attention in the follow-up of mastectomy patients since the second breast is subjected to essentially the same hormonal and etiological influences as the tumourous breast.

ER STATUS IN DYSPLASIAS ACCORDING TO AGE

AGE	ER +	ER -	TOTAL
20	1	1	2
21 - 30	7(33%)	14(67%)	21
31 - 40	13(29%)	32(71%)	45
41 - 50	12(26%)	34(74%)	46
51 - 60	4(31%)	9(69%)	13
61	0	5	5
TOTAL	37(28%)	95(72%)	132

TABLE 2

ER STATUS IN FIBROADENOMAS ACCORDING TO AGE

AGE	ER +	ER -	TOTAL
20	6(67%)	3(33%)	9
21 - 30	15(35%)	28(65%)	43
31 - 40	11(37%)	19(63%)	30
41 - 50	3(23%)	10(77%)	13
51	2(14%)	12(86%)	14
TOTAL	37(37%)	72(73%)	99

TABLE 3

ER STATUS IN CONTRALATERAL BREAST LESIONS

Histologic type	Predominant lesions		Accompanying lesions	
	ER +	ER −	ER +	ER −
Cystic disease	10 (27%)	27 (73%)		
Fibrosis	8 (22%)	29 (78%)		
Apocrine metaplasia	0	22 (100%)	5 (19%)	22 (81%)
Sclerosing adenosis	5 (28%)	13 (72%)	6 (22%)	22 (78%)
Typical ductal hyperplasia	1 (8%)	11 (92%)	28 (40%)	41 (60%)
Microcystic disease	3 (16%)	16 (84%)		
Typical lobular hyperplasia			2 (7%)	27 (93%)
Others	6 (16%)	31 (84%)	5 (9%)	51 (91%)
Total	33 (18%)	149 (82%)	47 (22%)	163 (78%)

TABLE 4

Over a 3-year period, we studied 180 biopsies from contralateral breasts and analyzed the predominant and the accompanying non-predominant histologic lesions encountered. The most frequent predominant lesions found in contralateral breasts were cystic disease and fibrosis. Most of the predominant lesions, in particular apocrine metaplasia (100%) and typical ductal hyperplasia (92%), were ER negative (82% negative versus 18% positive). There was a high incidence of ductal hyperplasia as an accompanying lesion (69/210 = 33%). The incidence of ER positiveness was significantly higher (40%) in this instance than when ductal hyperplasia existed as a predominant lesion (8%) (Table 4).

Whereas the incidence rate of estrogen-receptor-positive breast cancer tissues rose from premenopause (41%) to postmenopause (69%), hormonal status had no influence on benign lesions of the contralateral breast (15.5% ER+ in premenopause versus 17% in postmenopause (Table 5). An inverse relationship, however, was observed between ER-positive findings in the contralateral breast and the stage of the tumor in the involved

POSITIVE ESTROGEN RECEPTORS ACCORDING TO HORMONAL STATUS IN
CANCEROUS AND CONTRALATERAL BREASTS

	Cancerous Breast	Contralateral Breast	Number of cases
Premenopause	40 (41%)	15 (15.5%)	97
Perimenopause	7 (39%)	5 (28%)	18
Postmenopause	44 (69%)	11 (17%)	64
TOTAL	91 (51%)	31 (17%)	179

TABLE 5

POSITIVE ESTROGEN RECEPTORS IN CONTRALATERAL BREAST
ACCORDING TO TUMOR STAGE

Histology of the lesions in the contralateral breast	Tumor stage of the cancerous breast		
	I	II	III
Cystic disease	1/4	8/18	1/15
Microcystic disease	1/6	1/6	1/7
Apocrine metaplasia	0/2	0/14	0/6
Sclerosing adenosis	1/3	2/10	2/4
Ductal hyperplasia	1/1	0/5	0/6
Others	5/10	3/25	5/26
TOTAL	9/31 (29%)	14/78 (18%)	9/64 (14%)

TABLE 6

breast (29% ER-positive lesions in the contralateral breast in stage I carcinoma versus 14% ER+ in stage III carcinoma (Table 6).

Breast cancer

The determination of hormonal receptors is a very useful procedure for the choice of adjuvant treatments and for the therapeutic approach to recurrence and metastases. But there are some discrepancies and controversies concerning the prognostic value of these determinations.

In our study of 501 breast cancers, 218 were ER positive (43.5%) and 283 ER negative (56.8%) (Table 7). The percentage of positive cases was lower than the average reported in the literature (Blamey et al., 1980; Williams et al., 1985). This may be due to the fact that breast cancer in Latin America is often diagnosed late, when the disease is already in an advanced stage with a poor histologic grade. Under these circumstances, it is known the incidence of ER+ tumor is low. It may also be due to the presence of proteases such as plasminogen activators which may cleave receptors "in vitro" during the assay (Sherman et al., 1980; Thorsen, 1982). In our study, however, the distribution of ER-negative or positive tumors was not statistically related to the tumor stage.

An increase in the incidence of ER-positive tumors was observed from pre- (38%) to postmenopause (51%). Since the method used in this study assays only free receptors, this increase may be expected and explained by the fact that premenopausal patients have a great amount of endogenous estrogen

ER STATUS IN 501 BREAST CANCERS

	Total	Number of patients		
		Pre-menopause	Peri-menopause	Post-menopause
ER + fmol/mg (average)	218 (43.5%)	104 (38%) 123.6	14 (41%) 204.87	100 (51%) 175.46
ER -	283 (56.5%)	168 (62%)	20 (59%)	95 (49%)
TOTAL	501	272	34	195

TABLE 7

ER STATUS AND RECURRENCE ACCORDING TO THE CLINICAL STAGE

Stage	Number of Cases	Number of Recurrence	ER +	ER -	T	P value
I	77	4	1/29 (3%)	3/48 (6%)	0.51	0.56
II	228	42	15/99 (15%)	27/129 (24%)	1.29	0.20
IIIa	102	51	21/48 (44%)	30/54 (56%)	1.18	0.24
IIIb	24	14	5/13 (38%)	9/11 (82%)	2.14	0.04 *
Total	431	111	42/189 (22%)	69/242 (29%)	1.4	0.16

* Statiscally significant

TABLE 8

ER STATUS AND TYPE OF RECURRENCE

		ER +	ER −	Total
	Number of cases	189	242	431
RECURRENCE	Local	6 (3%)	15 (6%)	21
	Regional	4 (2%)	6 (2%)	10
	Distant	32 (17%)	48 (20%)	80
	Total	42 (22%)	69 (29%)	111 (26%)

TABLE 9

blocking the free receptors, whereas the opposite occurs in postmenopausal patients (Table 7).

Recurrences occurred in 111 of 431 patients (Tables 8 and 9) and were more frequent, both locally or systemically, in all clinical stages when tumors were ER negative. The disease-free interval and the survival, with or without disease, were slightly better in ER positive cases (Table 10), as has been observed by other authors (Williams et al., 1985).

Comparing patients who received post-surgical adjuvant treatment with those who did not, it was found that recurrences were more frequent in N+ / ER− cases than in N+ / ER+ cases but there was no significant difference in N0 cases, irrespective of whether the tumors were ER positive or negative (Table 11). This fact is of great clinical importance since some trials have shown fewer recurrences in N+ patients treated by chemotherapy than in untreated N0 patients, supporting the hypothesis that adjuvant chemotherapy is useful in N0 cases, particularly when the tissues are ER negative. This is further supported by the general acceptance that ER-negative tumors have a worse prognosis. Our results, however, demonstrating that the rate of recurrence is the same in N0 cases, regardless of whether ER negative or positive, disagree with this opinion and indicate that the selection of patients for adjuvant therapy must be carefully discussed.

In inflammatory breast carcinomas, there was a higher incidence of ER negative (57%) than ER positive tumors (49%) and the course of the disease in ER negative cases was more aggressive, with regional extensions and distant metastases. At the same time, the survival rate was better in estrogen-receptor positive cases (62%) than in receptor-negative cases (50%) (Table 12).

ER STATUS IN BREAST CANCER AND EVOLUTION OF THE DISEASE

ER	Number	alive without disease	alive with disease	dead from tumor	dead free of disease
Positive	218	158 (73%)	20 (9%)	37 (17%)	3 (1%)
Negative	283	194 (69%)	22 (8%)	62 (22%)	3 (1%)
Total	501	352 (70%)	42 (9%)	99 (20%)	6 (1%)

TABLE 10

RECURRENCE OF BREAST CANCER ACCORDING
TO ER STATUS, NODAL STATUS AND POSTSURGICAL ADJUVANT TREATMENT

	N + with postsurgical treatment	N 0 without postsurgical treatment
ER +	44/142 (31%)	5/55 (9%)
ER −	63/148 (43%)	12/102 (11%)
	T = 2.04 P. value = 0.04	T = 0.417 P. value = 0.68

TABLE 11

ER STATUS IN 49 INFLAMMATORY BREAST CANCERS

Extension of the disease	Number of cases	ER +				ER -			
		Total	Alive without disease	Alive with disease	Dead	Total	Alive without disease	Alive with disease	Dead
Local	10	6 (60%)	3	1	2	4 (40%)	2	1	1
Regional	34	15 (44%)	7	2	6	19 (56%)	7	2	10
Distant	4	0	0	0	0	4 (100%)	0	2	2
	48	21 (43%)	13/21 (62%)			27 (57%)	14/28 (50%)		

TABLE 12

This may be explained by the fact that cases with ER negative tumors are more severe, evolve more quickly from the outset, and, in addition, are frequently diagnosed late. Moreover, as previously stated, estrogen receptors disappear with the progression of the tumor by rupture of the receptor protein due to the increase in plasminogen activity.

REFERENCES

1. Allegra, J.C., Lippman, M.E., Green, L., Barlock, A., Simon, R., Thompson, E.B., Huff, K.K. and Griffin, W. Estrogen receptor values in patients with benign breast disease. Cancer, 44: 228-231, 1979.

2. Blamey, R.W., Bishop, H.M., Blake, J.R.S., Doyle, P.J., Elston, C.W., Haybittle, J.L. and Nicholson, R.I. Relationship between primary breast tumor receptor status and patient survival. Cancer, 46: 2765-2769, 1980.

3. Campbell, F.C., Blamey, R.W., Elston, C.W., Nicholson, R.J., Griffiths, K. and Haybittle, J.L. Estrogen receptor status and sites of metastasis in breast cancer. Br. J. Cancer, 44: 456-459, 1981.

4. Chamness, G.C. and McGuire, W.L. Scatchard plots: common errors in correction and interpretation. Steroids, 26: 538-542, 1975.

5. Christman, J.K., Silagi, S., Newcomb, E.W., Silverstein, S.C. and Acs, G. Correlated suppression by 5-bromodeoxyuridine of tumorigenicity and plasminogen activator in mouse melanoma cells. Proc. Natl.Acad. Sci.(USA), 72: 47-50, 1975.

6. Hahnell, R., Twaddle, E. and Vivian, A.B. Estrogen receptors in human breast cancer. II."In vitro" binding of estradiol by benign and malignant tumors. Steroids, 18: 681-708, 1971.

7. Hahnell, R. and Twaddle, E. Estimation of association constant of the estrogen receptor complex in human breast cancer. Cancer Res., 33: 559-566, 1973.

8. Jensen, E.V., DeSombre, E.R. and Jungblut, P.N. Estrogen receptors in hormone-responsive tissues and tumors. In: Endogeneous factors influencing host-tumor balance. R.W. Wissler, T.T. Dao and S. Wood Jr, eds, Univ. of Chicago, Press, 1967, p.p. 15-30.

9. Katzenellenbogen, B.S., Norman, M.J., Eckert, R.L., Peltz, S.W. and Mangel, W.F. Bioactivities, estrogen receptors interactions and plasminogen activator-inducing activities of tamoxifen and hydroxy-tamoxifen isomers in MCF-7 human breast cancer cells. Cancer Res., 44: 112-119, 1984.

10. Layne, E. Spectrophotometric and turbidimetric methods for measuring proteins. In: Methods in Enzymology, vol. 3, S.P. Colowick and N.O. Kaplan, eds, Academic Press, New York, 1957, p.p. 447-454.

11. Lowry, O.H.,.Rosenbrouch, N.J., Farr, A.L. and Randall, R.J. Protein measurement with the Folin phenolreagent. J. Biol. Chem., 193: 265-275, 1951.

12. Martin, P.M., Kuttenn, F., Serment, H. and Mauvais-Jarvis, P. Studies on clinical, hormonal and pathological correlations in breast fibroadenomas. J. Steroid Biochem., 9: 1251-1255, 1978.

13. Martin, P.M., Kuttenn, F., Serment, H. and Mauvais-Jarvis, P. Progesterone receptors in breast fibroadenomas. J. Steroid Biochem., 11: 1295-1298, 1979 a.

14. Martin, P.M., Rolland, P.H., Gammerre, M., Serment, H. and Toga, M. Estradiol and progesterone receptors in normal and neoplastic endometrium. Correlations between receptors, histopathological examinations and clinical responses under progestin therapy. Int. J. Cancer, 23: 321-329, 1979 b.

15. Mauvais-Jarvis, Kuttenn, F., Mowszowicz, I. and Sitrukware, R. Mastopathies bénignes: étude hormonale chez 125 malades. La Nouvelle Presse Médicale, 6: 4115-4118, 1977.

16. May-Levin, F., Contesso, G., Guerinot, F., Delarue, P. and Bohuon, C. Récepteurs des estrogènes et de la progestérone dans les affections non carcinomateuses du sein. Pathologie Biologie, 25: 233-239, 1977.

17. Melis, G.B., Guarnieri, G., Paoletti, A.M., Capelli, N., Selli, M., Petacchi, F.D., Ruju, A. and Fioretti, P. Caratteristiche endocrine delle donne con mastopatia fibrocistica. Minerva Ginecologica, 34: 897-901, 1982.

18. Mira-y-Lopez, R., Reich, E. and Ossowski, L. Modulation of plasminogen activator in rodent mammary tumors by hormones and other effectors. Cancer Res., 43: 5467-5477, 1983.

19. Mortel, R., Levy, C., Wolff, J.P., Nicolas, J.C., Robel, P. and Baulieu, E.E. Female sex steroid receptors in postmenopausal endometrial carcinoma and biochemical response to an antiestrogen. Cancer Research, 41: 1140-1147, 1981.

20. Ossowski, L., Biegel, D. and Reich, E. Mammary plasminogen activator. Correlation with involution, hormonal modulation and comparison between normal and neoplastic tissue. Cell, 16: 929-940, 1979.

172

21. Pinotti, J.A., Tolosa, H.A. de, and Sivini, F. Emprego experimental de um antiestrogênico no tratamento de casos de displasia mamária rebelde e outros processos terapêuticos - resultados preliminares. J. Bras. Gin., 87: 57-59, 1979.

22. Pinheiro, L.S. Perfis hormonais e anátomo-patológicos em pacientes portadoras de displasia mamária antes, durante e após tratamento com antiestrogênico (Tese de Doutorado apresentada ao Departamento de Ginecologia da FMRP-USP) Ribeirão Preto, SP, 1985.

23. Rosen, P.P., Menendez-Botet, C.J., Nisselbaum, J.S., Urban, J.A., Mike, V., Frachia, A. and Schwartz, M.K. Pathological review of breast lesions analyzed for estrogen receptor protein. Cancer Research, 35: 3187-3194, 1975.

24. Scatchard, G. The attractions of proteins for small molecules and ions. Ann. N.Y. Acad. Sci., 51: 660-672, 1949.

25. Sherman, M.R., Tuazon, F.E.B. and Miller, L.K. Estrogen receptor cleavage and plasminogen activation by enzymes in human breast tumor cytosol. Endocrinology, 106: 1715-1727, 1980.

26. Thorsen, T. Association of plasminogen activator activity and steroid receptors in human breast cancer. Eur. J. Cancer, Clin. Oncol., 18: 129-132, 1982.

27. Williams, M.R., Nicholson, R.I., Elston, C.W., Todd, J., Griffiths, K. and Blamey, R.W. Letters to the editor: estrogen receptors in primary breast cancer. Br. J. Cancer, 51: 907-908, 1985.

THE SPECTRUM OF APOCRINE CARCINOMA OF THE BREAST

M.G. CATTANI[1], P. GUGLIOTTA[2], M.P. FOSCHINI[1], V. EUSEBI[1]

1. Istituto di Anatomia e Istologia, Università di
    Bologna, 40138 Bologna, Italy
2. Istituto di Anatomia e Istologia Patologica, Università
    di Torino

Apocrine epithelium in the breast is commonly observed lining the cysts characteristic of cystic disease (Fig. 1) (Azzopardi, 1979). The cells are columnar to cuboidal, have eosinophilic cytoplasm and a round nucleus with a prominent nucleolus. After diastase digestion, the PAS method stains irregular coarse granules in the cell apices which ultra-structurally correspond to large osmiophilic electron-dense granules (Fig. 2) (Pier et al., 1970). In the literature, there are several conflicting opinions concerning the nature of this epithelium. Recently, definitive evidence that pink epithelium of the breast is apocrine in nature has been pro-vided by Mazoujian et al. (1983). These authors have immunocytochemically located an apocrine marker, GCDFP-15,

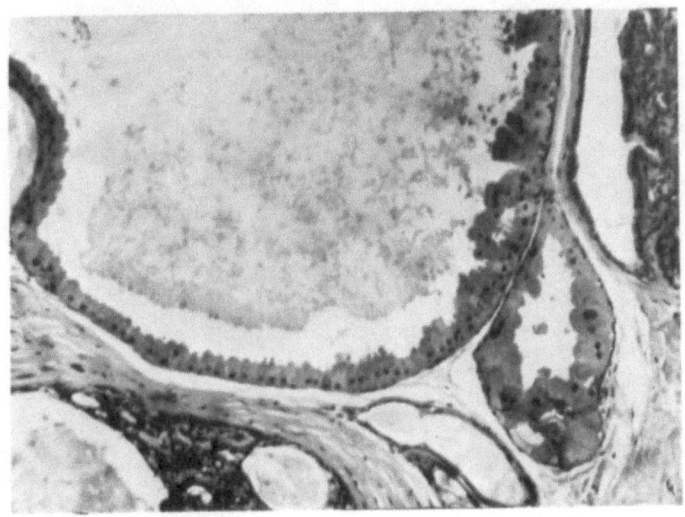

Fig. 1. Pink epithelium lining a lobular cyst (H&E x 60).

in this epithelium (Fig. 3). The same marker is also found in apocrine cells in other body sites. GCDFP-15 is a 15,000 dalton protein obtained from the fluid of tension cysts.

Whether apocrine changes represent a pathological process or are a sign of physiologic involution remains a moot question. The more important issue concerns the nature of cystic disease of the breast.

If we accept the view recently proposed by Love et al. (1982) that cystic disease of the breast is a normal phenomenon due to physiologic involution of the mammary gland, we must also accept apocrine changes as non-pathological modifications of the breast epithelium of the lobules.

Apocrine epithelium is seen in about 10% of fibroadenomas (Fig. 4). It is also rarely found in sclerosing adenosis and benign epitheliosis (Azzopardi, 1979). It is

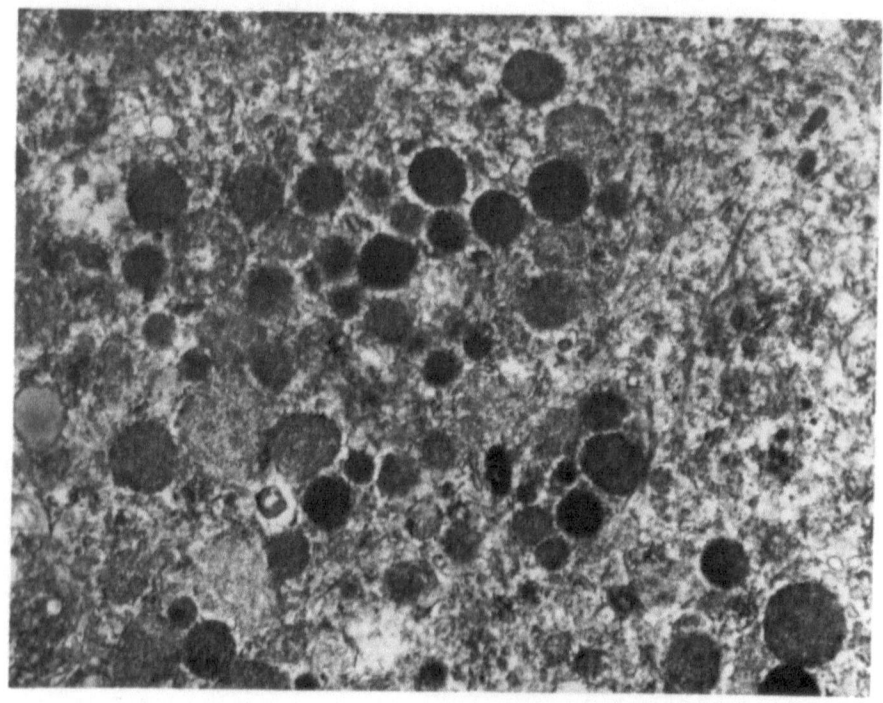

Fig. 2. Normal pink epithelium: numerous electron-dense granules are present through the cytoplasm (EM x 16.000).

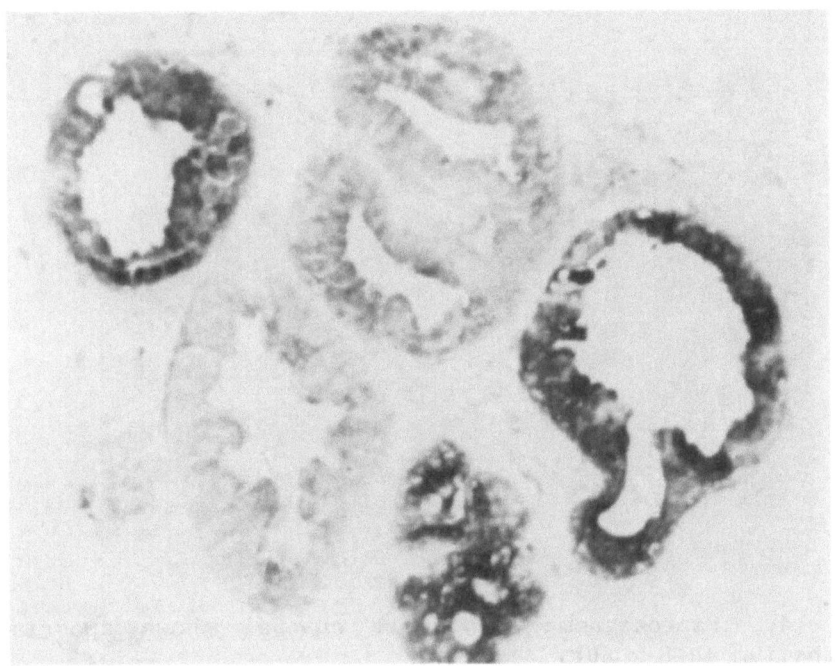

Fig. 3. The pink epithelium is immunoreactive with GCDFP-15 antiserum (Immuno-beta-galactosidase x 70).

commonly seen in solitary papillomas of larger ducts. According to McDivitt et al. (1968), these changes are very useful diagnostically for distinguishing papillary carcinomas which rarely, if ever, contain apocrine epithelium, from papillomas and other benign papillary proliferations. However, this view has been recently contradicted by us, as we have shown that 50% of papillary carcinomas harbour GCDFP-15 immunoreactive cells (Papotti et al., 1983).

The notable discrepancies in the literature concerning the morphological features of apocrine carcinoma of the breast have recently been stressed (Eusebi et al., 1984).

The definition and, consequently, the reported incidence of these tumours vary considerably. McDivitt et al. (1968) defined the tumour as "tubular or tubulo-alveolar cancer made of opaque, acidophilic cells resembling oncocytes," and included this entity in the group of relatively rare carcinomas.

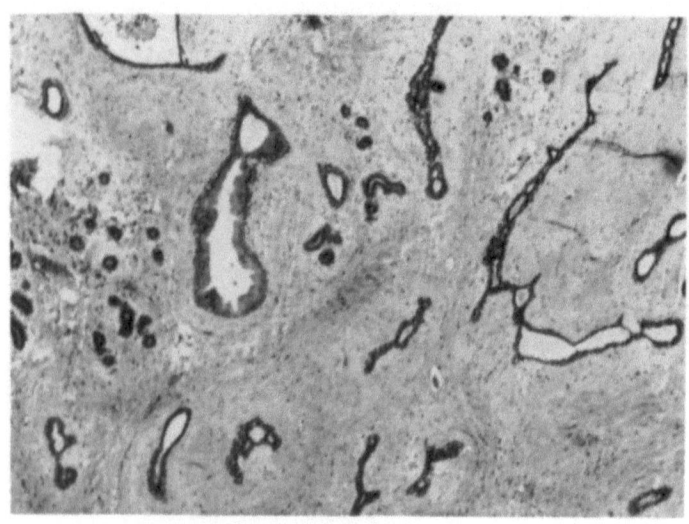

Fig. 4. Fibroadenoma. A small channel shows apocrine epithelium (H&E x 60).

Frable and Kay (1968), in a survey which covered a 16-year period, identified 19 patients with tumours containing cells which resembled "apocrine epithelium identical morphologically with apocrine glands normally seen in the axilla." These authors stated that apocrine carcinoma accounts for one per cent of mammary carcinomas. A lower incidence (0.3-0.4 per cent) was suggested by Azzopardi (1979) if only those carcinomas of the breast, largely composed of easily recognizable apocrine-type epithelium, are considered "apocrine" in nature (Fig. 5).

In their study of 1,000 cases of breast carcinoma, Fisher et al. (1975) did not find any pure cases considered worthy of the designation of apocrine carcinoma. They stated that "only 2.2 per cent of breast carcinomas contained varying numbers of cells with oxyphilic granular cytoplasm reminiscent of those of apocrine glands." In addition, they were inclined to consider that these changes represented oxyphilic rather than apocrine metaplasia, a view previously held by Hamperl (1977). Similarly, Bonser et al. (1961), who gave an incidence of 14.5 per cent, were not convinced that "pink cell carcinomas" could be equated with apocrine metaplasia. More recently, Haagensen et al.

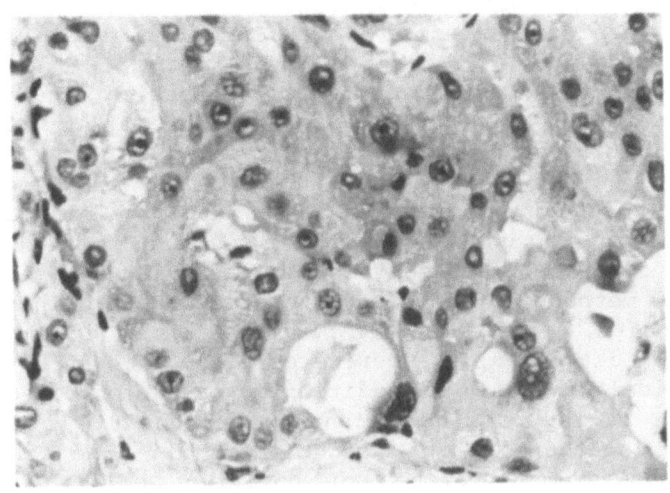

Fig. 5. Duct carcinoma composed of "easily recognizable epithelium" (H&E x 180).

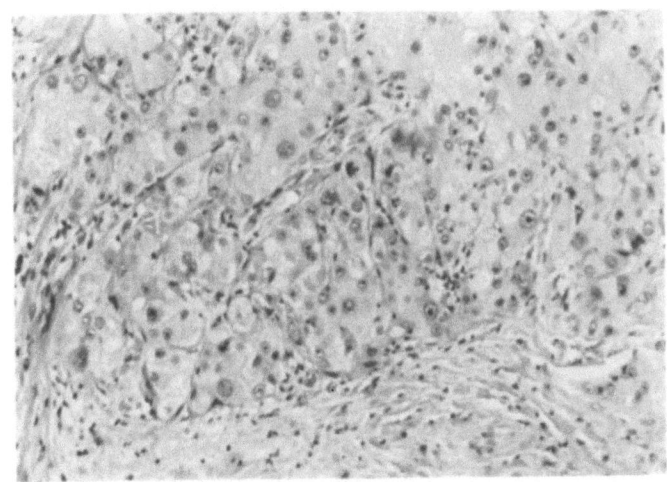

Fig. 6. Apocrine duct carcinoma. the neoplastic cells display a large, granular cytoplasm (H&E x 90).

(1981) suggested that the basic criteria for a diagnosis of apocrine carcinoma of the breast should include acidophilia of the cytoplasm, large size of the neoplastic cells, and cytoplasmic "snouts" projecting into the glandular lumina. Using these criteria, they found that no less than 60 per cent of carcinomas studied had apocrine features.

These very different views emphasize the lack of objective diagnostic criteria for reliable light microscopic identification of apocrine carcinomas.

As a result, in order to assess the real incidence and the mode of recognition of these tumours, we studied 100 consecutive cases of breast carcinomas using an immunocyto-chemical method for the detection of GCDFP-15. The presence of apocrine differentiation was confirmed in four cases initially diagnosed as apocrine carcinomas on structural and cytological grounds. In addition, 8 cases contained immuno-reactive cells: one case contained about 10% of positive elements scattered throughout the tumour. The other seven cases showed only patches of positive cells. In six of these tumours, the immunoreactive cells appeared different from the negative elements in that they showed either eosinophilic granular or foamy cytoplasm. The main histo-logically recognizable features of the immunoreactive

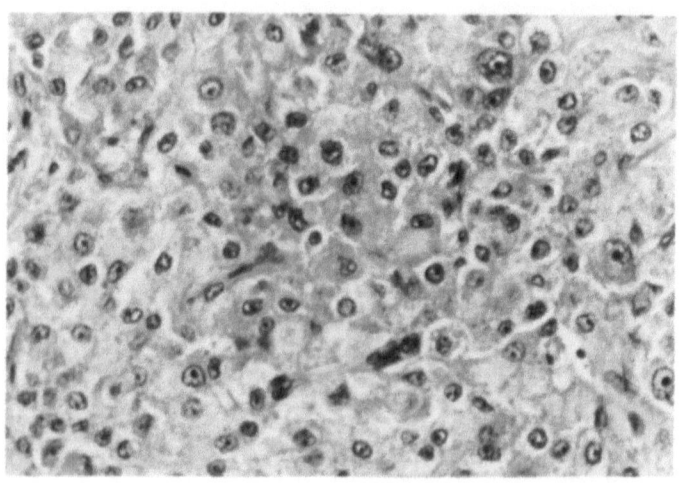

Fig. 7. Apocrine duct carcinoma: the neoplastic cells display round nuclei with prominent nucleoli (H&E x 105).

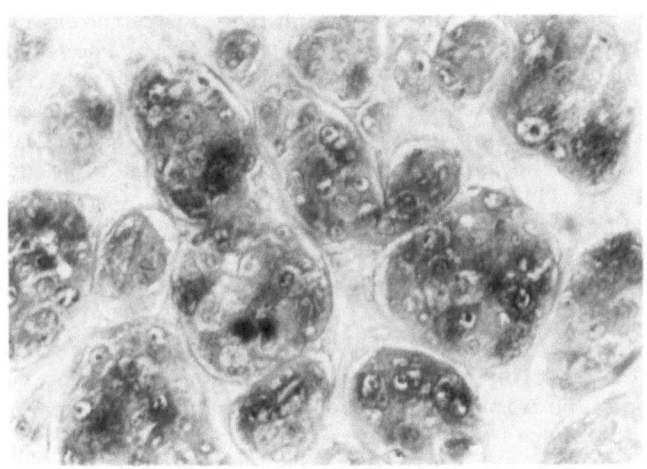

Fig. 8. Most of the cells are immunoreactive (anti-GCDFP-15 antiserum, immuno-beta-galactosidase x 105).

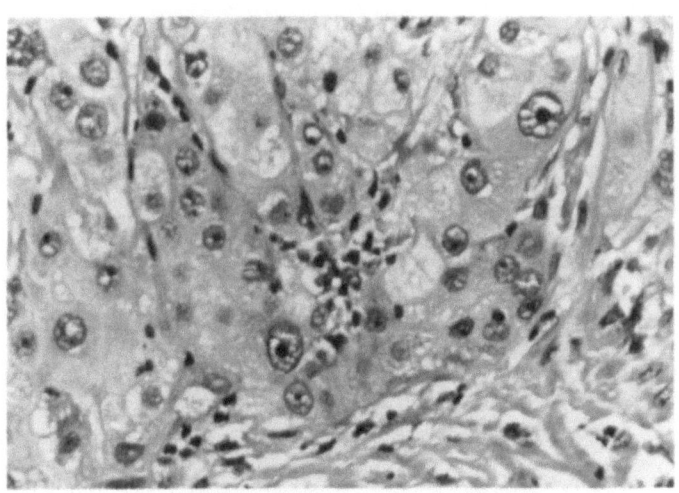

Fig. 9. Apocrine duct carcinoma: some of the neoplastic cells show a "clear" foamy cytoplasm (H&E x 280).

cases were the large eosinophilic granular cytoplasm (Fig. 6) coupled with rounded nuclei with prominent nucleoli (Fig. 7 and 8). In addition, among the eosinophilic elements, cells with foamy cytoplasm were also numerous (Fig. 9). These cells are immunoreactive with the apocrine marker, as recently shown by Eusebi et al. (1984). These authors described a case of atypical medullary carcinoma in which roughly one-third of total neoplastic proliferation consisted of an area with numerous foamy cells (Fig. 10). In this area, only the neoplastic foamy elements were GCDFP-15 positive (Fig. 11). Eusebi et al. (1984) were therefore convinced that foamy cells, together with elements having large eosinophilic granular cytoplasm and round nuclei with prominent nucleoli were the histologic hallmarks of apocrine carcinomas.

In a correlation between histologic and ultrastructural parameters of apocrine carcinomas, it was found that in the cytoplasm of apocrine elements, in addition to electron dense granules, large vesicles with a granular content were also consistently seen (Fig. 12). Therefore, it was stated that these same vesicles were an additional ultrastructural feature of apocrine elements. This is in agreement with the findings of Mazoujian et al. (1984), who located the apocrine marker GCDFP-15 in similar vesicles at the electron microscopic level, using an immuno-gold technique.

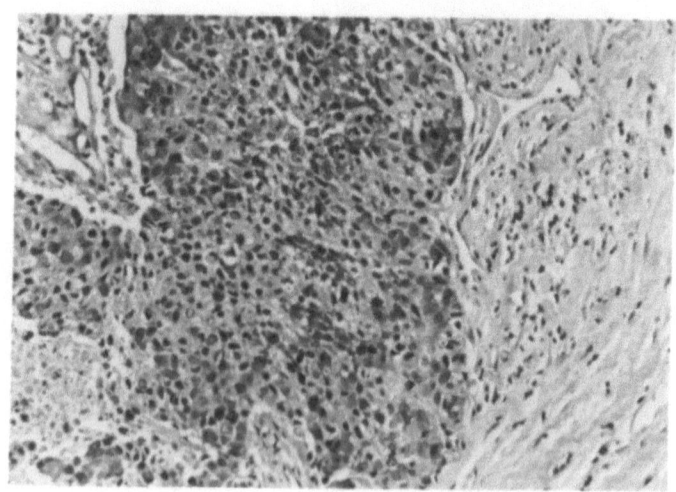

Fig. 10. Atypical medullary carcinoma: this area displays foamy neoplastic cells (H&E x 80).

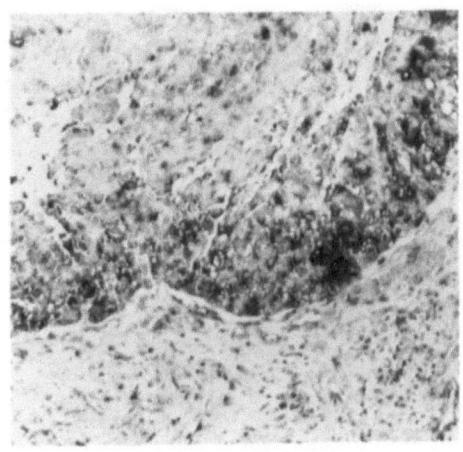

Fig. 11. The same area as Fig. 10 which is strongly positive for the apocrine marker (anti-GCDFP-15, immuno-beta-galactosidase x 60).

The fact that neoplastic apocrine epithelium can also display foamy cytoplasm has also been recently shown by us (Eusebi et al., 1984) in a series of invasive "histiocytoid" lobular carcinomas of the breast. It therefore appears that there is a large spectrum of apocrine carcinomas of the breast which ranges from the histiocytoid variant of lobular carcinomas possessing large eosinophilic cytoplasm, easily recognizable as apocrine epithelium. Recently, in a paper entitled "Glycogen-rich, clear-cell breast cancer," Fisher et al. (1985) questioned apocrine differentiation of histiocytoid invasive lobular carcinomas and criticized another well established entity referred to as lipid-rich carcinoma (Ramos and Taylor, 1974). These authors found that in 45 of their cases, the tumours were largely composed of clear cells containing glycogen. Seventy-eight per cent of these cases appeared to be ductal invasive, 11 per cent lobular invasive, 7 per cent a mixture of a ductal and tubular carcinoma, and one case each, medullary and tubular. These same authors stated that the literature concerning clear-cell neoplasm of the breast was not only confusing but also inconsistent.

We think that the alleged inconsistency found by these authors in the literature was partly due to a conceptual

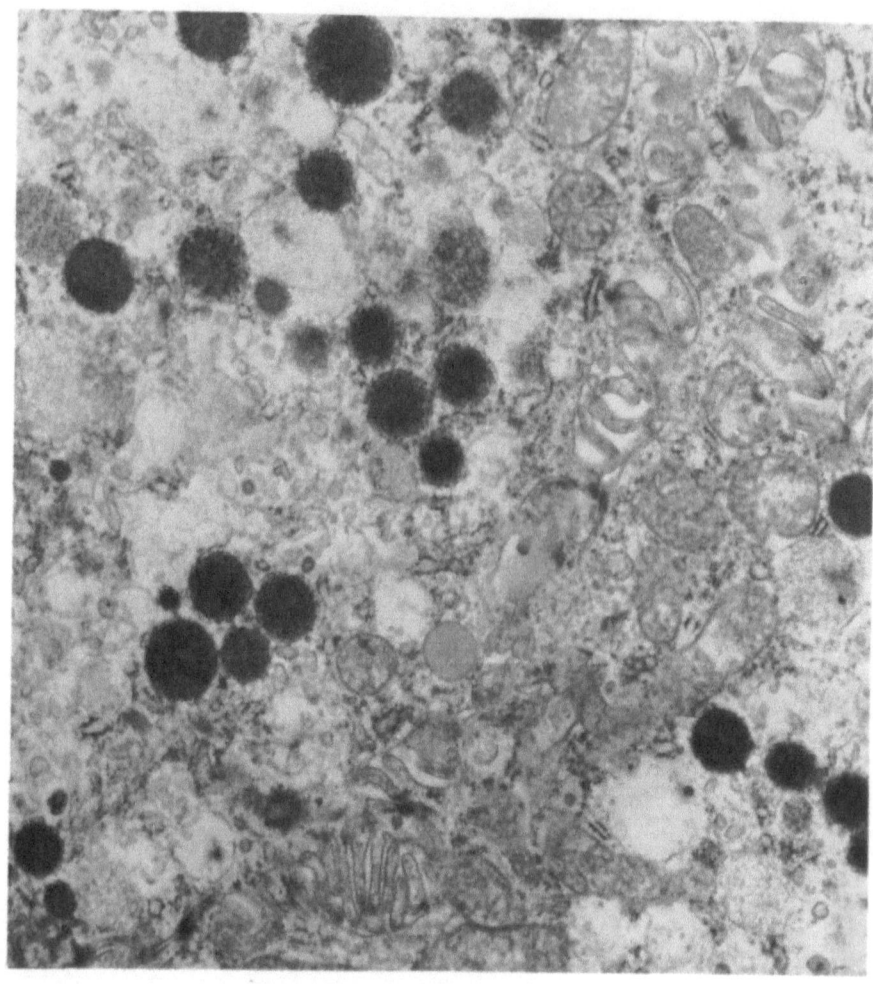

Fig. 12. Apocrine duct carcinoma: the cytoplasm contains large mitochondria as well as electron-dense granules and large granular vesicles (EM x 16.000).

definition of clear cells, which was lacking in their paper. This was inferred by the observation in Figure 4 of their paper in which a case of a poorly fixed invasive lobular carcinoma with extensive autolytic features was shown. Skorpil (1943) first described glycogen-rich clear cells in breast carcinoma. These cells were defined as lamprocytes from the ancient Greek. Therefore, the existence of glycogen-rich tumours has been recognized for a long period of time (Barwick et al., 19). It is also well-known that breast carcinomas can produce more than one substance, e.g., mucins (Gad and Azzopardi, 1975) and casein (Eusebi et al., 1977), lactalbumin (Walker, 1979), GCDFP-15 (Eusebi et al., 1984), polypeptides (Junitti and Berggren, 1983; Cross et al., 1985), as well as chromogranin (Bussolati et al., 1985). The finding of glycogen in breast carcinoma is therefore in keeping with this view and must be regarded as an additional cellular product of neoplastic cells. The colour of the cytoplasm of a given cell is due partly to cellular content and partly to the type of fixation. It has been shown, for instance, that lacunar cells in nodular sclerosis Hodgkin's lymphoma display clear cytoplasm when fixed in formalin, but not when Zenker fluid is used (Lukes, 1971). Thus, the presence of clear cells in a tumour may be the result of several endogenous products as well as of a fixation artifact.

In the series of 100 consecutive cases of breast car-cinomas recently studied, we did not find a statistically significant difference between positively and negatively staining tumours as far as their respective clinical, histo-pathological, and biochemical parameters were concerned. Mossler et al. (1980) found an absence of estrogen receptor activity in the apocrine carcinomas they studied. We were unable to confirm this in our series. Most of the apocrine tumours we examined exhibited ER activity and did not differ in this respect from the common run of breast carcinomas.

At the moment, therefore, apocrine differentiation of carcinomas of the breast must be regarded as a morphological and probably histogenetic finding, but further studies are needed in order to ascertain its biological significance.

ACKNOWLEDGEMENTS

Work supported by grants of MPI and CNR, Project "Oncologia" No. 85.02158.44.

184

REFERENCES

Azzopardi, J.G. Problems in breast pathology. In: Major
    Problems in Pathology, Volume 11, W.B. Saunders,
    London, 1979.
Barwick, K.W., Kashgarian, M., and Rosen, P.P. "Clear cell"
    change within duct and lobular epithelium of the human
    breast. In: Pathology Annual, Vol. 17, Part I,
    Sommers, S.C., and Rosen, P.P., eds.
    Appleton-Century-Crofts, Norwalk, Connecticut, 19 ,
    pp. 319-328.
Bonser, G.M., Dossett, J.A., and Jull, J.W. Human and
    experimental breast cancer. Pitman Medical, London,
    1961.
Bussolati, G., Gugliotta, P., Sapino, A., Eusebi, V., and
    Lloyd, R.V. Chromogranin-reactive endocrine cells in
    argyrophilic carcinomas ("carcinoids") and normal
    tissue of the breast. Am. J. Pathol. 120, 186-192,
    1985.
Cross, A.S., Azzopardi, J.G., Krausz, T., Van Noorden, S.,
    and Polak, J.M. A morphological and immunocytochemical
    study of a distinctive variant of ductal carcinoma in
    situ of the breast. Histopathology 9, 21-37, 1985.
Eusebi, V., Pich, A., Macchiorlatti, E., and Bussolati, G.
    Morpho-functional differentiation in lobular carcinoma
    of the breast. Histopathology 1, 301-314, 1977.
Eusebi, V., Betts, C.M., Haagensen, D.E., Gugliotta, P.,
    Bussolati, G., and Azzopardi, J.G. Apocrine
    differentiation in lobular carcinoma of the breast.
    Hum. Pathol. 15, 134-140, 1984.
Fisher, E.R., Gregorio, R.M., and Fisher, B. The pathology
    of invasive breast cancer. Cancer 36, 261-263, 1975.
Fisher, E.R., Tavares, J., Bulatao, I.S., Sass, R., and
    Fisher, B. Glycogen-rich, clear-cell breast cancer.
    Hum. Pathol. 16, 1085-1090, 1985.
Frable, W.J., and Kay, S. Carcinoma of the breast:
    histologic anc clinical features of apocrine tumors.
    Cancer 21, 756-763, 1968.
Gad, A., and Azzopardi, J.G. Lobular carcinoma of the
    breast: a special variant of mucin-secreting
    carcinoma. J. Clin. Path. 28, 711-716, 1975.
Haagensen, C.D., Bodian, C., and Haagensen, D.E. Jr. Breast
    carcinoma: risk and detection. W.B. Saunders,
    Philadelphia, 1981.
Hamperl, H. Das sogennante Schweissdrusencarcinoma der
    Mamma. Zeitschrift fur Krebsforschung 88, 105-119,
    1977.

Junitti-Berggren, L., Pitkanen, P., and Wilander, E.
    Argyrophil endocrine cells with ACTH and HCG
    immunoreactivity in a carcinoma of the breast.
    Virchows Arch. (Cell Pathol.) 43, 37-42, 1983.
Love, S.M., Gelman, R.S., and Silen, W. Fibrocystic
    "disease" of the breast - a nondisease? N. Engl. J.
    Med. 307, 1010-1014, 1982.
Lukes, R.J. Criteria for involvement of lymph-node, bone
    marrow, spleen, and liver in Hodgkin's disease. Cancer
    Research 31, 1755-1767, 1971.
Mazoujian, G., Warhol, H.J., and Haagensen, D.E. Jr. The
    ultrastructural localization of Gross Cystic Disease
    Fluid Protein (GCDFP-15) in breast epithelium. Am. J.
    Pathol. 116, 305-310, 1984.
Mazoujian, G., Pinkus, G.S., Davis, S., and Haagensen, D.E.
    Jr. Immunohistochemistry of a Gross Cystic Disease
    Fluid Protein (GCDFP-15) of the breast. Am. J. Pathol.
    110, 105-112, 1983.
McDivitt, R.W., Stewart, F.W., and Berg, J.W. Tumors of the
    breast. In: Atlas of Tumor Pathology, fascicle 2,
    Armed Forces Institute Pathology, Washington, D.C.,
    1968.
Mossler, J.A., Barton, T.K., and Brinkhous, A.D. Apocrine
    differentiation in human mammary carcinoma. Cancer 46,
    2463-2471, 1980.
Papotti, M., Gugliotta, P., Eusebi, V., and Bussolati, G.
    Immunohistochemical analysis of benign and malignant
    papillary lesions of the breast. Am. J. Surg. Pathol.
    7, 451-561, 1983.
Pier, W.J., Garancis, J.C., and Kuzma, J.F. The
    ultrastructure of apocrine cells. Arch. Path. 89,
    446-452, 1970.
Ramos, C.V. and Taylor, H.B. Lipid-rich carcinoma of the
    breast. A clinicopathologic analysis of 13 examples.
    Cancer 33, 812-816, 1974.
Skorpil, F. Uber das Vorkommen von sog.hellen Zellen
    (Lamprocyten) in der Milchdruse. Beitr. Pathol. Anat.
    Allg. Pathol. 108, 378-393, 1943.
Walker, R.A. The demonstration of α-lactalbumin in human
    breast carcinomas. J. Path. 129, 37-42, 1979.

SELECTED FREE PAPERS

BREAST CARCINOMAS WITH NEUROENDOCRINE ACTIVITY

JAHN M. NESLAND, RUTH HOLM AND JAN VINCENTS JOHANNESSEN

The Norwegian Radium Hospital and Institute for Cancer Research, Montebello, 0310 Oslo 3, Norway, and The Norwegian Cancer Society.

INTRODUCTION

In 1963 Feyrter and Hartmann described two cases of argyrophilic breast carcinomas and suggested that the tumors were derived from "das Helle-Zellen-Organ", a diffusely distributed system of argyrophilic clear cells described by Feyrter in 1938, and found to be present in the normal breast by Vogler in 1947. In 1977 Cubilla and Woodruff presented their series of 10 patients with similar tumours and demonstrated small electron dense membrane-bound granules in the 3 cases studied by electron microscopy. A number of hormones had already been detected in homogenates of breast carcinoma tissue or in serum from breast cancer patients, such as ACTH (Liddle et al 1965), PTH (Mavligit et al 1971, Melick et al 1972), HCG (Sheth et al 1974), calcitonin (Coombes et al 1975, Hillyard et al 1976). Interest in neuroendocrine breast tumours has been increasing by leaps and bounds recently, mainly due to the introduction of new techniques that enable the pathologist to localize hormones and peptides in sections prepared for light and electron microscopy.

DIAGNOSTIC CRITERIA

The argyrophilic reaction

The argyrophilic staining reaction has been widely accepted as a screening method for identifying endocrine tumors. In a large series of breast carcinomas (Azzopardi et al. 1982), 3-5% were argyrophilic when examined with the Grimelius technique (Grimelius 1968). Other silver impregnation methods such as the Bodian and Servier-Munger techniques are generally considered to be less reliable. Unfortunately, only a certain proportion of breast carcinomas with proven neuroendocrine differentiation are argyrophilic with the Grimelius technique, a technique that is full of pitfalls. Small variations in pH and temperature may influence the result and the staining result can be difficult to interpret. This latter can sometimes be improved by re-impregnation (Grimelius and Wilander, 1980).

The argentaffin reaction

The Masson technique, like the Grimelius method, stains secretory granules. Devitt's brief report in 1978 deals with an argentaffin breast carcinoid tumour, but no further details are given. Our experience is the same as Azzopardi's (1979) and Cubilla and Woodruff's (1977): that the argyrophilic breast carcinomas are nonargentaffin.

Biochemical analysis

The tumour tissue is homogenated before analysis of the hormone content and it is not possible therefore to evaluate the amount of connective tissue, normal epithelial constituents, etc. in the tissue analysed. ACTH (Liddle et al 1965), PTH (Mavligit et al 1971, Melick et al 1972), calcitonin (Hillyard et al 1976) have all been extracted from breast cancer tissue.

Electron microscopy

Small, membrane-bound electron dense granules are the diagnostic clue to endocrine tumours. The majority of carcinoid tumours and other carcinomas with neuroendocrine features have granules measuring about 100-300 nm in diameter with an electron dense core surrounded by a clear halo.

Several reports emphasize the diagnostic importance of such granules in endocrine tumours of the breast (Cubilla and Woodruff 1977, Devitt 1978, Kaneko et al 1978, Cohle et al 1979, Fisher, Palekar and NSABP collaborators 1979, Capella et al 1980, Chen 1981, Taxy et al 1981, Woodard et al 1981, Azzopardi et al 1982,). Ferguson and Anderson (1985) studied 114 specimens from benign and malignant breast lesions and noticed that dense core granules were present in about 50% of the benign breast lesions and in 80% of the malignant breast lesions. However, all types of secretory granules with an electron dense core were included in their study. Granules accumulated in the apical parts of the cells towards an intercellular lumen are usually of exocrine nature whereas neuroendocrine granules, if abundant, tend to be spread evenly in the cytoplasm of breast carcinomas. If only a few granules are seen, they are usually placed along the basal and lateral cell borders. We have found that electron dense granules of probable neuroendocrine nature are present in about 5-10% of breast carcinomas. (Nesland et al 1985, 1986) dependent on how many sections are studied. Only a few tumour cells may contain neuroendocrine granules, and neuroendocrine tumours may therefore remain undetected if electron microscopy is the only method used to make the diagnosis.

Immunocytochemistry

Several markers have been used to identify neuroendocrine tumours. The best way to recognize the endocrine nature of a tumour is by demonstrating peptide/hormone products within the cytoplasm of the tumour cells. The problem is that several hormones are produced in breast carcinomas (and in other neuroendocrine tumours). Immunoreactivity for ACTH (Cohle et al 1979, Woodard et al 1981, Juntti-Berggren et al 1983, Vinores et al 1984, Nesland et al 1985), bombesin (Memoli et al 1984, Nesland et al 1985, 1986), serotonin (Memoli et al 1984), HCG (Juntti-Berggren et al 1981, Raju and Fine 1983), prolactin (Raju and Fine 1983), gastrin (Nesland et al 1985), VIP (Nesland et al 1985), leu-enkephalin (Nesland et al 1986), pancreatic polypeptide (Nesland et al 1986), β-endorphin (Nesland et al 1986) and Sub-P (Nesland et al 1986) have all been reported. A large number of antibodies raised against different hormones are therefore necessary when breast tumours are screened for hormonal activity. Even a negative result does not exclude the possibility of neuroendocrine differentiation, since a hormone may be present in very low concentration, in an aberrant form, or be hitherto unknown and therefore undetectable by available antibodies.

Enolases belong to a group of cytoplasmic enzymes that participate in glycolysis. Four different isoenzymes have been detected and are formed by 2 of 3 subunits designated α, β and γ. The αα is the most common form and occurs in most tissues, ββ is present predominantly in muscle tissue and γγ enolase is characteristic for neurones and neuroendocrine tumours. In fact, γγ isoenzyme was first isolated in the brain, but its presence in neurones led to the designation "neuron-specific enolase" (NSE). Immuno-staining for NSE has been widely accepted as a good marker for neuro-endocrine tumours throughout the body (Schmechel et al 1978, Wharton et al 1981, Tapia et al 1981, Bishop et al 1982, Royds et al 1982, Gu et al 1983, Trojanowski and Lee 1983, Beemer et al 1984, Carlei et al 1984, Sheppard et al 1984, Springall et al 1984).

In the study by Vinores and coworkers (1984) 4 of 11 infiltrating ductal carcinomas and 2 of 11 fibroadenomas were positively stained for NSE, whereas all 7 intraductal carcinomas with structural and cytological features of endocrine differentiation studied by Cross and coworkers (1985) were positively stained with anti-NSE. Nesland and colleagues (1986) found immunoreactivity for NSE in 17 of 50 cases and immuno-reactivity for hormones in 12 of these 17. The specificity and usefulness of immunostaining with anti-NSE have however been questioned. Schmechel (1985) feels that the practical usefulness of the γ subunit of enolase needs investigation in each particular situation. The frequent immunostaining for NSE in breast carcinomas (Nesland et al, 1985, 1986 and submitted) raises doubts as to whether NSE is a specific marker of neuro-endocrine breast carcinoma or whether other cells are stained as well. Memoli et al (1984) and Nesland et al (1985 and 1986) emphasize that even normal and neoplastic myoepithelial cells stain weakly for NSE. Caution must therefore be exercised in the interpretation of NSE immunostaining in the breast even when careful testing of the NSE antibody is carried out before it is used for diagnosis.

The cytoplasmic enzyme NSE is not situated in the electron dense granules and a positive immunostaining with anti NSE is therefore rather diffuse.

Bussolati and coworkers (1985) obtained a positive immunostaining for chromogranin in 3 of 9 argyrophilic breast carcinomas and concluded that there were two possible interpretations:

a) argyrophilia in breast tumours might not be restricted to endocrine cells or
b) only part of the hormone-producing breast carcinoma is chromo-granin-reactive.

We do not consider immunostaining with antichromogranin to be the method of choice for detecting breast carcinomas with neuroendocrine differentiation (Nesland et al, submitted). The commercially available antibody that we used gave positive staining for chromogranin in both NSE-positive and NSE-negative tumours, in tumours with proven hormonal content and in tumours without detectable hormones.

Recently, several other markers for neuroendocrine tumours have been published. Monaghan and Roberts (1985) studied a group of breast carcinomas with the monoclonal antibody LICR-LON-E36 and obtained a positive staining in 34% of the 44 tumours studied. In the same series, anti-NSE stained 25% of the tumours, whereas only 8 tumours (18%) were stained with both antibodies.

Anti-P6P 9.5, an antibody raised against a soluble protein isolated from the brain, has been used in the study of neuroendocrine tumours outside the breast (Rode and coworkers (1985).

Antibodies against secretogranin I and II, two tyrosine-sulfated proteins occurring in a wide variety of endocrine and neuronal cells that pack peptides into secretory granules (Rosa et al 1985), may become useful markers for some neuroendocrine tumours. The secretogranins are immunologically and biochemically different from, but still related to, chromogranin A.

MORPHOLOGICAL CONSIDERATIONS

The morphology of breast carcinomas with neuroendocrine differentiation varies. Some tumours look like carcinoids (Cubilla and Woodruff 1977, Devitt 1978, Kaneko et al 1978, Fisher et al 1979, Raju and Fine 1983, Toyoshima 1983, Nesland et al 1985) and others like oat cell carcinomas (Wade et al 1983, Jundt et al. 1984). The majority of the carcinomas with neuroendocrine differentiation have the appearance of ordinary ductal carcinomas (Melick et al 1972, Sheth et al 1974, Coombes et al 1975, Hillyard et al 1976, Cubilla and Woodruff 1977 Partanen and Syrjänen 1981, Taxy et al 1981, Woodard et al 1981, Fetissof et al 1983, Juntti-Berggren et al. 1983, Toyoshima 1983, Memoli et al 1984, Cross et al 1985, Monaghan and Roberts 1985, Nesland et al 1985, 1986), lobular carcinomas (Cohle et al 1979, Gould and Chejfec 1980, Chen 1981, Fetissof et al 1983, Memoli et al 1984, Nesland et al 1985, Nesland et al 1986), apocrine carcinomas (Nesland et al 1985), mucinous carcinomas (Feyrter and Hartmann 1963, Fisher et al. 1979, Capella et al 1980, Chen 1981, Fetissof et al 1983, Toyoshima 1983, Nesland et al 1985) or tubular carcinomas (Nesland et al. 1986).

Recently published data indicate that with the diagnostic methods that are available today about 30% of all breast carcinomas have neuroendocrine features (Monaghan and Roberts 1985, Nesland et al. 1986, Nesland et al.submitted). The designation "carcinoid" seems meaningless for these tumours since the majority of them look and behave like ordinary ductal and lobular carcinomas. The term "carcinoid" should be restricted to tumours with a classic carcinoid appearance.

WHAT IS THE FUNCTION OF THE HORMONES PRODUCED?

Elevated serum level of hormones in patients with breast cancer has been reported (Feyrter and Hartmann 1963, Sheth et al. 1974, Hillyard et al 1976, Kaneko et al 1978, Cohle et al 1979, Woodard et al 1981, Monteiro et al 1984), but clinical symptoms related to hormone production have been reported in only two cases (Kaneko et al. 1978, Woodard et al, 1981).

An elevated blood pressure and norepinephrine excretion into the urine was noticed in the case reported by Kaneko and coworkers (1978). Biochemical analysis of tumour tissue was not performed, so final proof of hormone production in the tumour cells could not be obtained, but the autopsy did not reveal any other possible production site of the hormone.

Woodard and coworkers (1981) presented a case of infiltrating ductal carcinoma with an elevated serum ACTH content. The patient had clinical hypercortisonism related to the ectopic ACTH production. Immunostaining with anti-ACTH revealed immunoreactive products within nests of tumour cells.

What is the function of the clinically silent hormones? One explanation is that hormone production is just an aberrant cell product of no biological importance.

Some of the hormones produced are well known growth regulation factors. Some, like bombesin and insulin, are growth stimulating factors. Somatostatin, however, has an inhibitory effect on tumour growth. These hormones may therefore express a local effect and, according to the autocrine hypothesis, the cancer cell can stimulate its own growth by the production and secretion of a hormone-like substrate that can interact with specific membrane receptors on its surface and induce proliferation.

WHAT IS THE ORIGIN OF THE HORMONE-PRODUCING CELLS?

These hormone-containing cells are probably not derived from the neural crest. The tumours look like ordinary breast carcinomas and the hormone-producing cells have the same morphology as the rest of the tumour cells. We do not know whether the neuroendocrine activity of these hormone-producing cells is permanent or whether it is only present during a special period of the cell's development and is lost later in the course of tumour growth.

CONCLUSION

Neuroendocrine differentiation is not a rare phenomenon in breast carcinomas. About 30% of all breast carcinomas may present this feature and the tumours may be indistinguishable from ordinary ductal carcinomas, lobular carcinomas, etc. by light microscopy. More than 10 different hormones have been demonstrated in breast cancer cells, and these hormones probably have an autocrine function.

The ideal screening marker for detecting these tumours has not yet been found, but in addition to different monoclonal antibodies raised against specific peptides in neurogenic and neuroendocrine cells, staining with anti-NSE is a useful method.

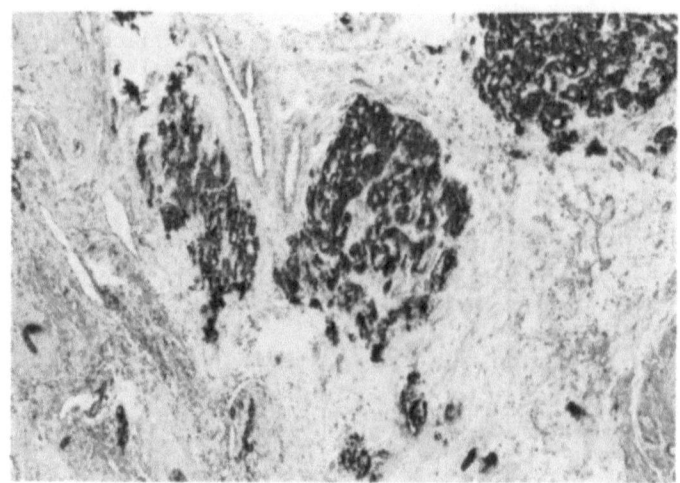

Fig. 1: <u>Immunostaining with anti-NSE</u>. All tumour cells are positively
stained (X 75).

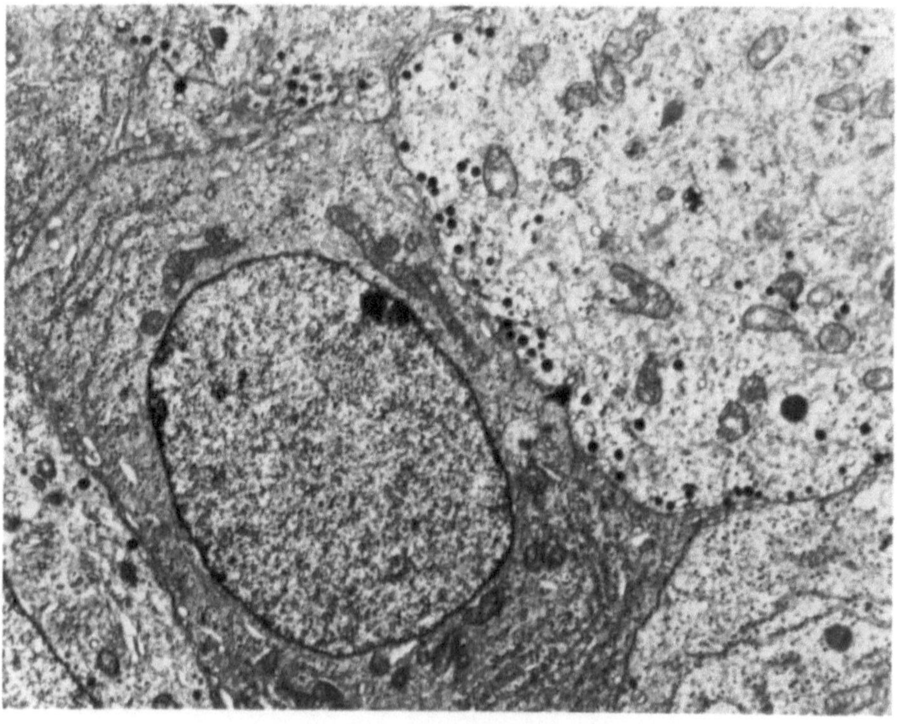

Fig. 2: Small membrane-bound electron dense granules of neuroendocrine
type are present in the periphery of the cells. (Uranyl acetate
and lead citrate X 8800).

REFERENCES

Azzopardi JG. Problems in Breast Pathology. Vol. 11 in the series Major Problems in Pathology (JL Bennington, ed.), W. B. Saunders, London, 1979.

Azzopardi JG, Muretto P, Goddeeris P, Eusebi V, Lauweryns JM. "Carcinoid" tumours of the breast: the morphological spectrum of argyrophil carcinomas. Histopathology 6: 549-69, 1982.

Beemer FA, Vlug AMC, van Veelen CWM, Rijksen G, Staal GEJ. Isozyme pattern of enolase of childhood tumors. Cancer 54: 293-296, 1984.

Bishop AE, Polak JM, Facer P, Ferri GL, Marangos PJ, Pearse AGE. Neuron-specific enolase: A common marker for the endocrine cells and innervation of the gut and pancreas. Gastroenterology 83: 902-925, 1982.

Bussolati G, Gugliotta P, Sapino A, Eusebi V, Lloyd RV. Chromogranin-reactive endocrine cells in argyrophilic carcinomas ("carcinoids") and normal tissue of the breast. Am J Pathol 120: 186-192, 1985.

Capella C, Eusebi V, Mann B, Azzopardi JG. Endocrine differentiation in mucoid carcinoma of the breast. Histopathology 4: 613-30, 1980.

Carlei F, Polak JM, Ceccamea A, Marangos PJ, Dahl D, Cocchia D, Michetti F, Lezoche E, Speranza V. Neuronal and glial markers in tumours of neuroblastic origin. Virchows Arch (Pathol Anat) 404: 313-324, 1984.

Chen KTK. Breast carcinomas with carcinoid features. Breast 7: 2-5, 1981.

Clayton F, Ordonez NG, Sibley RK, Hanssen G. Argyrophilic breast carcinomas. Evidence of lactational differentiation. Am J Surg Pathol 6: 323-33, 1982.

Cohle SD, Tschen JA, Smith FE, Lane M, McGavran MH. ACTH-secreting carcinoma of the breast. Cancer 43: 2370-76, 1979.

Coombes RC, Easty GC, Detre SI, Hillyard CH, Stevens U, Girgis SI, Galante LS, Heywood L, MacIntyre I, Neville AM. Secretion of immunoreactive calcitonin by human breast carcinomas. Br Med J 4: 197-99, 1975.

Cross AS, Azzopardi JG, Krausz T, Van Noorden S, Polak JM. A morphological and immunocytochemical study of a distinctive variant of ductal carcinoma in situ of the breast. Histopathology 9: 21-37, 1985.

Cubilla AL, Woodruff JM. Primary carcinoid tumor of the breast. Am J Surg Pathol 1: 283-92, 1977.

Devitt PG. Carcinoid tumour of the breast. Br Med J 2: 327, 1978.

Ferguson DJP, Anderson TJ. Distribution of dense core granules in normal benign and malignant breast tissue. J Pathol 147: 59-65, 1985.

Fetissof F, Dubois MP, Arbeille-Brassart B, Lansac J, Jobard P. Argyrophilic cells in mammary cancer. Hum Pathol 14: 127-34, 1983.

Feyrter F. Über den derzeitigen Stand der Lehre von den peripheren endo-
krinen (parakrinen) Drüsen. Acta Neuroveg (Wien) 25: 63-89, 1962.

Feyrter F, Hartmann G. Über die carcinoide Wuchsform des Carcinoma mammae,
insbesondere das Carcinoma solidum (gelatinosum) mammae. Frankfurter Z
Pathol 73: 24-39, 1963.

Fisher ER, Palekar AS, and NSABP collaborators. Solid and mucinous varieties of so-called mammary carcinoid tumors. Am J Clin Pathol 72: 909-16,
1979.

Gould VE, Chejfec G. Case 13. (Lobular carcinoma of the breast with secretory features). Ultrastruct Pathol 1: 151-156, 1980.

Grimelius L. A silver nitrate stain for A$_2$ cells of human pancreatic
islets. Acta Soc Med Upsaliensis 73: 243-270, 1968.

Grimelius L, Wilander E. Silver stains in the study of endocrine cells of
the gut and pancreas. Invest Cell Pathol 3: 3-12, 1980.

Gu J, Polak JM, van Noorden S, Pearse AGE, Marangos PJ, Azzopardi JG. Immunostaining of neuron-specific enolase as a diagnostic tool for Merkel
cell tumors. Cancer 52: 1039-1043, 1983.

Hillyard CJ, Coombes RC, Greenberg PB, Galange LS, MacIntyre I. Calcitonin
in breast and lung cancer. Clin Endocrinol 5: 1-8, 1976.

Jundt G, Schulz A, Heitz PhU, Osborn M. Small cell neuroendocrine (oat
cell) carcinoma of the male breast. Immunocytochemical and ultrastructural
investigations. Virchows Arch (Pathol Anat) 404: 213-221, 1984.

Juntti-Berggren L, Pitkänen P, Wilander E. Argyrophil endocrine cells with
ACTH and HCG immunoreactivity in a carcinoma of the breast. Virchows Arch
(Cell Pathol) 43: 37-42, 1983.

Kaneko H, Hojo H, Ishikawa S, Yamanouchi H, Sumida T, Saito R. Norepi-
nephrine-producing tumors of bilateral breasts. Cancer 41: 2002-7, 1978.

Liddle GW, Givens JR, Nicholson WE, Island DP. The ectopic ACTH syndrome.
Cancer Res 25: 1057-61, 1965.

Mavligit GM, Cohen JL, Sherwood LM. Ectopic production of parathyroid hormone by carcinoma of the breast. N Engl J Med 285: 154-56, 1971.

Melick RA, Martin TJ, Hicks JD. Parathyroid hormone production and malignancy. Br Med J 2: 204-205, 1972.

Memoli VA, Nesland J, Warren WH, Johannessen JV, Gould VE. Immunohistochemical and ultrastructural observations concerning the issue of neuroendocrine differentiation in breast carcinomas. Lab Invest 50: 39A, 1984.

Monaghan P, Roberts JDB. Immunocytochemical evidence for neuroendocrine
differentiation in human breast carcinomas. J Pathol 147: 281-289, 1985.

Monteiro JCMP, Ferguson KM, McKinna A, Greening WP, Neville AM. Ectopic production of human chorionic gonadotrophin-like material by breast cancer. Cancer 53: 957-962, 1984.

Nesland JM, Holm R, Johannessen JV. A study of different markers for neuroendocrine differentiation in breast carcinomas. Submitted for publication.

Nesland JM, Holm R, Johannessen JV, Gould VE: Neurone specific enolase immunostaining in the diagnosis of breast carcinomas with neuroendocrine differentiation. Its usefulness and limitations. J Pathol 148: 35-43, 1986.

Nesland JM, Memoli VA, Holm R, Gould VE, Johannessen JV. Breast carcinomas with neuroendocrine differentiation. Ultrastruct Pathol 8: 225-240, 1985.

Partanen S, Syrjänen K. Argyrophilic cells in carcinoma of the female breast. Virchow Arch (Pathol Anat) 391: 45-51, 1981.

Raju U, Fine G. The controversial mammary carcinoid tumor. Lab Invest 48: 69A, 1983.

Rode J, Dhillon AP, Doran JF, Jackson P, Thompson RJ. PGP9.5, a new marker for human neuroendocrine tumours. Histopathology 9. 147-158, 1985.

Rosa P, Hille A, Lee RWH, Zanini A, De Camilli P, Huttner WB. Secretogranins I and II: Two tyrosine-sulfated secretory proteins common to a variety of cells secreting peptides by the regulated pathway. J Cell Biol 101: 1999-2011, 1985.

Royds JA, Parsons MA, Taylor CB, Timperley WR. Enolase isoenzyme distribution in the human brain and its tumours. J Pathol 137: 37-49, 1982.

Schmechel DE. Gamma-subunit of the glycolytic enzyme enolase: nonspecific or neuronspecific. Lab Invest 52: 239-247, 1985.

Schmechel D, Marangos PJ, Brightman M. Neurone-specific enolase is a molecular marker for peripheral and central neuroendocrine cells. Nature 276: 834-836, 1978.

Sheppard MN, Corrin B, Bennett MH, Marangos PJ, Bloom SR, Polak JM. Immunocytochemical localization of neuron specific enolase in small cell carcinomas and carcinoid tumours of the lung. Histopathology 8: 171-181, 1984.

Sheth NA, Saruiya JN, Ranadive KJ, Sheth AR. Ectopic production of human chorionic gonadotrophin by human breast tumours. Br J Cancer 30: 566-70, 1974.

Springall DR, Lackie P, Levene MM, Marangos PJ, Polak JM. Immunostaining of neuron-specific enolase is a valuable aid to the cytological diagnosis of neuroendocrine tumours of the lung. J Pathol 143: 259-265, 1984.

Tapia FJ, Barbosa AJA, Marangos PJ, Polak JM, Bloom S, Dermody C, Pearse AGE. Neuron-specific enolase is produced by neuroendocrine tumours. The Lancet 1: 808-811, 1981.

196

Taxy JB, Tischler AS, Insalaco SJ, Battifora H. "Carcinoid" tumor of the breast. A variant of conventional breast cancer? Hum Pathol 12: 170-79, 1981.

Toyoshima S. Mammmary carcinoma with argyrophil cells. Cancer 52: 2129-38, 1983.

Trojanowski JQ, Lee VM-Y. Monoclonal and polyclonal antibodies against neural antigens: Diagnostic applications for studies of central and peripheral nervous system tumors. Hum Pathol 14: 281-285, 1983.

Vinores SA, Bonnin JM, Rubinstein LJ, Marangos PJ. Immunohistochemical demonstration of neuron-specific enolase in neoplasms of the CNS and other tissues. Arch Pathol Lab Med 108: 536-540, 1984.

Vogler E. Über das basilare Helle-Zellen-Organ der menschlichen Brustdrüse. Klin Med 2: 159-68, 1947.

Wade PHM, Millis SE, Read M, Could W, Lambert MJ III, Smith RE. Small cell neuroendocrine (oat cell) carcinoma of the breast. Cancer 52: 121-125, 1983.

Wharton J, Polak JM, Cole GA, Marangos PJ, Pearse AGE. Neuron-specific enolase as an immunocytochemical marker for the diffuse neuroendocrine system in human fetal lung. J Histochem Cytochem 29: 1359-1364, 1981.

Woodard BH, Eisenbath G, Wallace NR, Mossler JA, McCarty KS Jr. Adrenocorticotropin production by a mammary carcinoma. Cancer 47: 1823-27, 1981.

ESTROGEN RECEPTOR IMMUNOCYTOCHEMICAL ASSAY (ER-ICA) AND
LAMININ DETECTION IN 115 BREAST CARCINOMAS: A LIGHT AND
ELECTRON MICROSCOPY STUDY WITH A COMPUTERIZED (SAMBA 200)
QUANTITATIVE ANALYSIS ON TISSUE SECTIONS.

C. CHARPIN, P.M. MARTIN, J.C. LISSITZKY, J. JACQUEMIER,
F. KOPP, N. POURREAU, M.N. LAVAUT, M. TOGA.

Department of Pathology and Department of Experimental
Oncology, Faculty of Medecine, 27 Bd Jean Moulin,
13385 Marseille Cedex 5, France.

INTRODUCTION

Currently available histochemical or immunohistochemical
methods (Dandliker et al., 1978; Kurzon and Sternberger, 1978;
Lee, 1978; Nenci et al., 1976) have been shown to be unreliable
for ER detection (Chamness et al., 1980). Recently, specific
monoclonal antibodies against ER have been developed (Desombre
et al., 1984; Greene et al., 1984; King and Greene, 1984; King
et al., 1985; Press and Greene, 1984) making it possible to
carry out either ER enzyme immuno-assays (ER-EIA) or ER immunocytochemical assays (ER-ICA) based on ER antigenic site detection. We undertook a prospective study in a large series of
breast carcinomas using this new method with monoclonal anti-ER
antibody (H 222S p½) in conjunction with an immunoperoxidase
method. Our objective was to compare an ER immunocytochemical
assay with current biochemical assays, to study variations in ER
distribution in tumors using a computerized system for immunostaining analysis and, as accurately as possible, to delineate
intracellular distribution of immunoreactive ER using immunoelectron microscopy.

Laminin, a structural glycoprotein specific for basement
membranes, has been reported to play a role in the adhesion of
cells to the matrix (Liotta et al., 1983; Liotta, 1984, Terranova et al., 1980; Vlodavsky and Gospodarowicz, 1981). Because of
the functional and structural roles of basement membranes, the
immunohistochemical study (Albrechtsen et al., 1981; Barsky et
al., 1983; Burtin et al., 1982; Ekblom et al., 1984; Forster et
al., 1984; Gusterson et al., 1982; Kirkpatrick and d'Ardenne,
1984; Nielsen et al., 1983; Siegal et al., 1981) of laminin distribution in carcinomas constitutes a new approach to the understanding of tumor-cell invasion. Using fresh or frozen tissue
samples and well-characterized antibodies, the objective of this
study was to delineate the precise distribution of laminin by

light and electron microscopy under optimal technical conditions for antigen preservation.

MATERIALS AND METHODS

Materials

Samples of breast tissue which was surgically removed for cosmetic reduction (non-neoplastic breast) or for breast carcinoma were collected recently (1983 to 1985) from the pathology departments of Timone Hospital and the Institut Paoli Calmettes. Carcinomas were typed histologically according to the WHO classification (1981) and graded according to the Scarff-Bloom-Richardson grading system (1957) as used routinely. Cytosolic ER content was measured by the dextran-coated charcoal assay as previously described (Martin et al., 1978, 1979). Tumors with less than 10 fmol/mg protein were considered negative and, with 10 or more fmol/mg protein, positive.

Tissue and cells from other sources (thyroid, gastric mucosa, immature placenta and decidua) in which laminin staining had previously been reported (Charpin et al., 1985; Miettinen and Virtanen, 1984) served as positive tissue controls. MCF7 and basement membrane-producing PFHR9 cell lines were used as positive controls for ER and laminin detection respectively, in the electron microscope immunostaining procedure.

Tissue preparations

For light microscopy studies, the specimens were rapidly frozen (within 15 min in the operating room) in liquid nitrogen and stored embedded in OCT (Tissue-Tek, Miles) at -80°C. Tumor blocks were cut into 8 μm sections and then mounted on glass slides coated with the tissue adhesive provided in the ER-ICA kit. The sections were immediately fixed for 10 min. in 3.7% formaldehyde in phosphate-buffered saline (PBS), washed for 10 min. in PBS, subsequently fixed for 4 min. in methanol at -25°C and 2 min. in acetone at -25°C, then washed for 5 min. in PBS. One section from each block was processed. In 5 cases, 10 sections from the same tissue block were tested.

For electron microscopy, tumor fragments removed in the operating room were immediately cut into 5x5x2mm sections and fixed as described above. Thick sections of one hundred microns were cut with a Vibratome (Lancer 1000). The pre-embedding method was also applied to Vibratome sections obtained from frozen tissue blocks. Immunostaining was performed on free-floating sections in Petri dishes, using the same procedure as for light microscopy. The sections were then post-fixed in 1% osmium tetroxide solution (30 min.), dehydrated and embedded in araldite. Ultrathin sections were obtained using a diamond knife, then collected on 300-mesh copper grids and examined with a JEOL 1200 EX electron microscope.

Immunostaining procedure

For estrogen receptor detection, immunostaining was performed according to the method by King et al., (1985) using an
ABBOTT ER-ICA kit (ABBOTT Diagnostic Products GmbH, Wiesbaden-
Delkenheim, West Germany). Briefly, the sections were incubated
for 15 min. with the blocking reagent to suppress non-specific
binding, then, for 30 min. with monoclonal anti-ER antibody
H222SP' rinsed for 2x5 min. in PBS, then incubated for 30 min.
with the bridging antibody, rinsed for 2x5 min. in PBS and
incubated for 30 min. with the peroxidase anti-peroxidase
complex (PAP), rinsed in PBS, finally incubated for 6 min. in
chromogen (DAB and 0.06% hydrogen peroxide in PBS) and counterstained with Harris'hematoxylin. Negative controls were assessed using PBS and ER-ICA kit control serum (normal rat IgC) instead of the specific monoclonal anti-ER. MCF7 cells served as
positive controls.

For laminin detection, polyclonal and monoclonal anti-
laminin antibodies were used. Immunoperoxidase staining was
performed with avidin-biotin-peroxidase complex (ABC) kits
(Vector Laboratories, Institut Pasteur, Paris, France) as described previously (Charpin et al., 1982, 1985). Briefly, the
sections were incubated, first, with normal goat or rabbit serum, and then, with rabbit polyclonal or monoclonal antilamine
antibodies. The sections were subsequently incubated with biotin-labeled goat antirabbit IgG or biotin-labeled rabbit anti-
rat IgG. Endogenous peroxidase activity was blocked with a 0.3
per cent hydrogen peroxide solution for 20 min. before incubation with ABC and staining with 3-amino-9-ethyl carbazole
(Sigma). The slides were counterstained and mounted in an aqueous glycerine (80 per cent) and gelatin (4 per cent) solution.
Three types of negative controls were used: 1) PBS in place of
the specific antibody to eliminate false positivity due to the
ABC kit reagents, 2) substitution of irrelevant antisera for
the specific laminin antibody; and 3) rabbit and rat sera from
which the anti-laminin component had been removed by absorption
on a murine laminin Sepharose 4B affinity column.

For keratin detection, polyclonal anti-keratin antibody
(Labsystem) and Avidin Biotin Glucose Oxydase (Vector Laboratories) were used.

Immunostaining quantitative analysis

In each section a semi-quantitative method was used to
evaluate the immunocytochemical staining by means of a double
grading system: (a) staining intensity (SI): 0 to 3+, b) percentage of positive cells (PC) or areas: 1 = 1% to 30%, 2 = 31%
to 70%, 3 = 71% to 100%. This easily and routinely performable
semi-quantitative method of immunostaining evaluation was compared with a computerized system of image analysis in 20 tumors
and in MCF7 cytospins. This system, previously referred to as
SAMBA 200 (TITN) (Brugal, 1984; Seigneurin et al., 1984) provides the accurate percentages of positive areas and histograms of

200

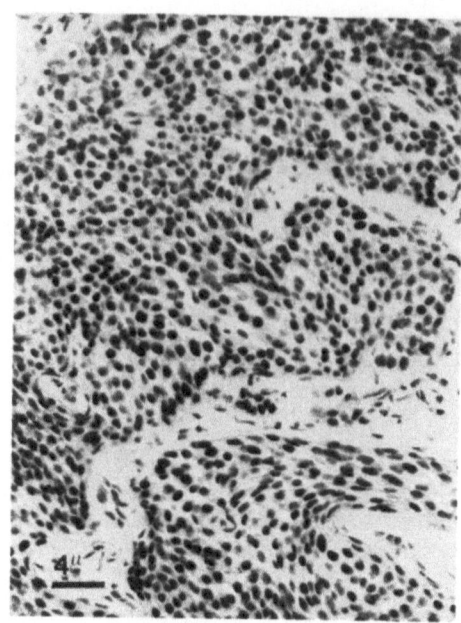

Fig. 1a: Immunostaining with monoclonal anti-ER antibodies
(ER-ICA, ABBOTT Lab.) Positive staining is observed
in tumor cell nuclei and is irregularly distributed
in tumors. In this case, 64% of ER-positive cell areas
are observed.

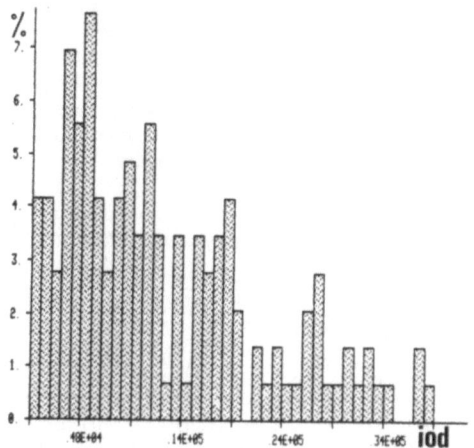

Fig. 1b: Histogram of Integral Optical Density (IOD) evaluated
by the computerized system of image analysis referred
to as SAMBA 200. IOD measures the staining intensity in
positive cells. The histogram corresponds to the case
illustrated above.

the staining intensity distribution (histograms of integral optical density, IOD). In this analysis, several fields on the same slide were examined to evaluate total cell areas (counterstained areas) and epithelial cell areas (positive keratin immunostained areas). For ER and laminin-positive immunostaining, thresholds were first determined on the TV screen and the count was then automatically performed.

RESULTS

1. ER IMMUNODETECTION

Positive immunostaining distribution

In positive tumors, the staining was observed in the nuclei of carcinomatous cells or of epithelial cells of non-tumorous adjacent breast tissue. Positive cells were heterogeneously distributed in the tissue sections in all cases. Staining intensity varied within a given tumor and the percentage of imlunostained cells varied among the positive cases (Fig. 1).

Immunoelectron microscopy provided more accurate data on intracellular immunoreactive ER distribution. This method consistently showed positive intranuclear immunostaining. Positive staining, consisting of osmiophilic black dots, was variable and irregularly distributed in the nuclei. It usually appeared diffusely spread throughout the nucleoplasm and did not involve the nucleolus. Positive cells were observed adjacent to completely negative cells, but generally positive cells were gathered in clumps or sheets.

Multiple sections from one tissue block displayed the same immunostaining pattern. No positive immunostaining was observed in negative controls, ruling out nonspecific reactions due to the kit reagents. Immunostaining intensity was unchanged when tumors were stored for more than a year (1 to 4 years).

Semi-quantitative evaluation

Among the 98 carcinomas tested, 70% were ER-ICA positive and 30% ER-ICA negative. The staining intensity (SI) in positive cases increased with cytosolic ER mean range levels: SI = 1 (31.5%) - ER mean: 63 fmol/mg prot.; SI = 2 (33%) - ER mean: 145 fmol/mg prot.; SI = 3 (35.5%) - ER mean: 246 fmol/mg prot.; correlation SI/ER, $p < 0.001$. Similarly, the percentage of positive cells (PC) increased significantly ($p < 0.01$) with ER levels: PC = 1 (19%) - ER mean = 33 fmol/mg prot.; PC = 3 (42%) - ER mean = 215 fmol/mg prot.

ER immunostaining and ER biochemical assay

Cytosolic ER levels were > 10 fmol/mg prot. in 74% of the tumors included in our series. This rate of positive ER tumors correlates with previous reports.

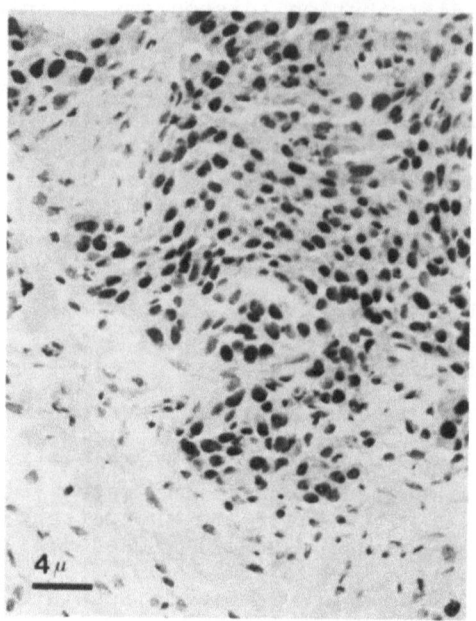

Fig. 1c: Immunostaining with monoclonal anti-ER antibodies;
34% of the cell areas are ER-positive.

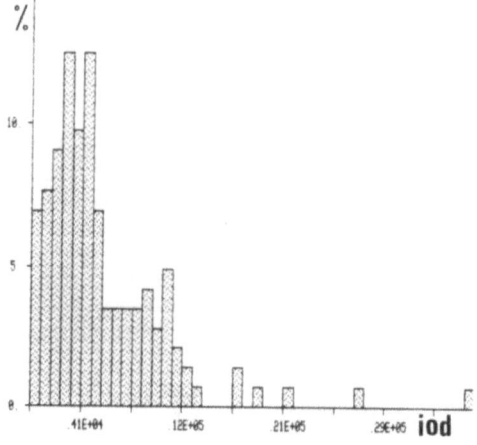

Fig. 1d: IOD histogram corresponding to Fig. 1c.

TABLE 1

Case number:		ER - ICA			
		Semi-quantitative		SAMBA 200	
		area	SI	area	IOD
1	:	++	+++	10%	4784
2	:	++	++	61%	54131
3	:	+++	+++	30%	21188
4	:	++	+++	13%	9186
5	:	+++	+++	89%	20442
6	:	+++	+++	64%	76179
7	:	+++	+++	34%	18459
8	:	++	++	17%	16122
9	:	++	+++	10%	4323
10	:	+	++	2%	14348

Area : percentage of immunostained areas (+ to +++; or %)
SI   : staining intensity (+ to +++)
IOD : integral optical density

In 88% of the cases, ER-ICA results correlated with binding assays but in 12% of the cases, this was not the case.
Reexamination of results suggests that discrepancies between
the methods could be attributed to the fact that the tumor fragments sampled for ER-ICA and biochemical assays were not the
same or that the tumor samples contained very few tumor cells
which could be detected by ER-ICA only.

ER computerized (SAMBA 200) quantitative analysis

MCF7 cytospins, which served as positive controls, were
first evaluated by this method. SAMBA 200 analysis showed that
the percentage of positive cells varied from 30% to 90% depending on the slides. Most of these variations were not correctly
evaluated by simple subjective semi-quantitative analysis. In
10 tumors, the histogram of integral optical density in an ER-
positive area was established, as shown in fig. 1. Also, the
percentage of ER-positive areas versus keratin-positive epithelial areas was compared to semi-quantitative analysis (Table 1).
Some discrepancies were consistently observed; in particular,
the percentage of positive cells evaluated by semi-quantitative
analysis was over-scored when staining intensity was high and
vice-versa.

2. LAMININ IMMUNODETECTION

Laminin distribution

In non-neoplastic breast tissue, only extracellular lami-

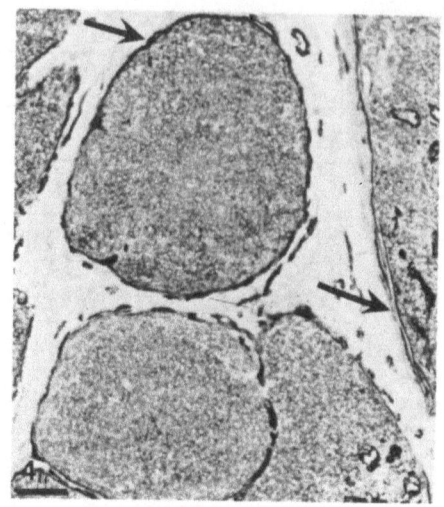

Fig. 2a: Double immunostaining procedure, anti-laminin with
avidin-biotin-peroxidase, and anti-keratin with avidin-
biotin-glucose-oxidase. Positive laminin staining is
observed in the basement membrane only and keratin
staining is observed in the cell cytoplasm.
In this case, positive laminin staining (33% laminin-
positive area versus keratin within epithelial cell
area) consists of a virtually continuous and often
thickened or multilayered linear structure (arrow) with
visible components of tumors around ducts.

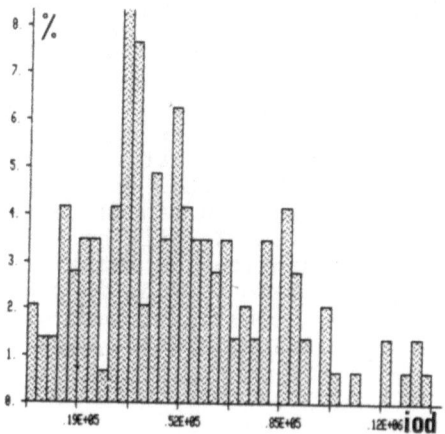

Fig. 2b: SAMBA analysis of Integral Optical Density (IOD) of
laminin immunostaining (IOD = 50589).

nin staining was visible as regular continuous linear structures in basement membranes around ducts and lobules. Staining was also observed in basement membranes around blood vessels. No intracellular staining was observed.

In carcinomas, laminin staining was also visible, but only
extra-cellularly. Staining, however, was irregular in distribution. In intraductal carcinomas and in the intraductal component of invasive carcinomas, laminin staining produced a continuous linear pattern around the involved ducts but, in contrast
to that seen in non-neoplastic breast tissue, it appeared irregular and thickened, as shown by darker staining. Staining occurred along the epithelial cell layers in contact with the stroma. No staining was observed in the deeper cell layers of the
involved ducts, although some staining was visible in the basement membranes of small blood vessels (Fig. 2).

In invasive carcinomas, the staining pattern was heterogenous, even within individual tumors. Staining was discontinuous
around the epithelial cells infiltrating the stroma, with gaps
and irregular thickening. Some areas were devoid of periepithe-
lial laminin positivity. In very rare cases, the tumors were
devoid of staining, except for the basement membranes of blood
vessels (Fig. 2).

In carcinomas of all types, intense immunostaining of the
blood vessels was seen with antilaminins. On high-power magnification, the basement membranes appeared thickened or multilayered and displayed a continuous linear or annular pattern.

The electron microscope study showed that in non-neoplastic breast tissue, laminin staining was regularly distributed
in the basement membranes, although some infolding was observed.
No intracellular staining was detected. Both epithelial and
vascular basement membranes were continuous and of consistent
thickness. In carcinomas gaps and breaches in laminin immunostaining were observed. The strong staining observed by light
microscopy corresponded clearly to basement membrane thickening
and multilayering. Although this pattern was visible mainly in
intraductal carcinomas, it was also observed in invasive carcinomas. Some tumor areas lacked laminin staining. No staining
was observed between or around individual tumor cells, or within the cytoplasm. Most blood vessels had abnormal basement membranes with a multilayered pattern, but no gaps or breaches in
the basement membrane were seen. Endothelial cells never displayed laminin intracellular positivity.

Laminin quantitative analysis

The semi-quantitative analysis of laminin staining was
compared with computerized analysis using the SAMBA (Table 2).
As described for ER-positive staining, laminin-positive areas
were compared to total cell areas (evaluated by the counterstain) and epithelial cell areas (keratin-positive areas). Comparison of the percentage of positive laminin areas and the
histograms (Fig. 2) of staining intensity evaluated by the

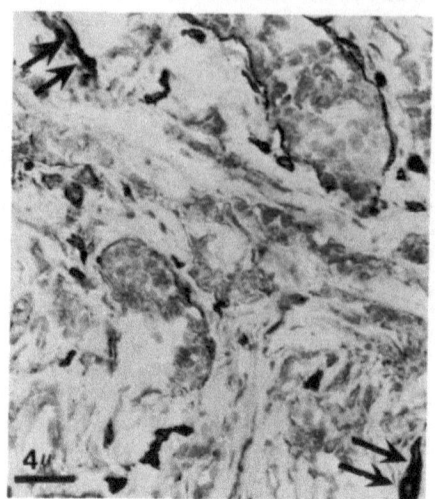

Fig. 2c: Double immunostaining procedure, as in fig. 2a.
In this invasive high-grade tumor laminin immunostaining is visible in a few places occurring in a discontinuous pattern (arrow). Note the strong immunostaining around vessels (double arrow). (6% laminin-positive
area, versus keratin-positive epithelial cell area).

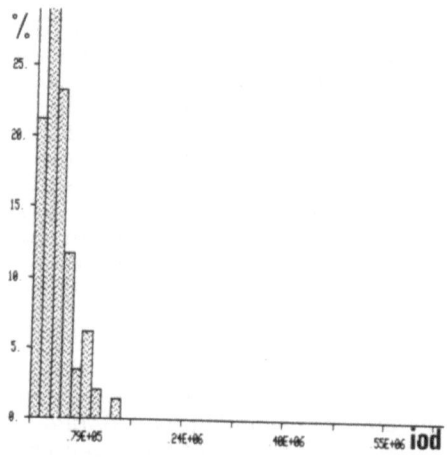

Fig. 2d: SAMBA analysis of Integral Optical Density of laminin
immunostaining (IOD = 1885).

TABLE 2

Laminin immunostaining analysis: comparison of semi-quantitative and computerized SAMBA 200 analysis in ten cases.

	LAMININ-POSITIVE IMMUNOSTAINING			
	Semi-quantitative analysis		SAMBA 200 analysis	
	area	SI	area	IOD
1	++	+	7%	3800
2	+++	+++	33%	50589
3	++	++	20%	17452
4	+	+	2%	2132
5	+	++	26%	2817
6	++	++	20%	5337
7	++	+++	12%	10609
8	+++	+++	39%	40972
9	++	++	55%	6174
10	+	++	6%	885

Area : percentage of immunostained area (+ to +++ ou %)
SI   : staining intensity (+ to +++)
IOD : Integral Optical Density

two methods (Table 2) showed that there was significant differences between cases which were not or erroneously detected by
the semi-quantitative analysis.

DISCUSSION

Until very recently, the information about subcellular estrogen receptor distribution and quantitative assays for ER were based on the binding of radioactively labeled steroids. The
recent development of a number of monoclonal antibodies
(Desombre et al., 1984; Greene et al., 1984; King and Greene,
1984; King et al., 1985) against ER provides a new approach to
the determination of ER based on the detection of antigenic
sites instead of the binding of the labelled hormone. Monoclonal antibodies make it possible to detect occupied and unoccu-
pied sites (Desombre et al., 1984) and are suitable for light
and electron microscope immunocytochemical assays. This is particularly useful to assess ER intracellular localization and ER-
positive cell distribution in tissues.

Also ER-ICA permits assessment of ER heterogeneity among
cells or regions within a tissue or lesion, in contrast to binding assays which measure only the average receptor level in
cell homogenates.

Breast carcinomas are heterogeneous within their histologic types and their degree of differentiation. Moreover, tumors enclose heterogeneous cell populations as demonstrated particularly by a variety of heterogeneously distributed epithelial cell-associated antigens: some clones enclose so-called differentiation antigens such as casein (Bussolati et al., 1975), lactalbumin (Bailey et al., 1982), gross cystic disease fluid protein (GCDFP) (Mazoujian et al., 1983). other clones contain CEA or lactoferrin (Walker, 1980; Wurster et al., 1980). Similarly, immunocytochemical assays showing that each tumor is a pool of ER+ and ER- cells, should permit a deeper insight into hormone responsiveness. The heterogeneous laminin distribution in tissue expresses the heterogeneity of tumors and the variable ability of tumor cells to produce basement membrane components. In all types of tumors, in situ or invasive, only some tumor cells are able to produce the basement membrane component. These cells, however, are consistently adjacent to the stroma. This appears to be a necessary factor for basement membrane synthesis. The presence of gaps or disruptions or the total lack of basement membrane in some areas of invasive carcinomas, may reflect decreased synthesis or decreased assembly of secreted components or, alternatively, proteolysis resulting from tumor cell-derived proteases, such as collagenase IV (Liotta et al., 1983; Siegal et al., 1981). Basement membrane synthesis and lysis result therefore from interactions of biochemical factors between epithelial cells and the interstitium.

Most of the histochemical or immunohistochemical techniques which have been used for ER detection (Dandliker et al., 1978; Kurzon and Sternberger, 1978; Lee, 1978; Nenci et al., 1976) in tissue sections have previously been shown to be inconsistent with the biochemical detection of estrogen receptors (Chamness et al., 1980). In contrast, ER-ICA correlates well with binding assays, suggesting its potential value for anti-estrogen response prediction. In our study, ER-ICA correlated with binding assays in 88% of the cases; this is similar to the findings of King et al., (1985) and Pertschuk et al., (1985) (84% and 86%, respectively). In our material, there was strong evidence that differences between both assays could result from inadequate tissue sampling indicating that ER-ICA reliability could be improved by rigorous quality control of tissue sampling.

Although the ER immunocytochemical assay basically constitutes a qualitative analysis of ER in tissues and is complementary to quantitative evaluation of binding assays, promising results may be achieved by improving this qualitative analysis by using immunocytochemical grades and scores which can serve as indices for correlation with biochemical assays and clinical data. Attention must be focused, however, on the fact that immunostaining quantification, even when performed by trained pathologists, is a method mainly involving subjective appraisal which may lead to erroneous and non-reproducible results. In this respect, the use of a computerized system of image analysis provides more accurate and reliable data as shown by our preliminary results with the SAMBA 200.

Similarly, no reliable correlation between laminin immunostaining and clinical data can be established without a reproducible and accurate method of evaluating staining results.
Nevertheless, computerized analysis of immunostained basement
membrane components and proteolytic enzymes in tumors using the
SAMBA 200, will ensure a better evaluation of the capacity of
tumor cells to diffuse and invade.

SUMMARY

An estrogen receptor immunocytochemical assay (ER-ICA) was
applied to 115 breast carcinomas and the results were compared
to those of steroid binding assays performed on cytosol extracts of the same tumors. Also laminin (lam) distribution was
studied in the same tumors. Immunoperoxidase (PAP) staining
was performed on frozen sections using mouse monoclonal antibody to estrogen receptor (H 226SPγ) whereas anti-laminin antibodies avidin-biotin-peroxydase complex, ABC kit were used for
lam detection. A pre-embedding method was selected for the im-
muno-electron microscope study. A semi-quantitative analysis
and a computerized image analysis system (SAMBA 200 TITN) were
used to evaluate positive ER and lam immunostaining. Positive
ER immunostaining was always observed in the nuclei of tumor
cells and of normal cells in adjacent breast tissue.The immunostaining pattern differed from one tumor to another, due to
variations in either the intensity or the percentage of positive cells. When immunohistochemical staining was compared to
biochemical assay, there was a 88% correlation, and staining intensity and the percentage of positive cells significantly increased (p $<$ 0.01) with cytosolic ER levels and were independent of cellularity. Lam was observed within vascular and epithelial basement membranes (BMs). Lam staining displayed a continuous linear pattern in intraductal carcinomas but was heterogeneously distributed with a discontinuous linear pattern in
invasive carcinomas. No intracellular lam staining was detected
The EM study showed lam immunostaining (LI) in the lamina densa
of BMs in non-neoplastic breast tissue. In tumors, LI often revealed abnormal multilayered BMs in blood vessels in the tumor
stroma. These results indicate that: (1) ER-ICA is the most reliable histochemical method to-date for ER detection and correlates in 88% of the cases with ER biochemical assays (2) ER-ICA
provides additional information on heterogeneous ER distribution within tumors (3) As a qualitative method, ER-ICA is unable
to replace quantitative ER determinations obtained by biochemical assay (4) ER-ICA, based on ER antigenic site detection, is
complementary to biochemical assay, based on ER functional site
determinations (5) laminin immunostaining constitutes a new approach to heterogeneous BM changes occurring in carcinomas and
permits a better understanding of cell diffusion processes and
of stroma-tumor cell interactions: the consistent extracellular
lam distribution in contact with the stroma, indicates that the
latter plays an important role in the assembly of BM components

210

(6) The SAMBA 200 provides a reliable, accurate method of evaluating the percentage of immunostained cells and areas.

ACKNOWLEDGEMENT

Supported by grants from INSERM and the University of
Marseille.

REFERENCES

1. Albrechtsen, R., Nielsen, M., Wewer, V., Engwall, E., and
Ruoslahi, E. Basement membrane changes in breast cancer de-
tected by immunohistochemical staining for laminin. Cancer
Res., 41: 5076-5081, 1981.

2. Barsky, S.H., Siegal, G.P., Jannotta, F. and Liotta, L.A.
Loss of basement membrane components by invasive tumors but
not by their benign counterparts. Lab. Invest., 49: 140-147,
1983.

3. Bailey, A.J., Sloane, J.P., Trickey, B.S. and Ormerod, M.G.
An immunocytochemical study of alpha lactalbumin in human
breast tissue. J. Pathology, 137: 13-23, 1982.

4. Bloom, H.J.G. and Richardson, W.W. Histological grading
and prognosis in breast cancer. Br. J. Cancer, 11: 359-367,
1957.

5. Burtin, P., Chavanel, G., Foidart J.M. et al. Antigens of
the basement membrane and the peritumoral stroma in human
colonic adenocarcinomas: an immunofluorescence study. Int. J.
Cancer, 30: 13-20, 1982.

6. Bussolati, G., Pich, A. and Alfani, V. Immunofluorescence
detection of casein in human mammary dysplastic and neoplastic tissues. Virchows Arch.(Path. Anat. and Histol.), 365:
15-21, 1975.

7. Brugal, G. Image analysis of microscopic preparations.In:
Methods and Achievements in Experimental Pathology. Jasmin,
G., Proschek, eds, S. Karger, Basel, 1984, p.p. 1-33.

8. Charpin, C., Bhan, A.K., Zurawski, V.R. and Scully, R.E.
Carcinoembryonic antigen (CEA) and carbohydrate determinent
(19-9) localization in 121 primary and metastatic ovarian
tumors: an immunohistochemical study with the use of monoclonal antibodies. Int. J. Gynecol. Pathol. 1: 231-245, 1982.

9. Charpin, C., Kopp, F., Pourreau-Schneider, N., Lissitzky,
J.C., Lavaut, M.N., Andonian, C., Martin, P.M. and Toga, M.
Laminin distribution in human decidua and immature placenta.
Am. J. Gynecol. Obstet. 151: 822-826, 1985.

211

10. Chamness, G.C., Mercer, W.D. and Mc Guire, W.L. Are histochemical methods for estrogen receptor valid? J. Histochem. Cytochem. **28**: 792-798, 1980.

11. Dandliker, W.B., Brauwn, R.J., Hsu, M.L., Brauwn, P.N., Levin, J., Meyers, C.Y. and Kolb, V.M. Investigation of hormone-receptor interactions by means of fluorescence labelling. Cancer Res., **38**: 4212-4218, 1978.

12. Desombre, E.R., Greene, G.L., King, W.J. and Jensen, E.V. Estrogen receptors, antibodies and hormone dependent cancer. In: Hormones and Cancer, Alan R. Liss, Inc., New York, 1984, p.p. 1-21.

13. Ekblom, P., Miettinen, M., Forsman, L. and Anderssen, L.C. Basement membrane and apocrine epithelial antigens in differential diagnosis between tubular carcinomas and sclerosing adenosis of the breast. J. Clin. Pathol. **37**: 357-363, 1984.

14. Forster, S., Talbot, I.C. and Critchley, D.R. Laminin and fibronectin in rectal adenocarcinoma: relationship to tumour grade stage and metastasis. Br. J. Cancer **50**: 51-61, 1984.

15. Greene, G.L., Sobel, N.B., King, W.J. and Jensen, E.V. Immunohistochemical studies of estrogen receptors. J. Steroid Biochem. **20**: 51-56, 1984.

16. Gusterson, B.A., Warburton, M.J., Mitchell, D., Elleson, M., Neville, A.M. and Rudland, P.S. Distribution of myoepithelial cells and basement membrane proteins in the normal breast and in benign and malignant breast diseases. Cancer Res. **42**: 4763-4770, 1982.

17. King, W.J. and Greene, G.L. Monoclonal antibodies localize estrogen receptor in the nuclei of target cells. Nature 307: 745-747, 1984.

18. King, W.J., Desombre, E.R., Jensen, E.V. and Greene, G.L. Comparison of immunocytochemical and steroid binding assays for estrogen receptor in human breast tumors. Cancer Res. **45**: 293-304, 1985.

19. Kirkpatrick, P. and d'Ardenne, A. Effects of fixation and enzymatic digestion on the immunohistochemical demonstration of laminin and fibronectin in paraffin embedded tissue. Clin. Pathol., **37**: 639-644, 1984.

20. Kurzon, R.M. and Sternberger, L.A. Estrogen receptor immunocytochemistry. J. Histochem. Cytochem. **26**: 803-809, 1978.

21. Liotta, L.A., Rao, C.N. and Barsk, S.H. Tumour invasion and the extracellular matrix. Lab. Invest, **49**: 636-649, 1983.

22. Liotta, L.A. Tumor invasion and metastases: role of the basement membrane. Am. J. Pathol. 117: 339-347, 1984.

23. Lee, Cytochemical study of estrogen receptor in human mammary cancer. Am. J. Clin. Pathol., 70: 197-203, 1978.

24. Martin, P.M., Rolland, P.M., Jacquemier, J., Rolland, A.M. and Toga, M. Routine analysis of multiple steroid receptors in human breast cancer. I. Technical features. Biomedecine 28: 278-287, 1978.

25. Martin, P.M., Rolland, P.M., Jacquemier, J., Rolland, A.M. and Toga, M. Multiples steroids receptors in human cancer. III. Relationship between steroid receptors and the activity of carcinomas throughout the pathological features. Cancer Chemoth. Pharmacol. 2: 115-120, 1979.

26. Mazoujian, G., Pinkus, G.S., Davis, S. and Haagensen, D.E. Immunohistochemistry of a gross cystic disease fluid protein (GCDFP 15) of the breast. A marker of apocrine epithelium and breast carcinomas with apocrine features. Am. J. Pathol. 110: 105-112, 1983.

27. Miettinen, M. and Virtanen, J. Expression of laminin in thyroid gland and thyroid tumors: an immunohistochemical study. Int. J. Cancer 34: 27-30, 1984.

28. Nenci, I., Beccati, M.D., Piffanelli, A. and Lanza, G. Detection and dynamic localization of estradiol receptor complexes in intact target cells by immunofluorescence technique. J. Steroid Biochem. 7: 505-511, 1976.

29. Nielsen, M., Christensen, L. and Albrechtsen, R. The basement membrane component laminin in breast carcinomas and axillary lymph node metastases. Acta Pathol. Microbiol. Immunol. Scand. 91: 257-264, 1983.

30. Press, M.F. and Greene, G.L. An immunocytochemical method for demonstrating estrogen receptor in human uterus using monoclonal antibodies to human estrophilin. Lab. Invest 50: 480-486, 1984.

31. Pertschuk, L.P., Eisenberg, K.B., Carter, A.C. and Feldman, J.G. Immunohistologic localization of estrogen receptors in breast cancer with monoclonal antibodies. Cancer 55: 1513-1518, 1985.

32. Seigneurin, D., Gauvin, C. and Brugal G. Quantitative analysis of human marrow granulocytic cell lineage using SAMBA 200 image processor. Analytical Quantitative Cytology 6: 168-177, 1984.

33. Siegal, G.P., Barsky, S.H., Terranova, V.P. and Liotta, L.A. Stages of neoplastic transformation of human breast tissue as monitored by dissolution of basement membrane components.

Invasion&Metastasis 1: 54-65, 1981.

34. Terranova, V.P. Rodubach, D.H. and Martin, G.R. Role of laminin in the attachment of PAM 212 (epithelial) cells to basement membrane collagen. Cell 22: 719-726, 1980.

35. Walker, R.A. Demonstration of carcino embryonic antigen in human breast carcinomas by the immunoperoxidase technique. J. Clin. Pathol., 33:356-360, 1980.

36. WHO., World Health Organization. International Tumor Classification of Breast Tumors, WHO, Second Ed. Geneva, 1981.

37. Vlodavsky, J. and Gospodarowicz, D. Respective roles of laminin and fibronectin in adhesion of human carcinomas and sarcoma cells. Nature 289: 304-307, 1981.

38. Wurster, K., Heberling, D. and Rapp, W. Carcinoembryonic antigen (CEA) and lactoferrin (LF) in benign and malignant disease of the breast. A contribution to the immunohistochemical demonstration of marker substances. Geburtshilfe Frauenheilk 40: 412-422, 1980.

ESTROGEN-RECEPTOR HISTOCHEMISTRY: A CRITICAL STUDY

L.J. VAN BOGAERT AND J. ABARCA

Avenue Capitaine Piret, 66, 1150 Brussels, Belgium

Estrogen-receptor (ER) assays are nowadays widely used over the world. They are carried out either by the dextran-charcoal (DCC) or by the sucrose-gradient sedimentation rate methods. False negative results have been reported by both techniques. On the other hand, it is well known that ER-positive breast tumors may be non-responders to hormone therapy, and that ER-negative cases have been shown to respond to anti-estrogens.

In front of these apparent contradictions, studies have shown that ER may be occupied by endogenous estrogens already bound to the receptor site. Moreover, it has been said that ER are "functional" only if they induce the synthesis of Progesterone-receptors (PgR). Hence, the ER complex must be translocated inside of the nucleus to become functional.

Parallely, immunocyto- and immunohisto-chemical approaches have been developped to demonstrate estrogen-binding-sites (EBS) in target tissues, especially breast tumors. At the present time, however, a lot of variations and differences do appear, not only insofar as methods, but also as results and their interpretation are concerned.

Thus, a critical immunohisto-chemical study was undertaken using 5 different kits of the same origin and 28 breast cancers, from which biochemical assays of ER and PgR were available. BT-20 breast cancer cells, known to be devoid of ER, and MCF-7 breast cancer cells, known to be ER-positive, were used as control. The originally recommended technical conditions were tested, but were also modified in order to improve the results (Tables 1 and 2). In the 4 first series different ER and PgR positive or negative tumors were used. In the fifth experiment, the 7 cancers with the highest ER content were selected, and controls were carried out by pre-incubation in the anti-estrogen tamoxifen.

The results are shown on Tables 3 to 7. The main conclusions which can be drawn from the results are the following: With the 3 first kits only cytoplasmic labeling was obtained. Immunostaining was heterogeneous with kit 1 and 3, faint with kit 1, or more or less intense with kit 2 and 3. Nuclear and cytoplasmic labeling were observed homogeneously with kit 4. No realationship was observed between immunostaining and biochemical assays. The fifth series consisted of tumors exhibiting the highest levels of ER. Tamoxifen was unable to block immunostaining. Labeling was intense but heterogeneous at the cytoplasmic level. Nuclear immunostaining was encountered in a few number of cells. MCF-7 nuclei were rather heterogeneously stained.

The main conclusion which can be drawn from these experiments is that immunostaining with the kits we used was dependent on the individual kit without clear relationship with the biochemical assessment of ER. Other experiments are under way to check the value of other kits from different factories. At the present time pathologists, should be careful and critical in the use of ER immunostaining.

ACKNOWLEDGMENTS

Supported by a grant from the Fondation Lefebvre.

REFERENCES

Van Bogaert, L.J., Present status of estrogen-receptor cytochemistry, Acta Histochem., 74, 37-43, 1984.

Van Bogaert, L.J., Present status of estrogen-receptor immuno-histochemistry, Acta Histochem., 76, 29-35, 1985.

Van Bogaert, L.J., and Abarca, J., Estrogen receptors in breast pathology, Path. Res. Pract., 180, 320, 1985 (abstract).

Van Bogaert, L.J., Estrogen-binding-sites and estrophilin histochemistry and their correlation with estrogen receptor biochemistry, submitted for publication.

PRELIMINARY STEPS

FIXATIVE	HEAT-FIXATION	REHYDRATATION	INHIBITION EPO	BACKGROUND INHIBITION
Bouin or formalin 10%	60' at 60°	toluol 5' methanol 100% 2x3' 95% 2x3'	H_2O_2 3.0% 5' at 20°C	normal sheep serum 20' at 20°C
formalin 4% (in PBS and sucrose)	idem	toluol 2x5' methanol 100% 2x3' 95% 2x3' tap water	H_2O_2 3.% 5' at 20 or 37°	normal serum 10'-20'-30' at 20 or 37°C or omitted
Bouin 2h at 37°C 2h at 20°C	idem	idem	idem	normal serum 20' at 37°C
Bouin 4h at 20°C	idem	idem	FRESH sol.	idem

TABLE 1

IMMUNOPEROXIDASE LABELING

SERIES	PRIMARY ANTIBODY	SECONDARY ANTIBODY	LABELING REAGENT	CONTRAST STAINING
1	20' at 203C	30' at 373C	AEC 40' at 203C	Haematoxylin 3' Tap water, PBS Glycerin jelly
2	30' at 373C	30' at 373C	AEC 30' at 373C	idem
3	15' at 373C 30' at 373C	15' at 373C 15' at 373C	AEC 5' at 373C DAB 5' at 203C	idem or without counterstain
4	15' at 373C	15' at 373C	DAB 5' at 203C	cfr (1)

TABLE 2

Kit 1 (Immulok Histoset)

CASE	ER*	PgR	LABELING		
BT-20	(-)		-/+	cytoplasm	heterogeneous
MCF-7	(+)		-/+	cytoplasm	heterogeneous
1	1,000	355.5(++)	-/+	cytoplasm	heterogeneous
2	62.61(++)	341.9(++)	-/++	cytoplasm	heterogeneous
3	(-)	89.6(+)	+	cytoplasm	heterogeneous
4	275(+++)	158.2(+)	-/+	cytoplasm	heterogeneous
5	946.6(+++)	1017.1(+++)	(-)		
6	(-)	121.2(+)	-/+	cytoplasm	heterogeneous
7	23.25(+)	194.3(+)	-/+	cytoplasm	heterogeneous
8	(-)	126.5(+)	-/+	cytoplasm	heterogeneous

* results in fmol/mg protein
  between brackets : significant +, highly significant +++

TABLE 3

Kit 2 (Histoset ORTHO 586025 E)

CASE	ER	PgR	LABELING		
MCF-7	(+)		+/++	cytoplasm	+/- homogeneous
9	294.2(+++)	144.5(+)	+/++	cytoplasm	homogeneous
10	6.2(+/-)	44.1(-)	+/++	cytoplasm	homogeneous
12	26.2(+)	304.6(++)	+/++	cytoplasm	homogeneous

TABLE 4

Kit 3 (Histoset ORTHO 586025 E)

CASE	ER	PgR	LABELING		
13	48.0(+)	100.4(+/-)	+/++	cytoplasm	+/- heterogen.
14	116.0(+++)	156.0(+)	+/++	cytoplasm	+/- heterogen.
15	5.0(+/-)	92.0(+/-)	++	cytoplasm	+/- heterogen.
16			+/++	cytoplasm	+/- heterogen.

TABLE 5

Kit 4 (Histoset ORTHO 586025 2E)

CASE	ER	PgR	LABELING	
17	2.89(-)	67.52(-)	nuclear + cyto.	homogeneous
18	12.86(+)	94.24(+/-)	nuclear + cyto.	homogeneous
19	9.21(+/-)	176.99(+)	nuclear + cyto.	homogeneous
20	33.60(+)	76.07(+/-)	nuclear + cyto.	homogeneous
21	14.40(+)	133.13(+/-)	nuclear + cyto.	homogeneous
22	63.54(++)	67.14(-)	nuclear + cyto. '	homogeneous
23*	?	?	nuclear + cyto.	homogeneous
24**	(-)		+/-, very heterogeneous	
25***	(+)		+/-, very heterogeneous	

* male breast cancer, ** BT-20, *** MCF-7

TABLE 6

Kit 5 (Immulok Histoset)

CASE	ER	PgR	LABELING		
1*	1000.		++	cytoplasm	heterogeneous
24	1041.	122.6(+/-)	++	cytoplasm	heterogeneous
5*	946.5	1017.1(+++)	++	cytoplasm	heterogeneous
			+/-	nucleus	
25	565.5	102.3(+/-)	+++	cytoplasm	heterogeneous
			+/-	nucleus	
26	768.8	76.7(+/-)	++	cytoplasm	heterogeneous
27	459.4	104.8(+/-)	++	cytoplasm	heterogeneous
			+	nucleus	
28	543.6	80.8(+/-)	++	cytoplasm	heterogeneous
MCF-7	(+)		+	nucleus	heterogeneous

* cases from kit series 1
(Tamoxifen pretreatment was devoid of blocking effect)

TABLE 7

TAMOXIFEN-INDUCED FLUORESCENCE   AS A PREDICTIVE TEST FOR

HORMONE RESPONSIVENESS OF BREAST CARCINOMA

J. MOURIQUAND[1], M.C. GENEVEY[2], H. BERIEL[2], R. PAYAN[3],
M.A. MERMET[4].

1.Laboratoire de Cytologie, Centre Hospitalier Régional de
  Grenoble, BP 217 X, 38043 Grenoble Cedex,
2.Laboratoire de Physiologie et Pharmacie, Faculté de Médecine,
  Domaine de la Merci, 38700 La Tronche,
3.Service de Gynécologie Obstétrique, Clinique Belledonne,
  Boulevard Gabriel Péri, 38400 Saint Martin d'Hères,
4.Laboratoire d'Histologie et d'Embryologie, Faculté de Médecine de Grenoble, Domaine de la Merci, 38700 La Tronche.

INTRODUCTION

In the past few years, the use of histochemical and immunohistochemical methods has been advocated to demonstrate steroid
receptors in breast tissue or mammary cells obtained by fine-
needle aspiration. These techniques have revealed the heterogeneity of tumor tissue with respect to cell hormone responsiveness (Greene et al., 1984; Lampertico, 1984; Lee, 1981, 1984;
Nenci, 1981; Pertschuk et al., 1981).

The prognostic value of these assays is still a subject of
debate (Mc Carty et al., 1984; Meijer et al., 1982; Penney and
Hawkins, 1982) since it has been shown, for instance, that only
53% of estrogen receptor (ER) positive tumors respond to endocrine therapy (Seibert and Lippman, 1982).

In this paper, we discuss a different predictive test for
hormone responsiveness in breast cancer. The test involves treating breast cancer patients prior to surgery with Tamoxifen,
an anti-estrogen molecule, which is metabolized by hormone responsive cells. The fluorescence of the Tamoxifen molecule or
its metabolites may be assessed from imprints of tumor tissue
at the time of surgery, thereby obtaining a quantitative evaluation of hormone responsive cells (Mouriquand et al., 1981 a,
1983 a, 1985).

MATERIALS AND METHODS

The study was based on 224 Tamoxifen-treated patients. Of
the number, 181 patients presented with operable breast carcinoma, and 16 with relapse of the disease during a long-course
of treatment with Tamoxifen. The latter group served as controls for unresponsive tumor cells. We also included 27 cases

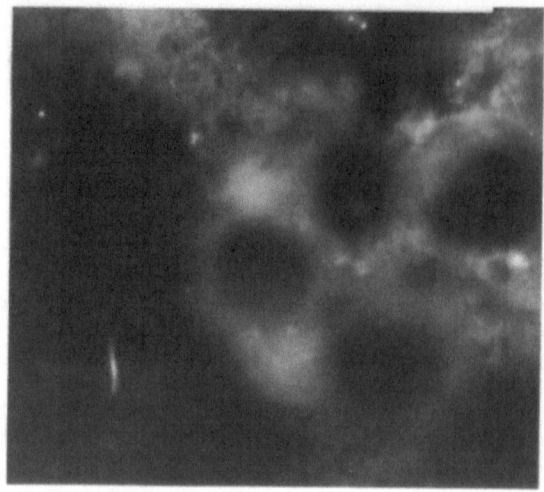

Fig. 1. Tamoxifen-treated breast tumor (21 days). GRADE II
Cytoprognostic classification. Fluorescence-negative
cells. x 1000.

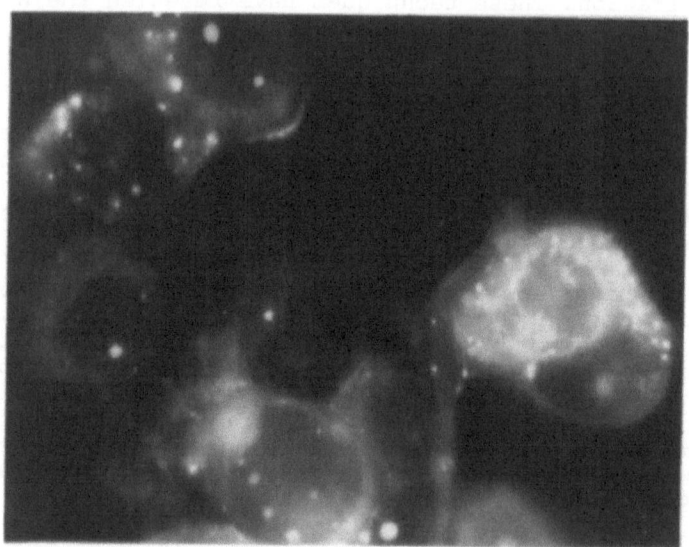

Fig. 2. Tamoxifen-treated breast tumor (14 days). GRADE II
Cytoprognostic classification. Fluorescence-positive
cells, some with intracytoplasmic fluorescent granules
with or without fluorescent nucleoli. x 1000.

of benign breast lesions given Tamoxifen to test the validity
of the method in benign hormone-responsive cells.

The operable breast cancer patients received Tamoxifen
(20 mg/day) from the time of the first, diagnostic, fine-needle
aspiration until surgery (average 10 days).

Twenty five of the 181 carcinomas were excluded from the
study: 4 colloid carcinomas with pronounced autofluorescence
of the colloid substance and 21 because of the small number of
cells on the imprints.

The remaining tumors were grouped according to cytoprognostic criteria (Mouriquand and Pasquier, 1980) Grade I, representing well-differentiated malignant cells (28 cases), Grade II, polymorphous tumor cells (45 cases) and Grade III, anaplastic cancer cells (83 cases). In addition, they were classified according to Bloom and Richardson (1957).

Fine-needle aspiration of breast tumor at the time of the
first examination of the patient was used as a diagnostic procedure and a fluorescence-negative control. At the time of surgery, tumor imprints and smears were prepared and immediately
fixed in equal parts of methanol and acetone and stained by a
hypochromic Papanicolaou staining procedure (Mouriquand et al.,
1981 b). Binding of Tamoxifen or its metabolites to eosin depends on the quality of Harris'hematoxylin and of the EA 50 solution (Merck) and requires differentiation in a hydrochloric
acid solution and omission of alkaline baths.

Cells were successively examined under ordinary light and
after UV excitation (excitation/emission wavelengths of 450-
490/515 nm) for a comparative evaluation. Poorly fixed cells
were rejected because of fluorescence artefacts. Smears were
considered positive when more than 25% of the cells showed yel-
low fluorescent granules within the cytoplasm, sometimes associated with fluorescent nucleoli. Negative cells were dark
green without fluorescent spots (Fig 1 and 2).

Binding of Tamoxifen or its metabolites to eosin was obtained in vitro by shaking two immiscible phases: a slightly
acid aqueous phase containing eosin and a chloroform phase containing Tamoxifen or its metabolites (4 hydroxytamoxifen and
N-desmethyltamoxifen, kindly supplied by ICI Pharma). The fluorescence spectrum was measured and negative controls were obtained for each measurement (Bartoli et al., 1982; Mouriquand
et al., 1983 b).

At the time of surgery, tumor samples were trimmed of fat
and stored in liquid nitrogen. The cytosol ER and PgR content
was determined within 3 months by the dextran-coated charcoal
assay (Saez et al., 1978).

For comparison between the groups, we used the Chi-square
test and the Student's test. Differences were considered significant at the $p \leq 0.05$ level.

CYTOPROGNOSTIC CLASSIFICATION	TAMOXIFEN FLUORESCENCE +	−	TOTAL
GRADE I	23 (82%)	5	28
GRADE II	24 (53%)	21	45
GRADE III	20 (24%)	63	83
TOTAL	67 (43%)	89	156

Table 1. Correlation between Tamoxifen Fluorescence and Cytoprognostic classification.

HISTOPROGNOSTIC CLASSIFICATION	TAMOXIFEN FLUORESCENCE +	−	TOTAL
GRADE I	22 (66%)	11	33
GRADE II	22 (42%)	30	52
GRADE III	2 (12.5%)	14	16
TOTAL	46	55	101

Table 2. Correlation between Tamoxifen Fluorescence and the Histoprognostic classification of Scarff and Bloom.

RESULTS

Benign breast lesions

Tamoxifen-induced fluorescence was strongly positive in benign hyperplastic epithelial cells and was observed in 20 out
of 27 benign breast lesions.

Breast cancer

Tamoxifen-induced cytoplasmic and nucleolar fluorescence
was observed in 67 out of 156 pre-treated primary cancers (43%)
whereas no fluorescence occurred in unresponsive (control) tumors of 16 patients in whom the disease recurred under therapeutic treatment with Tamoxifen.

A highly significant correlation ($p < 0.001$) was observed
between positive Tamoxifen-induced fluorescence and the degree
of cell differentiation as determined by cytological grading
(Table 1): 82% of well-differentiated grade I tumors were fluorescence-positive versus 24% of anaplastic grade III tumors.
There was also a significant correlation ($p < 0.01$) with histologic differentiation (Table 2).

The results of the biochemical assays are indicated in
Table 3.

The tumors of Tamoxifen-treated patients were more often
ER- negative than the control tumors of untreated patients

TABLE 3

HORMONE STATUS IN BREAST TUMORS OF 71 TAMOXIFEN-TREATED
PATIENTS AND 67 UNTREATED CONTROLS

PgR	TAMOXIFEN-TREATED PATIENTS (71)	CONTROLS UNTREATED PATIENTS (67)
PgR +	29 (41%) m.v. 675 fmol	24 (36%) m.v. 364 fmol
PgR -	42 (59%)	43 (64%)
ER +	12 (17%) m.v. 28 fmol	36 (54%) m.v. 122 fmol
ER -	59 (83%)	31 (46%)

m.v. mean value ; fmol per mg protein

F 1 PgR	+	-
= 0	8	31 (76%)
> 0	16 (67%) m.v. 706	10 m.v. 402
TOTAL	24	41

m.v. : mean value   fmol/mg protein

Table 5. Correlation between Tamoxifen fluorescence (Fl) and progesterone receptor content (PgR) of the 65 tumors.

(83% versus 46%). In the case of ER-positive tumors, values were low with a mean of 28 fmol versus 122 fmol in the untreated controls.

The incidence rates of PgR positivity was similar in treated and untreated cases (41% and 36%, respectively), but mean PgR values were significantly higher in tumors of Tamoxifen-treated patients than in the untreated patients (675 and 364 fmol , respectively).

Tissue PgR values were compared with the degree of tumor differentiation as defined by the cytoprognostic classification. (Table 4). In untreated patients, mean PgR values did not differ with tumor differentiation, whereas there was a highly significant difference in PgR values depending on the grade (from 176 fmol in grade III to 1410 fmol in grade I) in tumors of Tamoxifen-treated patients.

In these pretreated cases, positive Tamoxifen-induced fluorescence correlated with PgR status (Table 5).

227

CYTOPROGNOSTIC CLASSIFICATION	TAMOXIFEN-TREATED PATIENTS		MEAN VALUE	CONTROLS UNTREATED PATIENTS		MEAN VALUE
GRADE I						
PgR = 0	2			2		
PgR ∧ 0	8	20%	1410	6	25%	390
GRADE II						
PgR = 0	16			10		
PgR ∧ 0	11	59%	439	9	52.5%	330
GRADE III						
PgR = 0	24			31		
PgR ∧ 0	10	70.5%	176	9	77.5%	373
TOTAL	71		675	67		364

Progesterone receptors - fmol/mg protein

Table 4 - Progesterone receptors (PgR) content in Tamoxifen-treated patients and controls in correlation with the degree of cell differentiation according to the cytoprognostic classification.

228

DISCUSSION

A short pre-treatment of breast cancer patients with Tamoxifen (20 mg daily for 10 days preceding surgery) provides valuable information on tumor cell responsiveness to hormone treatment.

In this study, Tamoxifen-induced fluorescence was observed in the tumors of 43% of pre-treated patients, correlating with an average value of 40% hormone responsiveness in breast cancers. A significant correlation was found between Tamoxifen uptake and tumor cell differentiation, suggesting that the uptake of Tamoxifen by tumor cells represents a biochemical aspect of cellular differentiation.

In pre-treated tumors, moreover, a negative or reduced ER status corresponded to an increase in PgR values which, in turn, correlated with tumor cell differentiation and Tamoxifen uptake.

Thus, pre-treatment with Tamoxifen appears to be a valuable test (Namer et al., 1980; Robel et al., 1983, 1984; Waseda et al., 1981) in which results correlate with tumor cell differentiation and hormone responsiveness. The test is easy to perform and has been used in 215 pre- or post-menopausal patients without any adverse effects since 1980. Determining fluorescence induced by Tamoxifen or its metabolites in tumor cells is a procedure that may be routinely carried out in any cytology department.

REFERENCES

1. Alonso, K. and Brownlee, N.- Estrogen receptors by immuno-fluorescence comparison with a dextran-coated charcoal assay. Ann. Clin. Lab. Sc. 1981, 11, 132-137.

2. Bartoli, M.H., Rochat, J., Jacrot, M., Beriel, H. and Mouriquand,J.- La fluorescence du Tamoxifène comme marqueur de l'hormonodépendance : aspect physico-chimique. C.R. Acad. Sci. 295 (série III), 307-310, 1982.

3. Bloom, H.J.G. and Richardson, W.W.-Histological grading and prognosis in breast cancer. Br. J. Cancer, 11, 359-377, 1957.

4. Greene, G.L., Sobel, N.B., King, W.J. and Jensen, E.V.- Immunochemical studies of estrogen receptors. J. Steroid Biochem., 20, 51-56, 1984.

5. Jacobs, S.R., Wolfson, W.L., Cheng, L. and Lewin, K.J.- Cytochemical and competition protein binding assays for estrogen receptor in breast disease. Cancer, 51, 1621-1624, 1983.

6. Krishan, L. and Ganapethi, R.- Laser flow cytometric studies on the intra-cellular fluorescence of anthracycline.
   Cancer Res. 40, 3895-3400, 1980.

7. Lampertico, P.- Determination of hormone receptors in 13
   Pathology Laboratories in Italy. istocitopathologia, 6,
   47-54, 1984.

8. Lee, S.H.- Sex steroid hormone receptors in mammary carcinoma diagnostic immunohistochemistry. (Masson monographs in
   diagnostic pathology). R.A. Delellis, Ed. Masson Publishing,
   New York, 1981.

9. Lee, S.H.- Validity of estrogen receptor assay supported by
   the observation of a cellular response to steroid manipulation. J. Histo. Cytochem., 32, 901-906, 1984.

10. Mc Carty, K.S., Hiatt, K.B., Budwit, D.A., Cox, E.B.,
    Leight, G., Reintgen, D., Georgia de, G., Hilliard, F., and
    Durham, N.C.- Clinical response to hormone therapy correla-
    ted with estrogen receptor analysis. Arch. Pathol. Lab. Med.
    108, 24-26, 1984.

11. Meijer, C.J.L.M., Van Marle, J., Persijn, J.P., van Niewen-
    huizen, W., Baak, J.P.A., Boon, M.E. and Lindeman, J.-
    Estrogen.Receptors in Human Breast Cancer. II. Correlation
    between the histochemical method and biochemical assay.
    Virchows Arch (Cell Pathol.), 40, 27-37, 1982;

12. Mouriquand, J. and Pasquier, D.- Fine-needle aspiration of
    breast carcinoma; a preliminary cytoprognostic study. Acta
    Cytol., 24, 153-159, 1980.

13. Mouriquand, J., Mouriquand, C., Sage, J.C., Saez, S.,
    Jacrot, M. and Gabelle, Ph. La fluorescence du Tamoxifène
    comme marqueur de l'hormonodépendance: une étude cytologi-
    que sur des ponctions biopsie de tumeurs malignes du sein
    des femmes traitées. C.R. Acad. Sci. 283 (série III), 801-
    806, 1981 a.

14. Mouriquand, J., Mouriquand, C., Petitpas, E., Louis, J. and
    Mermet, M.A.- Differential nucleolar staining affinity with
    a modified Papanicolaou staining procedure. Stain. Tech.,
    56, 215-219, 1981 b.

15. Mouriquand, J., Jacrot, M., Louis, J., Mermet, M.A., Saez,
    S., Sage, J.C. and Mouriquand, C.- Tamoxifen induced fluo-
    rescence as a marker of a human breast tumor cell responsi-
    veness to hormonal manipulations correlation with progeste-
    rone receptor content and ultrastructural alterations. Can-
    cer Res., 43, 3948-3954, 1983 a.

16. Mouriquand, J., Bartoli, M.H., Rochat, J., Beriel, H. and
    Louis, J.- Tamoxifen induced fluorescence: spectrofluorime-
    tric study and clinical applications of the ion-pair eosin-

230

Tamoxifen. Proc. 10th Intern. Symp. on biological characterization of human tumors. Brighton 24-28 October 1983 b.

17. Mouriquand, J., Louis, J., Mermet, M.A., Sage, J.C.,
Payan, R. and Mouriquand, C.- Tamoxifen-induced fluorescence in shortly pre-treated surgical breast carcinoma: a predictive test to hormonal responsiveness. Breast disease, 1,
13-16, 1985.

18. Namer, M., Lallane, C. and Baulieu, E.E.- Increase of progesterone receptor by Tamoxifen as a hormonal challenge
test in breast cancer. Cancer Res., 40, 1750-1752, 1980.

19. Nenci, I.- Estrogen receptor cytochemistry in human breast
cancer: status and prospects. Cancer, 48, 2674-2686, 1981.

20. Penney, G.C. and Hawkins, R.A.- Histochemical detection of
estrogen receptors: a progress report. Br. J. Cancer, 45,
237-246, 1982.

21. Pertschuk, L.P., Tobin, E.H., Carter, A.C., Eisenberg, K.B.
Leo, V.C., Gaetjens, E. and Bloom, N.D.- Immuno-histologic
and histochemical methods for detection of steroid binding
in breast cancer: a reappraisal. Breast Can. Res. and
Treat., 1, 297-314, 1981.

22. Robel, P., Martel, R., Namer, M. and Baulieu, E.E.- Progesterone receptor as an indicator of the response of post
menopausal endometrial carcinoma and metastatic breast
cancer to an antiestrogen. In: Progesterone and Progestins.
C.W. Bardin, E. Milgromm and P. Mauvais-Jarvis, eds, Raven
Press, New York, 1983, P. 367.

23. Robel, P., Gravanis, A., Catelli, M.G., Binart, N., George,
M., Laval, C. and Baulieu, E.E.- Female sex steroid receptors in post-menopausal endometrial carcinoma. Biochemical
responses to anti-estrogen and progestin. In: Hormones and
Cancer. A.R. Liss, Raven Press, New York, 1984, pp. 167-
179.

24. Saez, S., Martin, P.M. and Chauvet, C.D.- Estradiol and
progesterone receptor levels in human breast adenocarcinoma in relation to plasma estrogen and progesterone levels.
Cancer Res., 38, 3468-3473, 1978.

25. Seibert, K. and Lippman,M.-Hormone receptors in breast cancer. In: Clinical Oncology, Vol. 1, N° 2, W.B. Saunders
Company Ed. 1982, pp. 735-794.

26. Waseda, N., Kato, Y., Imura, H. and Kurata, M.- Effects of
Tamoxifen on estrogen and progesterone receptors in human
breast cancer. Cancer Res., 41, 1984-1988, 1981.

27. Yanovich and Taub, R.N.- Digitized video fluorescence microscopy studies of adriamycin interaction with single P
388 leukemic cells. Cancer Res. , 42, 3583-3586, 1982.

HORMONAL RECEPTORS AND OTHER TUMOR PARAMETERS IN BREAST CANCER

N.J. AGNANTIS and C. PETRAKIS

Department of Pathology, Greek Anticancer Institute, Snt Savvas Hospital, 171, Alexandros avenue, Athens, Greece.

This report provides a pathological review of 250 breast cancers analyzed for estrogen (ER) and progesterone (PgR) receptors and correlates a series of parameters with ER and PgR results: histologic type, grade, tumor size and margin, lymphocytic infiltration, stromal fibrosis, patient age. The results were tested with the chi-square method and indicated as very highly statistically significant ($p < 0.001$), highly statistically significant ($p < 0.01$), statistically significant ($p < 0.05$) and of uncertain statistical significance ($p < 0.1$). A statistically significant difference is indicated as SSD.

Since the histologic features of breast cancer may vary from one section to another, only frozen sections adjacent to the tissue sample supplied for biochemical hormone receptor determination were used for diagnostic examination. Biochemically, estrogen (ER) and progesterone (PgR) receptors were determined by the dextran-coated charcoal (DCC) assay. Samples which contained more than 10 fmol/mg protein were considered positive.

On the basis of the ER and PgR content, the 250 breast carcinomas were classified in four groups:

1. ER+/PgR+ : 66.8%
2. ER+:PgR- : 15.6%
3. ER-/PgR+ : 7.6%
4. ER-/PgR- : 10.0%

Tumor type

There was no statistically significant difference (SSD) in the hormone receptor content in the different histologic types of breast cancer. Nevertheless, it was noticed that the tubular type of ductal carcinoma showed a high ER and PgR content, that medullary carcinoma had a low ER and PgR content, and that lobular carcinoma had a higher ER and PgR content than ductal carcinoma. These results are not statistically significant but support the findings of other authors. Thus, there is general agreement that medullary carcinomas have low levels of ER (Rosen et al., 1975, 1978; Martin et al., 1978; Parl and Wagner, 1980; Silfversward et al., 1980, Lesser et al., 1981). There is also some agreement that lobular carcinomas have more receptors than ductal carcinomas (Rosen et al., 1975, 1978; Antoniades and Spector, 1979; Howat et al., 1983). Tubular carcinomas are reported to be rich in ER (Rosen et al., 1975, 1978; Antoniades and Spector, 1979; Howat et al., 1983). High receptor levels are also described in papillary carcinoma, whereas other histologic types, like comedocarcinoma and colloid carcinoma, have rather low values (Silfversward et al., 1980).

Tumor grade

Positive ER values were found in 86.4% of grade I, in 89.3% of grade II and 56% of grade III tumors. No SSD was found between grade I and II tumors, but when grade I and II tumors together were compared with grade III tumors (GI + GII 89%, GIII 56%), a SSD clearly appeared (p $<$ 0.001). PgR results also showed a SSD (p $<$ 0.01) between grade I + II tumors versus grade III tumors (78% and 60% respectively).

These results are in agreement with those of Martin et al., (1978); Fisher et al., (1980); Mc Carty et al., (1980); Millis (1980); Parl and Wagner (1980); Silfversward et al., (1980); Lesser et al., (1981); Howat et al., (1983) and Blanco et al., (1984). They suggest a positive correlation between receptor content and degree of differentiation. Rosen et al., (1975, 1978) also found similar results, but they could not establish a significant statistical difference. Maynard et al., (1978) observed grade-related receptor differences only in postmenopausal women.

Tumor size

A significant statistical difference in ER values was observed between tumors less than 2 cm in diameter (91% ER+) and tumors larger than 2 cm in diameter (76% ER+). No SSD, however, was observed concerning the PgR content.

These findings differ from those of Rosen et al., (1975), 1978), Parl and Wagner (1980) and Howat et al., (1983) who did not find a correlation between receptor content and tumor size.

Tumor margin

Tumors with irregular margins had a higher percentage of ER (SSD, p $<$ 0.05) but no SSD was noticed for PgR.

These findings do not agree with those of Howat et al., (1983) who failed to detect a correlation for either ER or PgR.

Lymphocytic infiltration

Tumors with a low grade of lymphocytic infiltration had a higher ER content than tumors with a higher grade of lymphocytic infiltration. No SSD was noticed, however, between lymphocytic infiltration and PgR content.

A similar correlation between lymphocytic infiltration and ER content was already observed by Rosen et al., (1975, 1978); Millis, (1980); Parl and Wagner, (1980); Silfversward et al.,

233

(1980); Lesser et al., (1981); Chabon et al., (1982) and Howat
et al., (1983) who all noticed an increasing degree of lymphocytic infiltration in the tumor associated with a decreasing
incidence of ER activity. In addition, Howat et al., (1983)
found the same correlation for PgR, an observation which we
could not confirm.

Stromal fibrosis

Fibrosis was unrelated to the presence of ER and PgR, as
already observed by other authors (Rosen et al., 1975, 1978;
Masters et al., 1978; Martin et al., 1978; Parl and Wagner,
1980; Howat et al., 1983), although it is generally assumed
that tumors rich in connective tissue stroma should have a low
content of hormone receptors.

Patient age

The ER positivity increases from premenopause (75.9%) to
postmenopause (85.9%), (p < 0.05) as already observed by
Silfversward et al., (1980), Lesser et al., (1981), Howat et
al., (1983), Parl and Wagner (1980) but not by Rosen et al.,
(1975, 1978) and Howat et al., (1983).

However, no correlation was found between premenopausal
or postmenopausal status and PgR levels, as also reported by
Howat et al., (1983).

Generally, all the authors have found a high percentage
of ER in postmenopausal women. This fact can probably be explained by the absence of high levels of estrogen binding to
the hormone receptors, whereas in premenopausal women, ER receptors are blocked by circulating estrogens and thus not detectable.

In conclusion, the present study shows that:

1. with an increase in tumor grade, the ER and PgR content
   decreases,
2. with an increase in tumor size, the ER content decreases,
3. with an increase in tumor margin irregularity, the ER content increases,
4. with an increase in lymphocytic infiltration of the tumor,
   the ER content decreases,
5. with an increase in patient age, the ER content increases.

Thus, the results of our study are in agreement with those of other authors although we established the different histologic parameters exclusively on frozen sections adjacent to
the tumor sample subjected to hormone receptor determination,
a method we consider the most accurate for obtaining a reliable correlation.

ACKNOWLEDGEMENTS

The authors wish to express their thanks to Mrs Julia

234

Yioti-Galati for the preparation of the biochemical assays.

REFERENCES

1. Antoniades, K. and Spector, J., Correlation of estrogen receptor levels with histology and cytomorphology in human mammary cancer. Am. J. Clin. Pathol., 71, 497-503, 1979.

2. Blanco, G., Alavaikko, M., Ojala, A., Collan, Y., Heikkinen, M., Hietanen, T., Aine, R. and Taskinen, P.J. Estrogen and Progesterone Receptors in breast cancer: relationships to tumour histopathology and survival of patients. Ant. Res. 4, 383-390, 1984.

3. Brooks, S.C., Saunders, D.E., Singhakowinta, A. and Vaitkevicins, V.K., Relation of tumor content of estrogen and progesterone receptors with response of patient to endocrine therapy. Cancer, 46, 2775-2778, 1980.

4. Chabon, A.B., Goldberg, J.D. and Venet, L., Carcinoma of the breast: Interrelationships among histopathologic features, estrogen receptor activity and age of the patient. Human Pathol., 14, 368-372, 1982.

5. Fisher, E.R., Redmond, C.K., Liu, H., Rochette, H. and Fisher, B., Correlation of estrogen receptor and pathologic characteristics of invasive breast cancer. Cancer, 45, 349-353, 1980.

6. Howat, J.M.T., Barnes, D.M., Harris, M. and Swindell, R., The association of cytosol estrogen and progesterone receptors with histological features of breast cancer and early recurrence of disease, Br. J. Cancer, 47, 629-640, 1983.

7. Jonat, W., Maass, H., Stolzenbach, G. and Trams, G., Estrogen receptor status and response to polychemotherapy in advanced breast cancer. Cancer, 46, 2809-2813, 1980.

8. Kiang, D.T. and Kennedy, B.J., Factors affecting estrogen receptors in breast cancer. Cancer, 40, 1571-1576, 1977.

9. Lesser, M.L., Rosen, P.P., Senie, R.T., Duthie, K., Menendez-Botet, C. and Schwartz M.K., Estrogen and progesterone receptors in breast carcinoma. Correlations with epidemiology and pathology. Cancer, 48, 299-309, 1981.

10. McCarty, K.S., Barton, T.K., Fetter, B.F., Woodard, B.H., Mossler, J.A., Reeves, M., Daly, J., Wilkinson, W.E. and McCarty, K.S., Correlation of estrogen and progesterone receptors with histologic differentiation in mammary carcinoma. Cancer, 46, 2851-2858, 1980.

11. Maynard, P.V., Davies, C.J., Blamey, R.W., Elston, C.W., Johnson, J. and Griffiths, K., Relationship between estro-

gen-receptor content and histological grade in human primary breast tumors. Br. J. Cancer, 38, 745-748, 1978.

12. Martin, M., Jacquemier, J., Rolland, P.H., Rolland A.M. and Toga, M., Tumeurs mammaires humaines: Corrélations entre les récepteurs hormonaux stéroidiens et l'anatomie pathologique. Une hypothèse: valeur pronostique des récepteurs hormonaux. Bull. Cancer, 65 (4), 383-387, 1978.

13. Masters, J.R.W., Hawkins, R.A., Sangster, K. et al., Estrogen receptors, cellularity, elastosis and menstrual status in human breast cancer. Eur. J. Cancer, 14, 303-307, 1978.

14. Millis, R.R., Correlation of hormone receptors with pathological features in human breast cancer. Cancer, 46, 2869-2871, 1980.

15. Parl, F.F.and Wagner, P.K. The histopathological evaluation of human breast cancers in correlation with estrogen receptor values, Cancer, 46, 362-367, 1980.

16. Rosen, P.P., Menendez-Botet, C.J., Nisselbaum, J.S., Urban, J.A., Miké, V., Fracchia, A. and Schwartz, M.K., Pathological review of breast lesions analyzed for estrogen receptor protein.Cancer Res., 35, 3187-3194, 1975.

17. Rosen, P.P., Menendez-Botet, C.J., Senie, R.T., Schwartz, M.K., Schottenfeld, D., and Farr, G.H., Estrogen receptor protein (E.R.P.) and the histopathology of human mammary carcinoma. In : Hormones, Receptors and Breast Cancer, M.L. McGuire, ed, 1978, pp. 71-83.

18. Silfverswärd, C., Gustafsson, J.A., Gustafsson, S.A., Humla, S., Nordenskjöld, B., Wallgren, A. and Wrange, O. Estrogen receptor concentrations in 269 cases of histologically classified human breast cancer. Cancer, 45, 2001-2005, 1980.

RELATIONSHIP OF THE ESTROGEN RECEPTOR ACTIVATION TO THE HISTOLOGICAL

FINDINGS IN MAMMARY CARCINOMA

Markku HELLE[1], Jaakko ANTONEN[2] and Kai KROHN[2]

[1]Mikkeli Central Hospital, Mikkeli, Finland
[2]Institute of Biomedical Sciencies, University of Tampere, Tampere, Finland

INTRODUCTION

The morphological classifications of breast carcinomas have been inadequate in the assessment of response to the therapy or the prognosis of patients. Since the demonstration of a correlation of the estrogen receptor (ER) and the progesterone receptor (PR) status to the response to endocrine therapy (McGuire 1975), disease free interval and survival (Knight et al. 1977; Blamey et al. 1980) in breast cancer, attempts have been made to find correlations between the ER and PR status and the histology of breast carcinomas (review, Underwood 1983).

Monoclonal antibodies against human milk fat globule membranes have revealed differences in the differentiation, together with cellular heterogeneity, in breast carcinomas. This findings could have prognostic significance and even therapeutic implications in breast cancer. It has been shown, indeed, that the absence of staining with a monoclonal antibody, HMFG-1, was correlated with a poor prognosis while extracellular staining of HMFG-1 was associated with a favourable clinical course (Wilkinson et al. 1984). However, Berry et al. (1985) with the same antibody found no correlation to the survival, to the estrogen receptor status or to the histological grade of tumors.

We have previously described several monoclonal human milk fat globule membrane antibodies (Ashorn and Krohn 1985; Krohn et al. 1985) and shown that one of these, III D 5, correlates significantly to the estrogen receptor positivity of breast cancer (Krohn and Helle 1986). In this study we compared the correlation of the III D 5 reactivity, and the ER and PR status to histologic parameters which are known to be of prognostic significance in breast cancer.

MATERIAL AND METHODS

Tissue specimens

Biopsy specimens were collected from all infiltrating ductal and lobular breast cancer patients (N=85) operated upon at Mikkeli Central Hospital during years 1981-1983. At the operation, a tissue block from the cancer was sent to the pathological laboratory, where a part of it was trimmed for histology and immunohistochemistry and an adjacent piece taken for receptor assay. The histological examination, as well as immunohistochemistry were performed on routine paraffin embedded sections, after fixation in buffered formalin. Sections were stained with haematoxylin and eosin .

Steroid receptor assays

Receptor assays were performed at the hormone laboratory, Lauttasaaren Tutkimus, Helsinki, Finland from the cytosol using charcoal method (Korenman and Dukes 1970). Values <4 fmol/mg protein were classified as negative and >4 fmol/mg protein positive for both estrogen and progesterone receptors.

Immunohistochemistry

The generation and characterization of the monoclonal antibody III D 5 has been published previously (Krohn et al. 1985). In immunohistochemistry we used paraffin sections and indirect peroxidase method.

Histological classification of breast cancer

The tumors were classified using the WHO classification (WHO 1981). Only infiltrating ductal and lobular carcinomas were included. The histological grade was assessed according to the method described by Bloom and Richardson (1957). Nuclear grade, necrosis, stromal fibrosis and stromal cell reaction were graded after Fisher et al. (1975).

RESULTS

The presence of the estrogen and/or progesterone receptor (ER/PR) and positive staining with antibody III D 5 in pre- and postmenopausal patients are given in table 1. As can be seen, both III D 5 reactivity as well as ER positivity were more often seen in postmenopausal patients, the difference between these two age groups being highly significant for III D 5 reactivity (p< 0.005) and significant for the ER positivity (p<0.025). The progesterone receptor status, on the other hand, showed no relationship to the age of patients.

Table 1. Relationship of patient's age to ER, PR and III D 5 status of breast cancer (N=74)

Age (years)	ER positive N (%)	PR positive N (%)	III D 5 positive N (%)
under 49	6(35)	7(35)	11(48)
over 49	38(67)	21(39)	49(79)

The III D 5 positivity was significantly or highly significantly correlated with histological signs of the tumor differentiation. Thus, the III D 5 positivity was more often seen in tumors with histological grades I or II (p< 0.05) and nuclear grades II or III (p< 0.01) than with less differentiated grade. A similar correlation was noticed with the lymphoid infiltration or the necrosis of the tumor (p<0.05 and p<0.01 respectively).

The estrogen receptor positivity also showed correlation with the differentiation of the tumor, being more often seen in histological grades I and II (p< 0.05), in tumors with lymphoid infiltration (p<0.025) and necrosis (p<0.05) but not to the nuclear grade. The progesterone receptor, on the other hand, correlated strongly with the nuclear grade and the lymphoid infiltration of the tumor, but not to the histological grade or to the necrosis. III D 5, more than the presence of ER or PR, correlated also with the stromal fibrosis but this finding was not significant.

DISCUSSION

Several monoclonal antibodies against human milk fat globule membrane have been described (Taylor-Papadimitriou et al. 1981; Foster et al. 1982; Hilkens et al. 1984). Rasmussen et al.(1982) in preliminary studies showed that there was no relatioship between the reactivity with HMFG 1, HMFG 2 and Mam-3 antibodies and the menopausal status, the lymph node status or the estrogen receptor status of tumors. The highly differentiated tumors seem to be more often positively stained with these antibodies but the material was too small for statistical analysis. In the study of Wilkinson et al. (1984) the extracellular staining of HMFG 1 antibody was associated with the better prognosis of the patients, but the authors did not found a correlation with the differentiation of tumors.

In this study we found a significant correlation of the reactivity with monoclonal HMFG antibody III D 5 with the differentiation of breast cancer. Thus, the III D 5 reactivity correlated with the histological grade, the nuclear grade, the lymphoid infiltration and the necrosis of

240

mammary carcinoma. Furthermore, we have confirmed the correlation of the ER status with the differentiation of breast cancer (McGuire et al. 1978; Rich et al. 1978; Fisher et al. 1980; Osborne et al. 1980; Millis 1980; Westerberg et al. 1980; Fisher et al. 1981; Rasmussen et al. 1981; Underwood 1983; Alanko et al. 1984; Wittliff 1984). The progesterone receptors correlated only with the nuclear grade and the lymphoid infiltration of tumors.

Of the III D 5 correlated features, the histological grade, the nuclear grade, the lymphoid infiltration and the necrosis of the tumor are shown to be prognostic indicators in breast cancer (Bloom and Richardson 1957; Fisher et al. 1975; Haybittle et al. 1982).

We have previously shown a statistically highly significant association of the III D 5 positivity to the presence of ER in mammary carcinomas and also a relative correlation with the presence of PR. Thus, the heterogenic antigenic structure detected by III D 5 could indicate an intact estrogen receptor regulated protein synthesis and it is possible that III D 5 positivity could assign a better prognosis in mammary carcinoma.

In conclusion, the monoclonal HMFG antibody III D 5 is correlated with histological features known to be prognostic indicators in breast cancer. This together with the correlation of the III D 5 status with the presence of ER in tumors could serve as a prognostic indicator of mammary carcinoma and studies are presently undertaken to see, whether the reactivity with antibody III D 5 would also correlate with the biological behaviour of the tumors.

REFERENCES

Alanko A., Mäkinen J., Scheinin T.M., Tolppanen E-M., and Vihko R., Correlation of estrogen and progesterone receptor and histological grade in human primary breast cancer. Acta Pathol. Microbiol. Immunol. Scand. Sect.A, 92, 311-315, 1984.
Ashorn P., and Krohn K., Characterization and partial purification of human milk fat globule membrane antigens by a polyacrylamide gel electrophoreresis and immunoblotting using monoclonal antibodies. Int. J. Cancer, 35, 179-184, 1985.
Berry N., Jones D.B., Smallwood J., Taylor I., Kirkham N., and Taylor-Papadimitriou J., The prognostic value of the monoclonal antibodies HMFG1 and HMFG2 in breast cancer. Br. J. Cancer, 51, 179-186, 1985.
Blamey R.W., Bishop H.M., Blake J.R.S., Doyle P.J., Elston C.W., Haybittle J.L., Nicholson R.I., and Griffiths K., Relationship between primary breast tumor receptor status and patient survival. Cancer, 46, 2765- 2769, 1980.

Bloom H.J.G., and Richardson W.W., Histological grading and prognosis in breast cancer: a study of 1409 cases of which 359 have been followed for 15 years. Br. J. Cancer, 11, 359-401, 1957.

Fisher E.R., Gregorio R.M., and Fisher B., The pathology of invasive breast cancer. A syllabus from findings of the national surgical adjuvant breast project (protocol No.4). Cancer, 36, 1-85, 1975.

Fisher E.R,, Osborne C.K,, McGuire W.L., Redmond C., Knight III W.A., Fisher B., Bannayan G., Walder A., Gregory E.J., Jacobsen A., Queen D.M., Bennett D.E., and Ford H.C., Correlation of primary breast cancer histopathology and estrogen receptor content. Breast Cancer Res. Treat., 1, 37-41, 1981.

Fisher E.R., Redmond C.K., Liu H., Rockette H., Fisher B., and collaborating NSABP investigators, Correlation of estrogen receptor and pathologic characteristics of invasive breast cancer. Cancer 45, 349-353, 1980.

Foster C.S., Dinsdale E.A.,Edwards P.A.W., and Neville M.A., Monoclonal antibodies to the human mammary gland II.Distribution of determinants in breast carcinomas. Virchows Arch.(Pathol Anat) 394, 295-305, 1982.

Haybittle J.L., Blamey R.W., Elston C.W., Johnson J., Doyle P.J., Campbell F.C., Nicholson R.I., and Griffiths K., A prognostic index in primary breast cancer. Br. J. Cancer, 45, 361-366, 1982.

Hilkens J., Buijs F.,Hilgers J., Hageman Ph., Calafat J., Sonnenberg A., and van der Valk M., Monoclonal antibodies against human milk-fat globule membranes detecting differentation antigen of the mammary gland and its tumors. Int. J. Cancer, 34, 197-206, 1984.

Knight III W.A., Livingston R.B., Gregory E.J., and McGuire W.L., Estrogen receptor as an independent prognostic factor for early recurrence in breast cancer. Cancer Res., 37, 4669- 4671, 1977.

Korenman S.G., and Dukes B.A., Spesific estrogen binding by the cytoplasm of human breast carcinoma. J. Clin. Endocrinol. 30, 639-645, 1970.

Krohn K., and Helle M., Recognition with a monoclonal antibody of a cytoplasmic mammary carcinoma antigen,correlated to the estrogen receptor status. Int. J. Cancer, 37, 43-47, 1986.

Krohn K., Ashorn R., and Helle M., Generation of monoclonal antibodies to human milk fat globule membrane antigens, with special reference to a precipitable secretory product of breast and ovarian carcinomas. Tumor Biology, 6, 13-23, 1985.

McGuire W.L., Current status of estrogen receptors in human breast cancer. Cancer, 36, 638-644, 1975.

McGuire W.L., Horwitz K.B., Zava D.T., Garola R.E., and Chamness G.C. Hormones in breast cancer: Update 1978. Metabolism, 27, 487-501, 1978.

Millis R.R., Correlation of hormone receptors with pathological features in human breast cancer. Cancer 46, 2869-2871, 1980.

Osborne C.K., Fisher E., Redmond C., Knight III W.A.,
    Yochomowitz W.A., and McGuire W.L., Estrogen receptor, a
    marker for human breast cancer differentation and
    patient prognosis. Adv. Exp. Med. Biol., 138, 377-385,
    1980.
Rasmussen B., Hilkens J., Hilgers J., Nielsen H.H., Thorpe
    S.M., and Rose C., Monoclonal antibodies applied to
    primary human breast carcinoma: relationship to
    menopausal status, lymph node status, and steroid
    hormone receptor content. Breast Cancer Res. Treat., 2,
    401-405, 1982.
Rich M.A., Furmanski P., and Brooks S.C.,and the breast
    cancer prognostic study surgery and pathology
    associates., Prognostic value of estrogen receptor
    determinations in patients with breast cancer. Cancer
    Res., 38, 4296-4298, 1978.
Taylor-Papadimitriou J., Peterson J.A., Arklie J., Burchell
    J. and Ceriani R.L., Monoclonal antibodies to epithelium-
    spesific component on the human milk fat globule
    membrane: production and reaction with cells in culture.
    Int. J. Cancer , 28, 17-21, 1981.
Westerberg H., Gustafson S.A., Nordenskjöld B.,
    Silfverswärd C., and Wallgren A., Estrogen receptor
    level and other factors in early recurrence of breast
    cancer, Int. J. Cancer, 26, 429-433, 1980.
WHO, International histological classification of tumors.
    Histological typing of breast tumours, No 2, Geneva, 17-
    22, 1981.
Wilkinson M.J.S., Howell A., Harris M., Taylor-Papadimitriou
    J., Swindell R., and Sellwood R.A., The prognostic
    significance of two epithelial membrane antigens
    expressed by human mammary carcinomas. Int. J. Cancer,
    33, 299-304, 1984,
Wittliff J.L., Steroid-hormone receptors in breast cancer.
    Cancer, 53, 630-643, 1984.
Underwood J.C.E., Oestrogen receptors in human breast
    cancer: review of histopathological correlations and
    critique of histochemical methods. Diagnostic
    Histopathology, 6, 1-22, 1983.

HORMONE PATTERNS IN BREAST CYSTIC FLUID (BCF) IN PATIENTS WITH FIBROCYSTIC DISEASE (FCD).

Pietro TARTAGLIA and Mario Di MOLFETTA

Department of Obstetrics and Gynaecology, Ospedale per gli Infermi, 48018 - Faenza, Italy.

Only recently has there been widespread interest in the biochemical and hormonal composition of needle-aspirated cystic fluid in fibrocystic disease (FCD) (Angeli and Dogliotti, 1984; Angeli et al., 1982; Bradlow et al., 1979, 1983; Frairia et al., 1983; Orlandi et al., 1984).Although there have been few studies to-date and results have been contradictory, some interesting findings of prognostic and diagnostic value have emerged.

In this paper, we report the results of our studies on the hormone composition of needle-aspirated fluid from cysts (diameter >1 centimeter) in patients with FCD. For this purpose, a comparison was made with blood levels of these hormones in the same patients during the secreting phase of the menstrual cycle (18th-21st day of the cycle). Findings were examined with a view to determining what valuable information could be obtained concerning breast pathology in general, and cyst recurrence in particular.

Gross cystic disease (GCD), an ominous form of fibrocystic disease (FCD) is characterized by the presence of cysts of over 3 millimiters in diameter.

The study was based on 36 patients with Gross Cystic Disease (GCD), aged from 34 to 46 years, in which, according ultrasonographic findings, cysts were over 1 cm in diameter. The patients had regular menstrual cycles and had not been subjected to any hormone treatment, at least not during the six months prior to this study. Levels of the following hormones were determined: prolactin (PRL); 17-beta-estradiol (17-BE), progesterone (P), dehydroepiandrosterone (DHEA) and testosterone (T). The plasma and cystic fluid values of PRL, 17 BE, P, DHEA and T are indicated in Fig. 1-5.

A total of 15 patients relapsed following aspiration of the cysts. Relapse occurred 3, 6 and 9 months after the initial procedure in 8, 4 and 3 cases, respectively. Only two patients (cases N° 3 and n° 21) relapsed 3, then 9 months after initial aspiration. In the 13 remaining cases, cysts recurred in 6 cases after 3 months, in 4 cases after 6 months and in 3 cases after 9 months. Blood and cystic fluid hormone levels

244

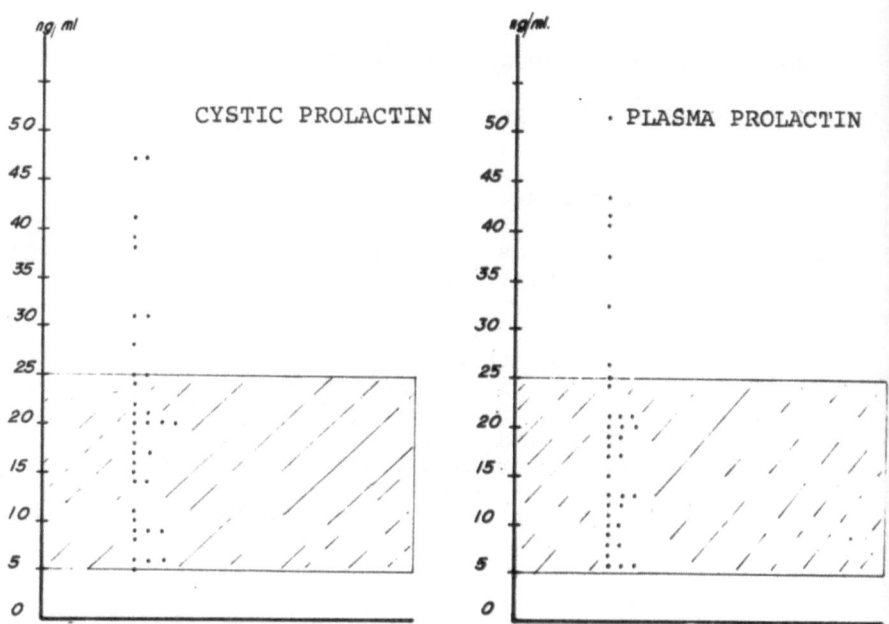

Fig. 1. Comparison of hormone levels occurring in the plasma
and cystic fluid of patients with GCD, P = 0.32,n.s.

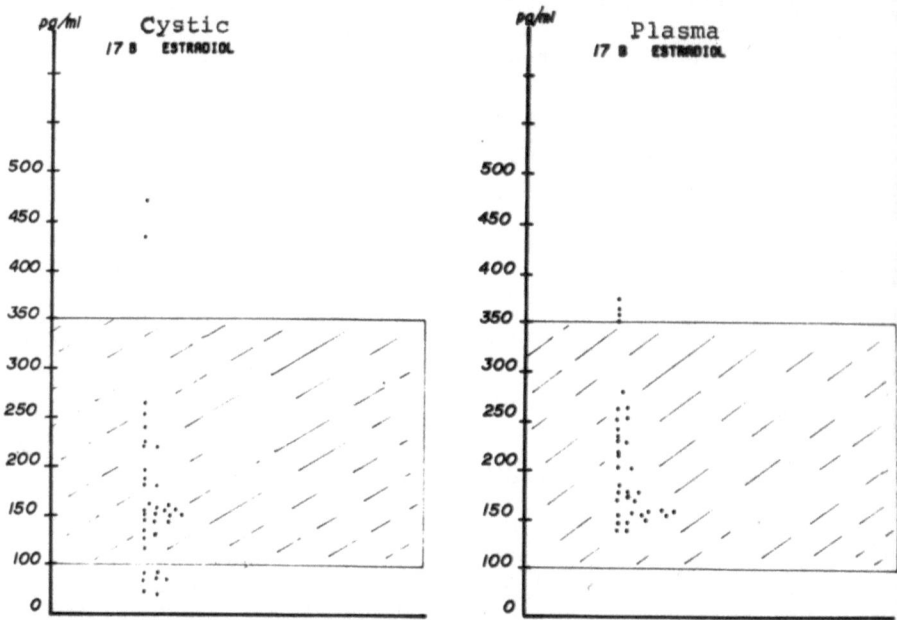

Fig. 2. Comparison of hormone levels occurring in the plasma
and cystic fluid of patients with GCD, P = 0.54,n.s.

were determined for a comparative study in these patients.
All cases, including patients with cyst recurrence, were examined clinically (palpation) and by ultrasonography and mammography.

Number of patients	36	
Relapses after 3 months	8	(22.2%)
Relapses after 6 months	4	(11.1%)
Relapses after 9 months	3	(8.3%)
Total number of relapses	15	(41.6%)

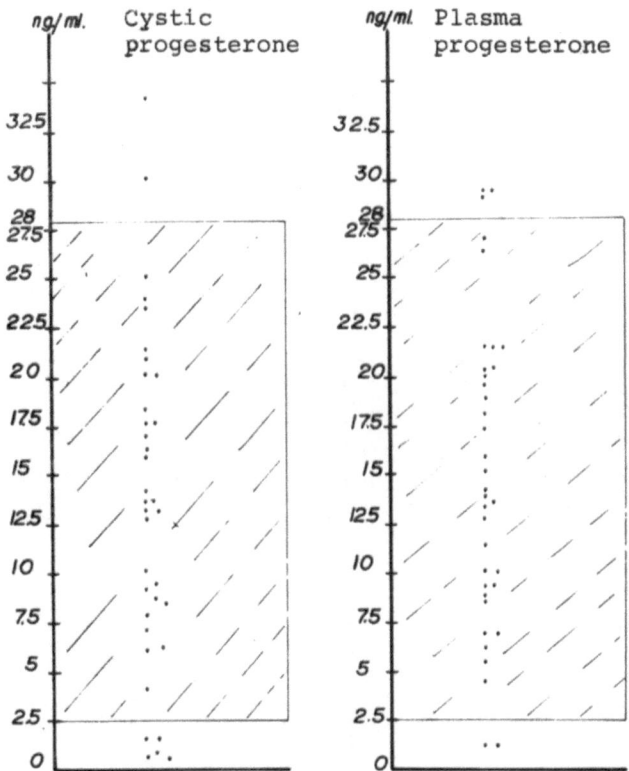

Fig. 3. Comparison of hormone levels occurring in the plasma
and cystic fluid of patients with GCD, P = 0.15, n.s.

RESULTS

The results were evaluated statistically (multiple linear suppression) and the following preliminary conclusions were drawn:

1. There was no significant correlation between plasma and cystic fluid levels of PRL (17 beta-estradiol, progesterone, testosterone and DHEA,

2. No clearcut differences were detected in relapsing patients during the period of observation.

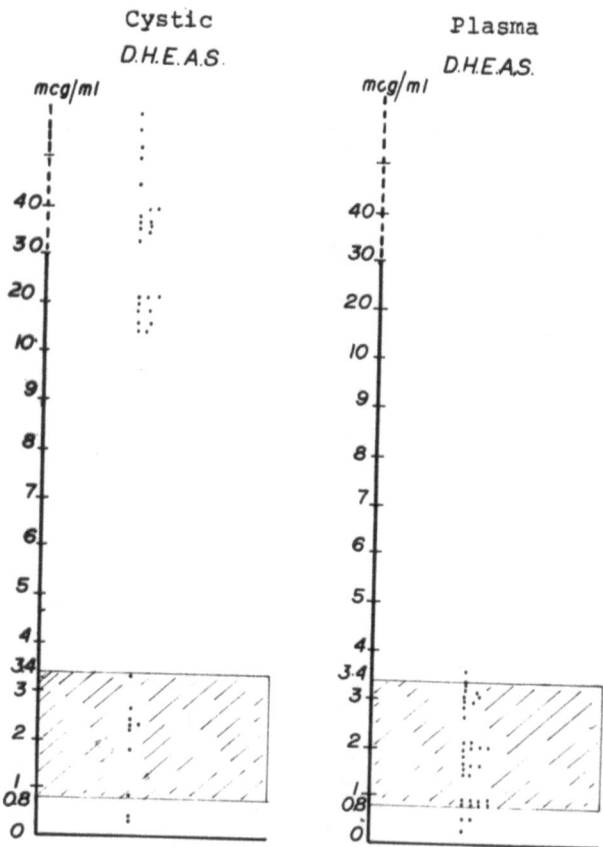

Fig. 4 : Comparison of hormone levels occurring in the plasma and cystic fluid of patients with GCD,
$P = 0.024 < 0.05$, s.

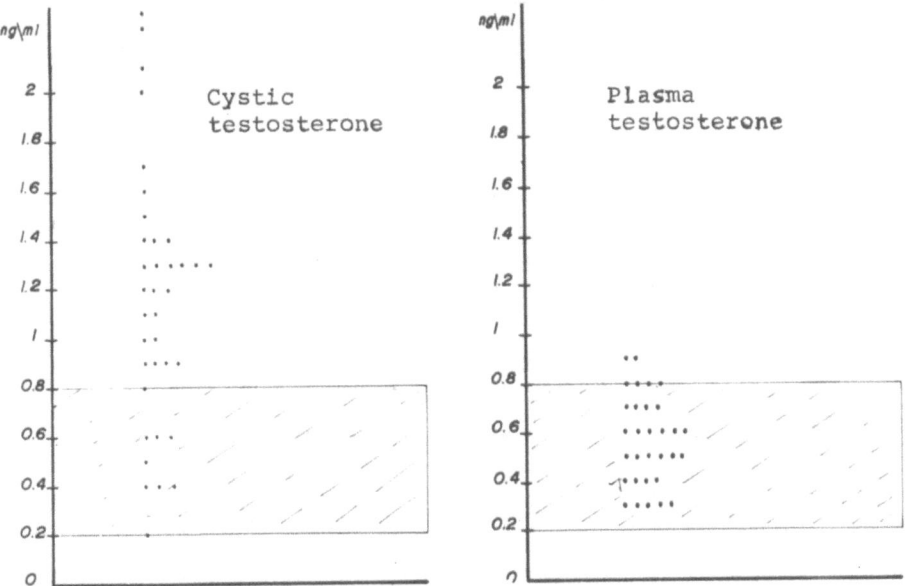

Fig. 5. Comparison of hormone levels occurring in the plasma
and cystic fluid of patients with GCD, P = 0.09, n.s.

A comparative analysis of the results recorded at the time
of the first observation and subsequently, at the time of relapse (using the same method), failed to reveal substantial
differences in hormone concentrations (Table 1).

We evaluated the possibility of a correlation between
hormone levels and the occurrence of a relapse in the group of
patients during the period of observation. For this purpose, we
resorted to multiple linear correlation analysis (Olivetti program "multivariate analysis code M2 400355") of initial findings. The data collected at the time of cyst recurrence were
subjected to reciprocal analysis. No correlation was detected
between symptomatology, and cyst diameter and number, on the
one hand, and hormone findings, on the other. There was some
correlation, however, between relapse and hormone data. Relapse and time of recurrence seemed to be particularly related to
cystic DHEA (coefficient 0.55) and cystic PRL (coefficient
0.54) levels.

These two results combined gave a correlation coefficient
of 0.68.

Although there was little correlation between plasma DHEA
levels and relapse, when plasma DHEA values were added, the

TABLE 1

FINDINGS IN 15 CASES	MEAN ± STANDARD DEVIATION INITIAL	DETERMINATIONS END	SIGNIFICANT DIFFERENCES IN %	
1. Cystic fluid prolactin (ng/ml)	27.0 ± 10.0	23.0 ± 13.0	-16.4%	t=1.2051
2. Plasma prolactin (ng/ml)	21.0 ± 13.0	19.0 ± 10.0	- 7.9%	t=0.6301
3. Cystic 17-beta-estradiol (ng/ml)	130.0 ± 82.0	112.0 ± 69.0	-13.8%	t=0.6832
4. Plasma 17-beta-estradiol (ng/ml)	136.0 ± 69.0	148.0 ± 46.0	8.1%	t=0.4358
5. Cystic progesterone (ng/ml)	10.4 ± 8.6	14.4 ± 7.0	39.2%	t=1.2505
6. Plasma progesterone (ng/ml)	10.9 ± 6.2	13.2 ± 5.9	21.0%	t=0.8997
7. Cystic fluid DHEA (mcg/ml)	28.8 ± 10.8	19.6 ± 13.2	-31.9%	t=2.0575
8. Plasma DHEA (mcg/ml)	2.3 ± 1.3	2.4 ± 0.9	4.1%	t=0.4160
9. Cystic testosterone (ng/ml)	1.4 ± 0.6	1.0 ± 0.4	-27.5%	t=1.8481
10. Plasma testerone (ng/ml)	0.6 ± 0.2	0.5 ± 0.2	- 9.6%	t=0.6359
11. Cyst diameter (cm)	2.3 ± 0.6	2.1 ± 0.5	- 5.9%	t=1.1687

Significant: $P < 0.05$

Highly significant: $P < 0.01$

correlation coefficient rose to 0.71 with P = 0.0001.

A multiple correlation coefficient of 0.79 was obtained by including the other findings, although, strictly speaking, they were not related to relapse.

In conclusion, it is clear that our understanding of the mechanisms underlying fibrocystic disease is in the initial stages, at least as regards the role played by hormones. At present, there is no known hormone profile capable of systematically and correctly characterizing this disease on the basis of plasma and cystic fluid findings.

Our date have shown that, with respect to recurrence, some hormones (cystic DHEA, cystic PRL and plasma DHEA), seem to play a significant role, especially when a synergistic effect is involved. Our study was too small for any definite conclusions to be drawn, but in the absence of reliable clinical and laboratory parameters, consideration should be given to further investigating the possibility of employing these or other hormone parameters for greater accuracy in clinically monitoring Gross Cystic Disease, in particular as regards the possible recurrence of cyst formation.

REFERENCES

1. Angeli, A. and Dogliotti, L.: Biochimica del liquido cistico. In: La Mastopatia Fibrocistica. Una revisione e Nuove Prospettive, Angeli A., Dogliotti L., eds, Excerpta Medica, 1984 pp. 40-48.

2. Angeli, A., Dogliotti, L., Borretta, G. and Violino, P.L.: Aspetti endocrinologici della mastopatia fibrocistica. Rec. Progr. in Med. 72, 49-51, 1982.

3. Bradlow, H.L., Schwartz, M.K., Fleisher, M., Nisselbaum, J.S. Boyar, R., O'Connor, J. and Fukushima, D.K.: Accumulation of hormones in breast cyst fluid, J. Clin. Endocrinol. Metab. 49, 778-782, 1979.

4. Bradlow, H.L., Schwartz, M.K., Fleisher, M., Rosenfeld, R.S. and Kream, J.: Hormone levels in human breast cyst fluid. In: Endocrinology of cystic breast disease, Angeli, A., Bradlow, H.L. and Dogliotti L., eds, Raven Press, New York, 1983, pp 59-75.

5. Frairia, R., Agrimonti, F., Fazzari, A.M., Barbadora, E.D., Boccuzzi, G. and Angeli, A.: Evidence for a transcortin-like component in human breast cyst fluid. Clin. Chim. Acta, 131, 15-27, 1983.

6. Orlandi, F., Dogliotti, L., Boccuzzi, G., Buzzi, G., Naldoni, C., Torta, M. and Angeli, A.: Cations, prolactin and dehydro-isoandrosterone sulfate in human breast cyst fluid. J. Endocrinol. Invest., 7 (suppl. 1), 166, 1984.

METASTASIS

CONSIDERATIONS OF CLINICAL RELEVANCE ON THE METASTATIC PROCESS: A WORKING

HYPOTHESIS

PIETRO M. GULLINO

Istituto Anatomia Patologica, University of Torino, Via Santena 7, 10126 Torino, Italy, and Laboratory of Pathophysiology, National Cancer Institute, Bethesda, USA

The ability to predict whether or not, where and when metastasis will occur, is a major challenge for the oncologist who in most cases can successfully remove the primary tumor. The assumption that the more we know about the biology of metastasis the more likely we are to give patients an optimal treatment seems reasonable. The possibility of obtaining reliable quantitative data in humans is limited by ethical considerations and technical difficulties, therefore animal and in vitro models are mostly utilized in the study of the metastatic process. The suitability of these models to improve our knowledge of metastasis in humans worries the experimentalist and fosters perplexity in the clinician. At this time there are no better alternatives than sorting out similarities and contradictions between the experimental findings and the clinical reality. One can at least hope that the experimental data on the biological characteristics of metastasis will help to prevent ineffectual or dangerous treatments based on misconceptions. The objective of this presentation is to discuss some experimental findings that may help in reaching this goal and to present a working hypothesis on conditions that may favour metastatic growth as surmised from our work on angiogenesis.

THE PRESENCE OF NEOPLASTIC CELLS IN THE BLOOD STREAM AND THE ONSET OF METASTASIS

For many years the opinion prevailed that circulating cancer cells were equivalent to metastatic spread. This opinion was founded on the belief that formation of a tumor was a localized event and metastatic spread occurred when the tumor reached a certain size. Indeed, the finding of neoplastic cells in circulation is easier in subjects bearing large rather than small tumors (Gazet, 1966, Anderson et al. 1974, Meyvisch et al. 1980). However, a correlation between onset of metastasis and number of neoplastic cells in the peripheral blood has not been established (Melamed et al. 1962, Malmgren 1967, Stein-Werblowsky 1980).

This is in part dependent upon the difficulty of detecting neoplastic cells in the blood stream. The following experimental data appear to be relevant for an interpretation of the clinical value of neoplastic cells in the blood stream.

(a) Three to four million neoplastic cells were released into the blood stream every hour by one gram of a rat mammary carcinoma grown with a procedure that ensured the collection of the blood flowing out of the whole tumor and only from the tumor (Butler and Gullino 1975). Despite this extensive release, metastatic foci were not observed in this experimental model.

(b) A fibrosarcoma implanted in the femoral region of C57BL mice was perfused with an oxygenated, cell-free medium that permitted the count of tumor cells, singly or in clumps. Approximately 5 days after transplantation, neoplastic cells could be found in the perfusate. A linear relationship was found between the density of the perfused vessels and the concentration of cells in the perfusate. Moreover, the increment in the number of lung metastases was following the increase in the number of clumps (4 or more neoplastic cells) found in the perfusate (Liotta et al. 1974). These findings have been interpreted to indicate that as soon as the vascular network of the tumor is formed, neoplastic cells penetrate through the vascular wall and can therefore be easily "washed out" by the perfusing fluid.

(c) Neoplastic cells injected intravenously showed signs of degeneration very rapidly (Takahashi 1915), suggesting that the blood stream is an unfavourable milieu for neoplastic cell survival.

The experimental evidence is therefore suggesting to the clinician that neoplastic cells are released into the blood stream as soon as the vascular network of the primary tumor is formed i.e. in the great majority of cases before the tumor is clinically detectable. Presence of neoplastic cells in the blood stream does not mean metastatic spread but only probability of it. This probability should increase with the increase in tumor size since the vascular network becomes larger and more cells are passing into the blood stream. However, the assumption that tumors give metastases only when they reach a large size is incorrect.

The observations that cell-clumps are more efficient in inducing metastasis and that tumor manipulation increases the number of these clumps (Liotta et al. 1976), suggest caution in handling the primary tumor during diagnostic as well as therapeutic procedures.

METASTASIZING CAPACITY AND ORGANOTROPISM OF NEOPLASTIC CELL POPULATIONS

The probability that cells able to form a metastatic colony were different from the rest of the tumor cell population became more compelling after the presence of circulating neoplastic cells was demonstrated to be a necessary but not sufficient condition for the onset of metastasis.

Strong support for the hypothesis was obtained from the application of the clonal selection technique in vivo. Neoplastic cells were dissociated from solid tumors, grown in culture, detached from the culture dish and reinjected i.v. into the appropriate host. The solid metastases from the lung were removed, the cells were dissociated and carried through another cycle. For B16 melanoma of the C57BL mouse the repetition of this procedure for 5 cycles yielded a cell subline that produced about 7-fold more lung metastases than the initial line upon i.v. injection (Fidler 1973). Similar results were obtained with a uv-induced sarcoma of C3H mice (Raz et al. 1981) and mammary carcinomas in Fisher rats (Neri et al. 1982). These findings are interpreted to indicate that the organotropism was dependent upon the prevalence of a clone with high metastasizing capacity already present in the initial tumor (Nicolson et al. 1978, Nicolson and Custead 1982). It must be emphasized that the cloning selection in vivo applied to liver metastasis in the B16 melanoma model yielded a subline with only a relative but not exclusive liver preference (Tao et al. 1979) and for the brain it failed to yield any population with brain organotropism. The clonogenic nature of the metastasizing cell population is, however, an important finding because it facilitates the analysis of two fundamental aspects of metastasis, the nature of the metastasizing cells and the type of selective pressures necessary to isolate them.

The search for peculiarities that may help in distinguishing cells with high versus low metastasizing capacity, has accumulated a large number of observations pointing out differences between the two populations (Fidler 1973). In general these differences are clear, but their relevance to the metastasizing capacity is less convincing.

Glycoconjugates of the cell surface for instance are believed to play a major role in promoting metastasis. Two examples may suffice to sustain this statement. Rat mammary carcinomas with high metastasizing capacity have been found to be poorer in ruthenium red stainable glycocalyx than mammary carcinomas with low metastasizing capacity (Kim et al. 1975, Gosh et al. 1980). The difference was due to high production of glycoconjugates by metastasizing cells that released them into the blood stream and low production by non metastasizing cells that retained the glycoconjugates on the cell surface.

The sialic acid content of murine tumors with high metastatic capacity was about 1.5 greater than the content of tumor lines with low with the degree of sialylation of galactosyl and N-acetyl galactosamyl residues in the glycoconjugates of the cell surface (Yogeeswaran and Salk, 1980, 1981).

Presently one can propose three interpretations for the difference in the content of glycoconjugates between cells metastasizing or not. (a) Shedding of glycoproteins from the cell surface may alter the antigenic properties of the neoplastic cells, therefore the increased metastasizing capacity could be the consequence of an "escape" from the host's immunological control (Kim 1970). (b) Sialolipoproteins can aggregate platelets (Karpatkin et al. 1981) and production of high quantities of glycoconjugates may enhance the frequency of clump formation and therefore metastasis (Fidler and Zeidman 1972, Liotta et al. 1976). Indeed, it is well known that inhibitors of platelet aggregation reduce the frequency of metastasis. (c) A third interpretation is suggested by the recently observed effect of gangliosides on mobilization of capillary endothelium (Alessandri et al. 1986) as discussed more extensively in the final section.

If the metastatic foci are clonogenic in nature the high production and shedding of glycoconjugates might have prognostic value provided that it is a property common to several tumor types.

The ability to solubilize collagen appears to be another property of the metastasizing cell population that might have prognostic value.

Media from cultures of highly metastatic murine tumors has been shown to contain proteolytic activity with preference toward type IV collagen. The proteolytic activity has been purified, it is a protein with molecular weight of about 65000 daltons which does not appreciably degrade type I, II, III or V collagens, nor non-collagenous proteins (Jones and DeClerck 1980, Liotta et al. 1980). Similar data were obtained with human neoplastic lines. Production of type IV collagenase is particularly important in facilitating the passage of neoplastic cells across the vascular wall. Indeed, the neoplastic cells washed out of the tumor vascular system, i.e. already penetrated across the capillary wall, solubilized collagen to a significantly higher degree than cells from the primary tumor or from non neoplastic tissues such as spleen or liver (Liotta et al. 1977). Moreover, in several mouse neoplastic lines the frequency of metastasis correlated positively with the amount of basement membrane degraded enzymatically (Liotta et al. 1980) and the ability of B16 melanoma cells to adhere to the subendothelial basement membrane of intact blood vessels related directly to their metastatic capacity (Poste and Fidler 1980).

There is good evidence in support of the hypothesis tnat the metastasizing cells are indeed a population with some peculiar characteristics as compared to the general cell population of the tumor. High production of glycoconjugates and collagenase type IV appear to be two characteristic features that might be exploited for clinical purposes.

STIMULATION OF METASTATIC GROWTH

Removal of the primary tumor in almost all patients occurs after millions of neoplastic cells have lodged in the host tissues. In most cases the appearance of metastasis some months or a few years after the removal of the primary tumor is simply a case of "lead-time bias", i.e. the interval necessary for the microscopic foci to become clinically detectable (Bailar 1976).

There are, however, observations that do not appear to be justified by this explanation. For instance, the death from metastasis of patients operated for primary breast cancer 20 years earlier was found to be still 16 times more frequent than would be expected in a normal population with a comparable overall death-rate (Brinkley and Haybittle 1975). In these cases the assumption that some event occurred to "awake" silent metastasis seems reasonable, although difficult to pin point at this time.

Tissue damage:

Fisher has given one of the first experimental demonstrations of the role that tissue damage might have on the occurrence of metastatic foci (Fisher and Fisher 1959). Only 50 cells of Walker carcinoma were injected into the vena porta in rats that 3 months later were subjected to repeated laparatomies and liver manipulations at 7-day intervals. All treated animals had tumors within a few weeks in contrast to untreated animals which had none. Indeed, contact with dead cells or fragments thereof appeared to have a determinant effect on the growth of silent metastasis in this experimental model (Fisher and Fisher 1963, Fisher et al. 1967).

There are at least 4 clinical events that may be relevant to the interdependence of tissue damage and metastasis formation. Palpation of tumors is obviously a necessary manipulation for diagnostic and therapeutic purposes. The procedure is known to increase the number of cells released into circulation by the tumor (Romsdahl et al. 1965) in particular cell-clumps that enhance frequency of metastasis rather than single cells (Liotta et al. 1976). Warren (1981) has called attention to the possible danger of microinjuries produced by these clumps liberated by repeated palpations, particularly in relation to the sensitivity to damage of capillary endothelium of certain organs (Dingemans 1973).

Increasing attention is being paid to hyperthermia as a possible form of cancer therapy but experimental observations of enhanced dissemination of metastasis following hyperthermia is another event to be considered under the heading of tissue injuries. Dickson and Ellis (1974) observed an unexpectedly large dissemination of cells by Yoshida sarcoma following inadequate heating at 42 °C. Yerushalmi (1976) reported a similar finding for the Lewis lung carcinoma but only following whole-body hyperthermia. Walker et al. (1978) also observed a dramatic promotion of metastasis in a poorly metastatic carcinoma of C3H mice following local heating sufficient to eradicate the primary tumor. In our experience with rat mammary carcinomas (Gullino et al. 1982), the temperature gradients within a heated tumor are surprisingly large. Differences of 1-2 °C among regions separated only by a few mm of tissue are quite frequent. These differences are difficult to predict or control and may very well determine whether the treatment is adequate or in danger of producing metastasis.

A large amount of work has been done on another agent that can intensify metastatic growth: x rays. Lungs of normal mice or rats irradiated for a few hours to several days before an intravenous injection of neoplastic cells, have been repeatedly shown to have more metastasis than non irradiated lungs (Brown 1973b, Peters 1974). Within a 200-2000 rads range the increase is dose dependent, transitory in nature and probably due to the elevated number of neoplastic cells trapped in the lungs (Fidler and Zeidman 1972, Brown 1973a,). Similar conclusions were reached for UV irradiation in C3H mice bearing fibrosarcomas (Kripke and Fidler 1980). A large number of metastases was also observed in the lungs of C3H male mice receiving intravenous injections of mammary carcinoma cells 9.5 months after irradiation (250 rad). The growth rate of foci in the fibrotic tissue was enhanced as compared to non irradiated animals (Thompson 1974).

Attention should be called to an experiment in which 500-2000 rad administered to rats 4 to 30 days after inoculation of a mammary carcinoma cell suspension did not significantly increase the number of lung metastases (Dao and Yogo 1967). Neoplastic cells that circulate after the tissue has been damaged seems to be a necessary condition to enhance the frequency of metastatic foci.

Radiotherapists are fully aware of the possible implications that these experimental data may have for human therapy. In view of the obvious clinical benefits derived from the irradiation procedures, the experimentalists have the responsability to elucidate the mechanism(s) involved in the laboratory results before firm conclusions on the limits between benefits and potential hazards may be drawn.

Another clinical event that possibly may be involved in stimulating metastatic growth is the incisional biopsy. The reason obviously is related to the release of neoplastic cells and clumps into circulation. The question has been hotly debated by clinicians. The experimental animal models have given both negative (Maun and Dunning 1946, Paslin 1973) and positive (Riggins and Ketcham 1965, Keller 1981,) answers to the possibility that an incisional biopsy enhances the frequency of metastasis. Clinical experience rather than the experimental models must provide the answer to this question.

Removal of primary tumor:

The extent of metastatic spread should be expected to be directly related to the survival of the host. Indeed this has been shown in 3 experimental systems. When the primary tumor was amputated the survival was longer but the metastatic pattern changed only in that metastasis were fewer and mostly confined to the lungs of the model studied (Wexler et al. 1965, Suit et al. 1970,).

The experiments concerned with metastatic pattern and survival of the host, bring out the question of growth acceleration of metastasis after removal of the primary tumor (Schatten and Kramer 1958, De Wys 1972, Gorelick et al. 1980, Ohl et al. 1980,). For a mammary carcinoma grown in C3H mice as multiple foci it has been observed that removal of one tumor was followed by an increase in labeled mitoses in the remaining foci and a shortening of the cell-doubling time (Gundoz et al. 1979).

Hindrance of metastatic growth by the primary tumor is believed to be one aspect of concomitant immunity. In a homotransplantable lymphoma, for instance, Gershon and Carter (1970) observed that a second transplant of the tumor in the same hamster was rejected in a way reminiscent of a homograft reaction. A comparable inhibitory influence on metastatic growth had been observed by Greene et al. (1960) in a transplantable hamster lymphoma. Enhancement of metastatic growth resulted either after primary tumor removal or after depression of the host immunological competence by injection of anti-lymphocyte serum. Similar data were obtained by Schatten and Kramer (1958) and Deodhar (1971) using sarcoma 180 in Swiss mice as a model.

On the contrary, Gorelick et al. (1980) using the Lewis lung carcinoma model, could also observe acceleration of metastatic growth after removal of the primary tumor, however, this occurred in tumors grown in immunosuppressed C57BL mice. Indeed, the rejection response to a second implant followed the same sequence and had the same general characteristics in normal and in immunodepressed mice. The authors suggest that suppression of metastatic growth by the primary tumor as well as rejection of a second graft depend upon a non immune mechanism. Possibly the tumor may generate factors that depress cell proliferation in general and not only the proliferation of metastatic foci. The well known atrophy of the bone marrow in tumor bearing patients could be an example.

At this time it seems reasonable to conclude that some evidence exists to suggest an influence of the primary tumor on the growth rate of metastasis, however the nature of this influence, if any, is unknown.

Immunocompetence:

Mammary carcinomas can be easily induced in female W/Fu rats by 3-methylcholanthrene. These tumors do not metastasize. However, if the animals are thymectomized and/or splenectomized and subjected during the early period of carcinogenesis to immunoselective pressure such as injections of BCG, metastasizing mammary carcinomas are produced (Kim et al. 1975).

This is one example of several types of experiments pointing to the determinant influence of the host on the metastasizing capacity of neoplastic cell populations. The nature of this influence is not clear. Macrophages and T-lymphocytes of the host appear to play a major role. For instance, tumors heterotransplanted into 3 week old athymic-nudes give frequent metastases. At this age the animals are poor in functional T-lymphocytes and have low natural-killer activity. However, if the 3 week old nudes are treated with corynebacterium parvum or polyinosinic-polycytidylic acid that enhance NK cells activity, the frequency of lung metastases is sharply reduced (Hanna and Fidler 1981).

The most perplexing aspect, however, is the behaviour of the metastatic cell population. Sugarbaker and Cohen (1972) for instance, tested the antigenicity of 7 pulmonary metastases of a highly immunogenic sarcoma induced by methylcholanthrene in syngenic C57BL mice. The 7 metastatic cell populations were transplanted into C57BL mice immunized against the primary tumor. Two implants were rejected, indicating that these cell populations shared transplantation antigens with the primary tumor. The remaining 5 implants grew uninhibited in the immunized host. Two of the 5 implants were immunogenic i.e. were able to induce rejection of a second implant, but the other 3 were not.

The diversity in the immunological behaviour of cell populations derived from the same tumor can be manifested within a single host. 14 out of 20 tumors that had been heterotransplanted subcutaneously in immunosuppressed hamsters metastasized into the lung, but in 12 of them the subcutaneous implant was later rejected while the lung metastasis continued to grow (Cobb 1972).

While it is clear that the immunological status of the host does profoundly influence the frequency and the rapidity of metastatic growth, our present knowledge of this area does not go beyond a very large accumulation of observations obtained with a variety of approaches applied to diverse experimental systems. Efforts to coordinate all these observations into a biologically meaningful system have not yet fully succeeded, therefore the possible clinical applications are still at an infant stage.

SUPPRESSION OF METASTATIC GROWTH

The existence of "dormant" metastasis is a well known event (Wheelock et al. 1981) but the reasons for this latency are poorly understood. The increase in volume of metastasis or the lack of it has long been assumed to depend on conditions affecting the growth fraction of the cell population.

Cytolysis:

The L5178y lymphoma of DBA/2 mice is one of the best models available to sustain the hypothesis that the dormant state of metastasis can be maintained by a cytolytic action of the lymphocytes against the neoplastic cells (Wheelock et al. 1980). L5178y lymphoma injected i.p. grows rapidly; however, when the host is previously challenged by a subcutaneous implant, the cell population of an intraperitonal implant is kept in zero net growth for weeks by the lytic action of T-lymphocytes. The lysis does not hit all cells. The ones that escape destruction have a decreased expression of tumor associated antigens (Wheelock et al. 1981).

This kind of observation suggested that potentiation of the lymphocyte action should control or depress metastatic growth. Accordingly, immunorestorative drugs have been used as an adjunct to surgery and thiobendazole given in the preoperative period has been reported to improve the cytotoxic response and decrease pulmonary metastases (Lundy et al. 1979). The inability to obtain complete destruction of the metastatic foci is usually ascribed to antigenic differences of metastatic cell populations as illustrated above.

The killing of neoplastic cells is not a prerogative of lymphocytes. Macrophages activated by cultivation in media to which supernatants of B16 melanoma cultures had been added were able to kill neoplastic cells in vitro and reduce the number of metastases when injected in vivo (Fidler 1976). The presence of macrophages in tumors is well recognized and Machinami (1973) demonstrated that foci of 6-12 cells produced in the lung after i.v. injection of Hepatoma AH7974 were already surrounded by macrophages.

The possibility that tumor macrophages derive from monocytes may have clinical implications. Fidler (1980) observed that i.v. injection of liposomes containing lymphokines substantially reduced the number of metastases and circulating monocytes are known to incorporate most of the injected lyposomes (Poste et al. 1982). If circulating monocytes accumulate within the tumor they could be carriers of antineoplastic effectors.

Besides acting as a cytotoxic cell, the macrophage is involved in the process of antigen recognition by lymphocytes. The role of this property in influencing the ability of macrophages to block cell growth is not clear.

One should not lose sight of the fact that in vivo tumors continue to grow relentlessly despite the high content of macrophages. Whether the antigens shed by the tumor form adducts with antibodies as well as with cytotoxic cells and neutralize their capacity to kill the neoplastic cells remains an unproven hypothesis. The basic question: why do antigenic tumors grow relentlessly and metastasize in hosts able to mount an immunological response to transplantation-type, tumor-specific antigens? remains unanswered. In a way the answer is clouded by a large volume of experimental data whose relevance to the human tumors and to the in vivo reality is questioned so that the whole concept of surveillance of neoplastic growth by the immune system of the host is now in dispute (Schwartz 1975, Möller and Möller 1976,).

Angiogenesis:

The assumption that control of metastatic growth requires death of the neoplastic cells is probably too limited. Formation of a tumor requires not only a cell population that grows continuously but also a vascular stroma that supplies and appropriately distributes the nutrients. One can surmise that lack of the vascular network produced by the host can prevent formation of a tumor. The most convincing experiment in support of this concept is the implantation of V2 carcinoma cells (Brem et al. 1976) in the center of the avascular corpus vitreous of a rabbit's eye. The cells grow to form a nodule about 1 mm in diameter or less, then stop growing and the nodule remains practically unchanged for weeks. However, if at the time of implantation a few neoplastic cells within the tunnel left by the needle migrate toward the vascularized retina, a network of vessels is formed to sustain a rapidly growing tumor. In this experiment presence or absence of angiogenesis conditions tumor formation (Brem et al. 1976). In fact, neoplastic tissues have high angiogenic capacity (Folkman 1974, Gullino 1978) and in the course of neoplastic transformation, the capacity to induce new formation of vessels is a property acquired by cell populations before the relentless growth is manifested (Ziche and Gullino 1982).

Blocking of angiogenesis should arrest the growth of a tumor. Indeed, a substantial reduction in the growth of V2 carcinoma was obtained by continuous infusion of a cartilage fraction with antiangiogenic activity (Langer et al. 1980). Alteration of tumor vascularization was considered the cause of inhibition of tumor growth in hamsters receiving high doses of selenium in drinking water (Jacobs et al. 1980, Watrach et al. 1982) or in mice treated with ICRF 159, a compound believed to influence the tumor vascular system (Salsbury et al. 1970, 1974; Atherton 1975).

Cell Hybridization:

Another possibility of blocking metastatic growth without killing the growing cells is indicated by the experiments of Standbridge and Ceredig (1981). HeLa-fibroblast hybrid cells were found unable to form tumors in athymic nude mice when injected subcutaneously, or intravenously, or when the animals were new-borns or heavily irradiated. Only rarely tumorigenic segregants arose spontaneously and they were chromosomally and biochemically very similar to their non-tumorigenic hybrid counterparts. Tumorigenic and non-tumorigenic populations were very sensitive to NK activity in vitro, however, both grew well in athymic nudes with high NK activity stimulated by corynebacterium parvum in vivo. Both tumorigenic and non-tumorigenic populations were indistinguishable in their proliferative behaviour and morphology during the first 3 to 4 days following transplantation. By day 4, however, the non-tumorigenic line terminated the mitotic activity and assumed a fibroblastic morphology; the tumorigenic line, on the contrary, went on growing to form a tumor. Cells obtained from the non-tumorigenic hybrids could be re-established in culture 15 days after transplantation when mitotic activity and growth had long ceased. Thus, viability was preserved and the HeLa-fibroblast hybrid cells were probably prevented from proliferating by factor(s) that inhibited mitotic activity without destroying the cells subjected to growth inhibition. No lymphoid infiltration was seen around either cell populations suggesting that cellular immune responses were not involved.

A comparable form of growth control has been observed by Stiles et al. (1976). Several years ago, Stoker et al. (1966) reported growth inhibition of polyoma transformed BHK21 cells by confluent fibroblasts not dividing and in contact or in close proximity to the BHK21 cells.

Anticoagulants:

A special position in the control of metastatic growth is occupied by treatment with anticoagulants. The assumptions on which the treatment was founded started from the observation that neoplastic cells injected i.v. usually acquire a tail of platelets supported by fibrin. Prompt and selective localization of fibrin around embolic tumor cells was detected in the capillaries examined with the transparent ear chamber technique. Cell aggregation followed by microemboli and destruction of endothelium and penetration of the neoplastic cells beyond the capillary wall occurred in rapid sequence (Wood 1964). Accordingly, drugs preventing platelet aggregation or platelet-release reactions (Gasic et al. 1968, Kolenich et al. 1972, Mussoni et al. 1978, Kohga et al. 1981,), drugs inactivating plasma clotting factors and thrombin generation (Boeryd 1966, Hilgard et al. 1972, Tsubura et al. 1977, Kobayashi et al. 1979, Williamson et al. 1980, Owen 1981, 1982,), drugs influencing fibrin deposition (Austin and Glaser 1969, Hagmar 1972) or fibrinolysis (Johnson and Wood 1963, Cederholm-Williams 1980,) were used under a variety of conditions. The rationale of the anticoagulation treatment in cancer relies mostly on the assumption that neoplastic cells are prevented from lodging within the capillaries and the prolonged permanence in the circulation enhances the chances of their destruction. Some direct effects of anticoagulants on the neoplastic cells have also been observed. On the whole, however, the clinical results of anticoagulation have been less convincing than the premises on which the treatments were grounded. A re-evaluation of these premises is now underway.

PRODUCTION OF GLYCOCONJUGATES, METASTASIZING CAPACITY AND ANGIOGENESIS

As mentioned in a previous section, several investigators have observed that metastasizing capacity is higher in neoplastic cell populations producing large quantities of glycoconjugates as compared to low producers (Kim et al. 1975, Yogeeswaran and Salk 1981).

The interpretation that an elevated synthesis and release of glycoconjugates alters the antigenic properties of the tumor cells and therefore subtracts them from immunological control is appealing, however convincing data do not exist to explain how this could occur. Good documentation is available for the interpretation that high production of glycoconjugates increases cell agglutination and formation of clumps, known to increase substantially the metastasizing capacity (Liotta et al. 1976). However, the increased facility for clumping only explains a higher possibility of microemboli, not their advantage for survival and growth into solid tumors.

We have observed that motility of endothelium is substantially improved (5 fold) by incubation of capillary endothelium with gangliosides, particularly GT1. The cells incorporated the ganglioside and increased their binding to fibronectin which appears to be the best substratum for supporting endothelial cell motility. Moreover, when an angiogenesis effector was utilized to induce neovascularization of the rabbit cornea in vivo, the area to be colonized by the capillaries became richer in sialic acid than the contralateral cornea treated with a non-angiogenic stimulus (Alessandri et al. 1986). Thus, in vivo also an increased concentration of gangliosides might precede neovascularization.

Formation of a vascular network by the host is necessary for the growth of a solid tumor (Folkman 1974) and in avascular organs like the corpus vitreous (Brem et al. 1976) or in perfused organs where the endothelium is unable to proliferate (Folkman et al. 1968), neoplastic cells form only a tiny nodule. like an in vitro spheroid, but not a solid tumor.

Evidence has been obtained to indicate that most tumors have angiogenic capacity (Folkman 1974) which is a property acquired in the course of neoplastic transformation (Ziche and Gullino 1982). One can hypothesize that the formation of a new vascular network is due to an "angiogenesis factor" that triggers and controls neovascularization or that angiogenesis is an end point in a sequence of several events that should occur in a given order. Following this second approach we observed that pericellular stroma fragmented by lytic enzymes acquired the ability to stimulate motility of capillary endothelium (Ungari et al. 1985) i.e. to initiate the first step in the new formation of a vessel.

Components of this stroma are fibronectin and heparin derivatives which constitute a substratum that best facilitates the mobilization of capillary endothelium when anchored to collagen (Alessandri et al. 1986). Since elevated production of lytic enzymes (Liotta et al. 1980) and gangliosides (Yogeeswaran and Salk 1980, 1981) are two well recognized properties of highly metastasizing cell populations, the previous observations are compatible with the following hypothesis: high production of glycoconjugates favours clumping, i.e. microembolism and "stickiness" to endothelium, but also creates in vivo a microenvironment similar to our in vitro incubation of endothelium with gangliosides. This event coupled with lysis of fibronectin, heparan sulfate of the basement membrane and hyaluronic acid of the interstitium (West et al. 1985) favours mobilization of capillary endothelium, i.e. the neovascularization that permits tumor growth. At this time the most satisfactory explanation of the high metastatic capacity of neoplastic

264

cell populations with high production of glycoconjugates and lytic enzymes, brings angiogenesis into consideration.

The obvious corollary to this working hypothesis is that by knowing more about the mechanism of angiogenesis we might be able to interfere with metastatic growth, particularly at the time of clinically silent metastasis.

CONCLUDING REMARKS

How much help has the experimentalist given to the clinician in the field of metastasis? A fair answer is probably: not much.

Growth, apparently unrestrained, is the major symptom of the neoplastic diseases and the prevalent thrust of the research effort is oriented towards an understanding of events that control cell growth. The experimentalist, lacking, at this time, a sufficient knowledge of cell proliferation and therefore a possibility of blocking growth, offers the clinician only a set of data that may help in avoiding misconceptions by increasing our knowledge of the metastatic process. To this end the following points, derived from experimental work, have been emphasized: (a) spreading of neoplastic cells occurs almost in all cases long before the primary tumor is clinically detected; (b) not every neoplastic cell is necessarily able to form a metastasis. The one that does, appears to be endowed with some peculiarity that is not clearly defined at this time; (c) a set of events may enhance onset and growth of metastasis. A clinician must be aware of them even if clinical necessities sometimes force him to ignore them; (d) the efforts at suppressing metastatic growth are at an infancy stage; (e) a working hypothesis linking production of glycoconjugates, metastasizing capacity and angiogenesis has been presented.

ACKNOWLEDGEMENTS

Part of the experimental work reported in this paper has been supported by the Associazione Italiana Ricerche Sul Cancro, and CNR (ITALY) P.F. Oncologia Grant n° 84.00478.44

REFERENCES

Alessandri, G., Raju, K.S., Gullino, P.M., Interaction of gangliosides with fibronectin in the mobilization of capillary endothelium: possible influence on the growth of metastasis. Invasion Metastasis, 134 (in press), 1986.

Anderson, J.C., Fugmann, R.A., Stalfi, R.L., Martin, D.S., Metastatic
     incidence of a spontaneous murine mammary adenocarcinoma. Cancer
     Res., 34, 1916-1920, 1974.
Atherton, A., The effect of (+)1, 2-bis(3,5-dioxopiperazin-1-yl) propane
     (ICRF 159) on liver metastases from a hamster lymphoma. Eur. J.
     Cancer, 11, 383-388, 1975.
Austin, J.P., Glaser, E.M., Inhibition of experimental tumours by
     defribinogenation. Clin. Sci., 37, 878, 1969.
Bailar, J.C., Mammography: a contrary view. Ann. Int. Med., 84, 77-84,
     1976.
Boeryd, B., Effect of heparin and plasminogen inhibitor (EACA) in brief
     and prolonged treatment on intravenously injected tumour cells.
     Acta. Pathol. Microbiol. Scand., 68, 347-354, 1966.
Brem, S., Brem, H., Folkman, J., Finkelstein, D., Patz, A., Prolonged
     tumor dormancy by prevention of neovascularization in the vitreous.
     Cancer Res., 36, 2807-2812, 1976.
Brinkley, D., Haybittle, J.L., The curability of breast cancer. Lancet,
     2, 95-97, 1975.
Brown, J.M., The effect of lung irradiation on the incidence of pulmonary
     metastases in mice. Br. J. Radiol., 46, 613-618, 1973 a.
Brown, J.M., A study of the mechanism by which anticoagulation with
     Warfarin inhibits blood-borne metastases. Cancer Res., 33,
     1217-1224, 1973 b.
Butler, T.P., Gullino, P.M., Quantitation of cell shedding into efferent
     blood of mammary adenocarcinoma. Cancer Res., 35, 512-516, 1975.
Cederholm-Williams, S.A., Molecular mechanism of fibrinolysis and its
     potential role in metastasis. In: Metastasis, clinical and
     experimental aspects; proceedings of the EORTC Metastasis Group
     International Conference, K. Hellmann, P. Hilgard and S. Eccles,
     eds., Martinus Nijhoff, The Hague, 1980, pp. 95-99.
Cobb, L.M., Metastatic spread of human tumour implanted into thymec-
     tomized, antithymocyte serum treated hamsters, Br. J. Cancer, 26,
     183-189, 1972.
Dao, T.L., Yogo, H., Enhancement of pulmonary metastases by x-irradiation
     in rats bearing mammary cancer. Cancer, 20, 2020-2025, 1967.
Deodhar, S.D., Enhancement of metastases by L-asparaginase in a mouse
     tumor system. J. Reticuloendothel. Soc., 10, 212-222, 1971.
De Wys, W.D., Studies correlating the growth rate of a tumor and its
     metastases and providing evidence for tumor-related systemic
     growth-retarding factors. Cancer Res., 32, 374-379, 1972.
Dickson, J.A., Ellis, H.A., Stimulation of tumour cell dissemination by
     raised temperature (42°C) in rats with transplanted Yoshida
     tumours. Nature, 248, 354-358, 1974.
Dingemans, K.P., Behaviour of intravenously injected malignant lymphoma
     cells; a morphologic study. J. Natl. Cancer Inst., 51, 1883-1895,
     1973.
Fidler, I.J., Zeidman, I., Enhancement of experimental metastasis

by x-ray: a possible mechanism. J. Med., 3, 172-177, 1972.

Fidler, I.J., The relationship of embolic homogeneity, number, size and viability to the incidence of experimental metastasis. Eur. J. Cancer, 9, 223-227, 1973.

Fidler, I.J., Selection of successive tumour lines for metastasis. Nature (New Biol.), 242, 148-149, 1973.

Fidler, I.J., Macrophage deficiency in tumor bearing animals: control of experimental metastasis with macrophages activated in vitro. In : The macrophage in neoplasia, M.A. Fink, ed., Academic Press, New York, 1976, pp. 245-257.

Fidler, I.J., Therapy of spontaneous metastases by intravenous injection of liposomes containing lymphokines. Science, 208, 1469-1471, 1980.

Fisher, B., Fisher, E.R., Experimental evidence in support of the dormant tumor cell. Science, 130, 918-919, 1959.

Fisher, B., Fisher, E.R.. Local factors affecting tumor growth. I. Effects of tissue homogenates. Cancer Res., 23, 1651-1657, 1963.

Fisher, B., Fisher, E.R., Fiduska, N., Trauma and the localization of tumor cells. Cancer, 20, 23-30, 1967.

Folkman, J., Tumor angiogenesis. Adv. Cancer Res., 19, 331-358, 1974.

Folkman, J., Winsey. S., Cole, P., Hodes, R., Isolated perfusion of thymus. In: Organ perfusion and preservation, J.C. Norman, ed., Appleton-Century-Crofts, New York, 1968, pp. 759-766.

Gasic, G.J., Gasic, T.B., Stewart, C.C., Antimetastatic effects associated with platelet reduction. Proc. Natl. Acad. Sci. USA, 61, 46-52, 1968.

Gazet, J-C., The detection of viable circulating cancer cells. Acta Cytol. (Balt.), 10, 19-25, 1966.

Gershon, R.K., Carter, R.L., Facilitation of metastatic growth by anti-lymphocyte serum. Nature, 226. 368-370, 1970.

Ghosh, L., Nassauer, J., Faiferman, I., Ghosh, B.C., Ultrastructure study of membrane glycocalyx in primary and metastatic human breast carcinoma. Clin. Oncol., 6, 21-24, 1980.

Gorelick, E., Segal, S., Feldman, M., Immunological and non-immunological mechanisms in the interactions between the local tumor and its metastasis. In: Metastatic tumor growth, E. Grundmann, ed., Gustav Fischer, New York, 1980, pp. 159-166.

Greene, H.S.N., Harvey, E.K., The inhibitory influence of a transplanted hamster lymphoma on metastasis. Cancer Res., 11, 460-462, 1960.

Gullino, P.M., Angiogenesis and oncogenesis. J. Natl. Cancer Inst., 61, 639-643, 1978.

Gullino, P.M., Jain, R.K., Grantham, F.H.,Temperature gradients and local perfusion in a mammary carcinoma. J. Natl. Cancer Inst., 68, 519-533, 1982.

Gundoz, N., Fisher, B., Saffer, E.A., Effect of surgical removal on the growth and kinetics of residual tumor. Cancer Res., 39, 3861-3865, 1979.

Hagmar, B., Defibrination and metastasis formation: effects of Arvin on experimental metastases in mice. Eur. J. Cancer, 8, 17-28, 1972.

Hanna, N., Fidler, I.J., Expression of metastatic potential of allogenic and xenogenic neoplasms in young nude mice. Cancer Res., 41, 438-444, 1981.

Hilgard, P., Beyerle, L., Hohage, R., Hiemeyer, V., Kubler, M., The effect of heparin on the initial phase of metastasis formation. Eur. J. Cancer, 8, 347-352, 1972.

Jacobs, M.M., Shubik, P., Feldman, R., Influence of selenium on vascularization in the hamster cheek pouch. Cancer Lett., 9, 353-357, 1980.

Johnson, J.H., Wood, S. Jr., An in vitro study of fibronolytic agents on V2 carcinoma cells and intravascular thrombi in rabbits. Bull. Hopkins Hosp., 113, 335-346, 1963.

Jones, P.A., DeClerck, Y.A., Destruction of extracellular matrices containing glycoproteins, elastin, and collagen by metastatic human tumor cells. Cancer Res., 40, 3222-3227, 1980.

Karpatkin, S., Pearlstein, E., Salk, P.L., Yogeeswaran, G., Role of platelets in tumor cell metastases. Ann. N.Y. Acad. Sci., 370, 101-118, 1981.

Keller, R., Induction of macroscopic metastases via surgery; the site of the primary tumor inoculum is critical. Invasion Metastasis, 1, 136-148, 1981.

Kim, U., Metastasizing mammary carcinomas in rats: induction and study of their immunogenicity. Science, 267, 72-74, 1970.

Kim, U., Baumler, A., Carruthers, C., Bielat, K., Immunological escape mechanism in spontaneously metastasizing mammary tumors. Proc. Natl. Acad. Sci. USA, 72, 1012-1016, 1975.

Kobayashi, M., Yamashita, T., Tsuburu, E., Inhibition of blood-borne pulmonary metastasis by sulfated polysaccharides; correlation between antimetastatic and anticoagulative activity. Tokushima J. Exp. Med. 26, 41-51, 1979.

Kolenich, J.J., Mansour, E.G., Flynn, A., Haematological effects of aspirin. Lancet, 2, 714, 1972.

Kohga, S., Kinjo, M., Tanaka, K., Ogawa, H., Ishira, M., Tanaka, N., Effects of 5-(2-chlorobenzyl)-4,5,6,7-tetrahydorthieno[3,2-C] pyridine hydrochloride (ticlopidine), a platelet aggregation inhibitor, on blood-borne metastasis. Cancer Res., 41, 4710-4714, 1981.

Kripke, M.L., Fidler, I.J., Enhanced experimental metastasis of ultra-violet light-induced fibrosarcomas in ultraviolet light-irradiated syngenic mice. Cancer Res., 40, 625-629, 1980.

Langer, R., Conn, H., Vacanti, J., Haudenschild, C., Folkman, J., Control of tumor growth in animals by infusion of an angiogenesis inhibitor. Proc. Natl. Acad. Sci. USA, 77, 4331-4335, 1980.

Liotta, L.A., Kleinerman, J., Saidel, G.M., Quantitative relationships of intravascular tumor cells, tumor vessels, and pulmonary metastases following tumor implantation. Cancer Res., 34, 997-1004, 1974.

Liotta, L.A., Kleinerman, J., Saidel, G.M., The significance of hematogenous tumor cell clumps in the metastatic process. Cancer Res.,
36, 889-894, 1976.

Liotta, L.A., Kleinerman, J., Catanzaro, P., Rynbrandt, D., Degradation
of basement membrane by murine tumor cells. J. Natl. Cancer Inst.,
58, 1427-1431, 1977.

Liotta, L.A., Tryggvason, K., Garbisa, S., Gehron Robey, P., Murray,
J.C., Interaction of metastatic tumor cells with basement membrane
collagen. In: Metastatic tumor growth, E. Grundmann ed., Gustav
Fischer, New York, 1980, pp. 21-30.

Liotta, L.A., Tryggvason, K., Garbisa, S., Hart, I., Foltz, C.M.,
Shafie, S., Metastatic potential correlates with enzymatic
degradation of basement membrane collagen. Nature, 284, 67-68,
1980.

Lundy, J., Lovett, E.J., Wolinsky, S.M., Conran, P., Immune impairment
and metastatic tumor growth; the need for an immunorestorative drug
as an adjunct to surgery. Cancer, 43, 945-951, 1979.

Malmgren, R.A., Studies of circulating cancer cells in cancer patients
In: Mechanisms of invasion in cancer, P. Denoix, ed.,
Springer-Verlag, New York, 1967, pp. 108-117.

Machinami, R., A study on the invasive growth of malignant tumors.
II. Ultrastructural features of the metastatic growth of Yoshida
ascites hepatoma 7974 in the rat brain. Acta Pathol. Jap., 23,
261-278, 1973.

Maun, M.E., Dunning, W.F., Is the biopsy of neoplasms dangerous? Surg.
Gynecol. Obstet., 82, 567-572, 1946.

Melamed, M.R., Cliffton, E.E., Seal, S.H., Cancer cells in the peripheral
venous blood: a quantitative study of cells of problematic origin.
Am. J. Clin. Pathol., 37, 381-388, 1962.

Meyvisch, C., Van Hoorde, P., Mareel, M., Invasiveness and the metastatic
potential of tumour cells, In: Metastasis, clinical and
experimental aspects: proceedings of the EORTC Metastasis Group
International Conference, K. Hellmann, P. Hilgard and S. Eccles,
eds., Martinus Nijhoff, The Hague, 1980, pp. 33-37.

Möller, G., Möller, E., The concept of immunological surveillance against
neoplasia. Transplant Rev., 28, 3-15, 1976.

Mussoni, L., Poggi, A., DeGaetano, G., Donati, M.B., Effect of ditazole
an inhibitor of platelet aggregation, on a metastasizing tumour in
mice. Br. J. Cancer, 37, 126-129, 1978.

Neri, A., Welch, D., Kawaguchi, T., Nicolson, G.L., Development and
biologic properties of a metastatic tumor cell variant involving
selective and nonadaptive processes. J. Natl. Cancer Inst., 68,
507-517, 1982.

Nicolson, G.L., Brunson, K.W., Fidler, I.J., Specificity of arrest,
survival, and growth of selected metastatic variant cell lines,
Cancer Res., 38, 4105-4111, 1978.

Nicolson, G.L., Custead, S.E., Tumor metastasis is not due to adaptation of cells to a new organ environment. Science, 215, 176-178, 1982.

Öhl, S., Schüning, F., Schmidt, C.G, Growth inhibition of simulated metastases by a large primary tumor. In: Metastasis, clinical and experimental aspects: proceeding of the EORTC Metastases Group International Conference, K. Hellmann, P. Hilgard, S. Eccles, eds., Martinus Nijhoff, The Hague, 1980, pp. 65-68.

Owen, C.A., Effect of Walker 256 tumor or turpentine on hemostatic factors locally and generally in rats. Eur. J. Cancer Clin. Oncol., 17, 919-924, 1981.

Owen, C.A., Hypersensitivity to Warfarin in rats with Walker 256 carcinoma (41297), Proc. Soc. Exp. Biol. Med., 169, 1-3, 1982.

Paslin, D.A., The effects of biopsy on the incidence of metastases in hamsters bearing malignant melanoma. J. Invest. Dermatol., 61, 33-38, 1973.

Peters, L.J., The potentiating effect of prior local irradiation of the lungs on the development of pulmonary metastases. Br. J. Radiol., 47, 827-829, 1974.

Poste, G., Fidler, I.J., The pathogenesis of cancer metastasis. Nature, 283, 139-145, 1980.

Poste, G., Bucana, C., Raz, A., Bugelski, P., Kirsch, R., Fidler, I.J., Analysis of the fate of systemically administered liposomes and implication for their use in drug delivery. Cancer Res., 42, 1412-1422, 1982.

Raz, A., Hanna, N., Fidler, I.J., In vivo isolation of a metastatic tumor cell variant involving selective and nonadaptive processes. J. Natl. Cancer Inst., 66, 183-189, 1981.

Riggins, R.S., Ketcham, A.S., Effect of incisionmal biopsy on the development of experimental tumor metastases. J. Surg. Res., 5, 200-206, 1965.

Romsdahl, M.M., McGrath, R.G., Hoppe, E., McGrew, E.A., Experimental model for the study of tumor cells in the blood. Acta Cytologica, 9, 141-145, 1965.

Salsbury, A.J., Burrage, K., Hellmann, K., Inhibition of metastatic spread by I.C.R.F. 159: selective deletion of a malignant characteristic. Br. Med. J., 4, 344-346, 1970.

Salsbury, A.J., Burrage, K., Hellmann, K., Histological analysis of the antimetastatic effect of (+)-1, 2-bis (3,5-dioxopiperazin-1-yl) propane. Cancer Res., 34, 843-849, 1974.

Schatten, W.E., Kramer, W.M., An experimental study of postoperative tumor metastases. II. Effects of anesthesia, operation, and cortisone administration on growth of pulmonary metastases. Cancer, 11, 460-462, 1958.

Schwartz, R.S., Current concepts; another look at immunologic surveillance. New Engl. J. Med., 293, 181-184, 1975.

Stanbridge, E.J., Ceredig, R., Growth-regulatory control of human cell hybrids in nude mice. Cancer Res., 41, 573-580, 1981.

Stein-Werblowsky, R., On the prevention of haematogenous tumor metastases in rats: the role of the proteinase inhibitor "Trasylol." J. Cancer Res. Clin. Oncol., 97, 129–135, 1980.

Stiles, C.D., Desmond, W., Chuman, L.M., Sato, G., Saier, M.H., Jr., Growth control of heterologous tissue culture cells in the congenitally athymic nude mouse. Cancer Res., 36, 1353–1360, 1976.

Stoker, M.G.P., Shearer, M., O'Neill, C., Growth inhibition of polyoma-transformed cells by contact with static normal fibroblasts. J. Cell Sci., 1, 297–310, 1966.

Sugarbaker, E.V., Cohen, A.M., Altered antigenicity in spontaneous pulmonary metastases from an antigenic murine sarcoma. Surgery, 72, 155–161, 1972.

Suit, H.D., Sedlacek, R.S., Gillette, E.L., Examination for a correlation between probabilities of development of distant metastasis and of local recurrence. Radiology, 95, 189–194, 1970.

Takahashi, M., An experimental study of metastasis. J. Pathol. Bacteriol., 20, 1–13, 1915.

Tao, T.W., Matter, A., Vogel, K., Burger, M.M., Liver-colonizing melanoma cells selected from B-16 melanoma. Int. J. Cancer, 23, 854–857, 1979.

Thompson, S.C., Tumour colony growth in the irradiated mouse lung. Br. J. Cancer, 30, 337–341, 1974.

Tsubura, E., Yamashita, T., Kobayachi, M., Higuchi, Y., Isobe, J., Inhibitory mechanism of blood-borne pulmonary metastasis by sulfated polysaccharides. In: Cancer metastasis; approaches to the mechanism, prevention, and treatment. P.G. Stansly and H. Sato, eds., University of Tokyo Press, Tokyo, 1977, pp. 147–161.

Ungari, S., Raju, K.S., Alessandri, G., Gullino, P.M., Cooperation between fibronectin and heparin in the mobilization of capillary endothelium. Invasion Metastasis, 5, 193–205, 1985.

Walker, A., McCallum, H.M., Wheldon, T.E., Nias, A.H.W., Abdelaal, A.S., Promotion of metastasis of C3H mouse mammary carcinoma by local hyperthermia. Br. J. Cancer, 38, 561–563, 1978.

Warren, B.A., Cancer cell-endothelial reactions: the microinjury hypothesis and localized thrombosis in the formation of micrometastases. In: Malignancy and the hemostatic system. M.B. Donati, J.R. Davidson and S. Garattini, eds., Raven Press, New York, 1981, pp. 5–25.

Watrach, A.M., Milner, J.A., Watrach, M.A., Effect of selenium on growth rate of canine mammary carcinoma cells in athymic nude mice. Cancer Lett., 15, 137–143, 1982.

West, D.C., Hampson, I.N., Arnold, F., Kumar, S., Angiogenesis induced by degradation products of hyaluronic acid. Science, 228, 1324–1326, 1985.

Wexler, H., Minton., J.P., Ketcham, A.S., A comparison of survival time and extent of tumor metastasis in mice with transplanted, induced and spontaneous tumors. Cancer, 18, 985–994, 1965.

Wheelock, E.F., Weinhold, K.J., Goldstein, L.T., Tumor dormancy in animals and man. In: Metastatic tumor growth, E. Grundmann, ed., Gustav Fischer, New York, 1980, pp. 123-130.

Wheelock E.F., Weinhold K.J., Levich, J., The tumor dormant state. Adv. Cancer Res., 34, 107-135, 1981.

Williamson, R.C.N., Lyndon, P.J., Tudway, A.J.C., Effects of anti-coagulation and ileal resection on the development and spread of experimental intestinal carcinomas. Br. J. Cancer, 42, 85-94, 1980.

Wood, S. Jr., Experimental studies of the intravascular dissemination of ascitic V2 carcinoma cells in the rabbit, with special reference to fibrinogen and fibrinolytic agents. Bull. Schweiz Akad. Med. Wiss., 20, 92-121, 1964.

Yerushalmi, A., Influence on metastatic spread of whole-body or local tumor hyperthermia. Europ. J. Cancer, 12, 455-463, 1976.

Yogeeswaran, G., Salk, P.L., Cell surface sialylation of metastatic variant murine tumor cell lines. In: Clinical and experimental aspects: proceedings of the EORTC Metastasis Group International Conference, K. Hellmann, P. Hilgard and S. Eccles, eds., Martinus Nijhoff , The Hague, 1980, pp. 422-426.

Yogeeswaran, G., Salk, P.L., Metastatic potential is positively correlated with cell surface sialylation of cultured murine tumor cell lines. Science, 212, 1514-1516, 1981.

Ziche, M., and Gullino, P.M., Angiogenesis and neoplastic progression in vitro. J. Natl. Cancer Inst., 69, 483-487, 1982.

THE AXILLA IN BREAST CANCER

F. Hartveit

Department of Pathology, The Gade Institute, University of Bergen,
5000-Bergen, Norway.

INTRODUCTION

Interest in the axilla in breast cancer focuses on its lymphatic component. It is the lymph vessels and their glands that demand attention. The latter lie on the drainage route between the breast and venous return to the heart. They show marked changes in the presence of an infiltrating carcinoma of the breast. These changes and their interpretation will form the subject of this paper. To illustrate them I shall draw heavily on material collected over the past 5 years from this Department.

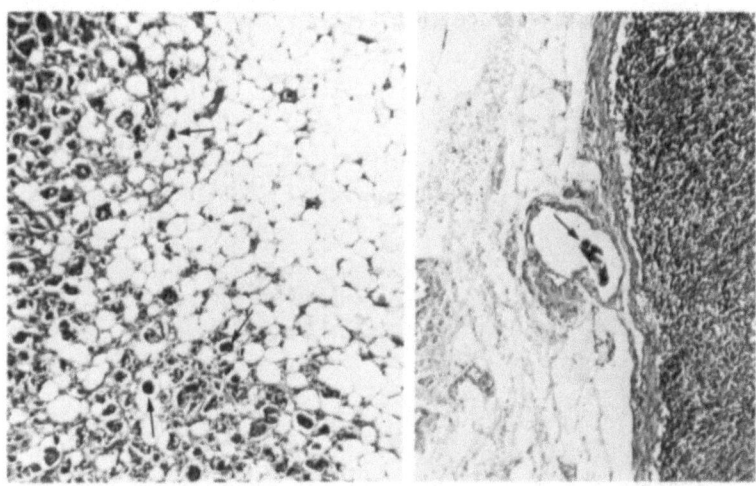

Fig.1: a) Section from the edge of a breast carcinoma (H&E x 70) showing infiltrating of tumour cells, alone and in groups (arrowed), in the adjacent fatty tissue.

b) Section from an axillary node from the same patient (H&E x 70) showing embolic tumour cells in an afferent lymphatic vessel (arrow).

The very nature of infiltrative growth implies that tumour cells spread from the primary tumour mass out into the surrounding host tissue. They may leave the company of their companions, as individuals or groups of individual cells (Fig. 1a) and are then free to wander in the interstitial fluid. In the natural course of events this fluid drains into the rich lymphatic plexus of the breast. Over 98% of the lymph leaving the breast drains to the axilla (Hultborn et al., 1955), through its nodes and on via lymphatic collecting trunks to the superior vena cava. There is thus an established pathway for the passage of fluid and of cells that are free to wander, from the breast to the blood stream. Tumour cells take advantage of this route of spread. These tumour emboli travelling with the stream of lymph, reach the axillary nodes(Fig. 1b).

So far the picture is clear; from here on we approach the frontiers of our knowledge.

The nodes themselves.

The nodes themselves are said to develop along the course of the lymphatic vessels before birth. Lymphoid cells accumulate in a supporting cellular matrix; the whole being surrounded by a fine fibrous capsule (Arno, 1980). In the human this leads to the formation of a structure, a "node" or "gland", in which many afferent vessels enter on the convex side. The lymph is dispersed within the node, to be collected again in the efferent vessels, which are few in number, and leave the node at its hilum on the concave surface (Fig.2).

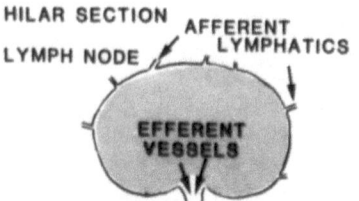

Fig. 2: Diagram of a hilar section of a lymph node, i.e. one passing through the hilum, where the efferent vessels leave the node, and through its greatest circumference. The afferent lymphatics enter the node here in this plane of section.

NODAL NUMBER IN AXILLARY SPECIMENS

		No. of specimens	No. of nodes Mean ± SD
Autopsy controls	right	40	7 ± 5
	left	40	7 ± 4
Breast cancer patients	node neg.	40	15 ± 7
	tumour > 1cm	5	12 ± 3
	1 — 2cm	10	15 ± 7
	2 — 4cm	13	19 ± 8

Table: Note: The number of nodes in the controls was similar on right and left (Hartveit and Samsonsen, 1985). The number in breast cancer patients was twice as high (Hartveit, 1981a), and increased with tumour diameter (Hartveit et al., 1982a).

How many nodes are formed? We have no basic information here, but can approach it by asking, "How many nodes are found?" In breast cancer patients the number of nodes recovered from the axillary specimen varies greatly, from patient to patient, and from centre to centre (Durkin and Haagensen, 1980; Fisher and Slack, 1970). This could be an indication of true individual differences, and/or of differences in technique; both surgical and pathological.

Using methods that should give an optimal yield, i.e. wide dissection and clearance of the specimen in cedarwood oil, the number of nodes recovered from the axillae of women without breast cancer varies from none to twenty or more (Hartveit and Samsonsen, 1985). In the autopsy material quoted about 7 nodes were recovered using the dissection commonly used with a modified radical mastectomy. The number on the right and left was similar (Table). This suggests that their number under normal circumstances may be regulated by systemic rather than local factors.

Twice as many were found in corresponding specimens from breast cancer patients using the same method of investigation (Hartveit, 1981a). Their number increased with tumour diameter up to 4 cm in node-negative patients (Hartveit et al., 1982a). It is unlikely that the number of nodes in fact increases. The seeming increase can be explained on the basis of increase in size of small "nodelets" that would not otherwise be picked up by the method used. Such small nodes are seen on microscopy of macroscopically node-free fatty tissue (Hartveit, 1981a). The increase in nodal number with increasing tumour diameter is, on this basis, evidence of progressive interaction of the nodal lymphoid tissue and the breast tumour. Similarly the difference in number of nodes from patient to patient in the absence of cancer could reflect the patient's previous overall immunological experience.

276

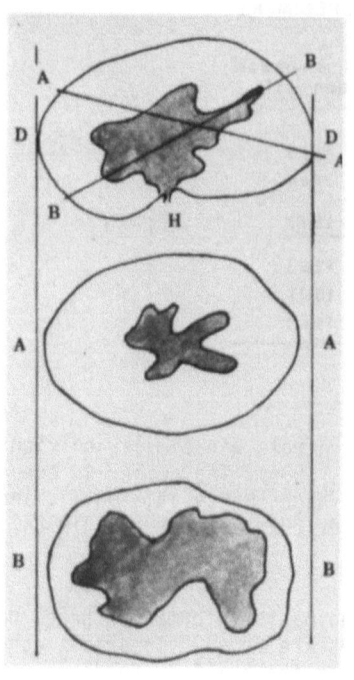

Fig. 3
Diagrammatic representation of a
standard (hilar) nodal section,
top, passing through the hilum and
the greatest nodal diameter. It has
thus three fixed points, D, H, D,
and is reproducible; in contrast to
the random sections AA and BB. In
A the cortex is overrepresented, in
B the medulla (Hartveit, 1982).

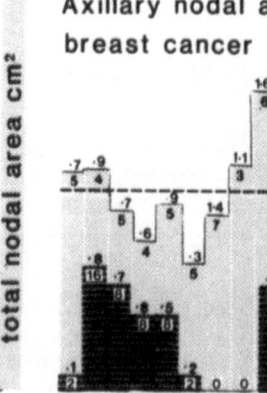

Fig. 4
Mean nodal lymphatic tissue area
(cm^2) from the axillae of node-
negative breast cancer patients
compared to that from non-cancer
autopsy controls.

Note: the greater area in the cancer
patients, that is most marked in the
second part of the year. The number
of cases is given for each month on
the histograms, the figures above
the line marking the mean are the
corresponding SD (Hartveit et al.,
1985).

In contrast the increase in nodal size, in the absence of tumour spread, is due to proliferative changes in the lymphoid tissue. If a node is under 3 mm in diameter when fixed, there is a 50/50 chance that one will not be able to recognize any particular histological pattern in it, compared to one in 10 of those over 3 mm (Hartveit, 1981a). These nodes may thus have been unstimulated at the time of the harvesting.

In a series of over 600 axillary nodes from 40 node-negative breast cancer patients 5 histological patterns were recognized in the lymphoid tissue (Hartveit, 1981a). The mean number of nodes recovered was 15 ± 7/case. The factor most frequently recorded was a diffuse follicular pattern, seen in about half the nodes. This was followed by germinal centres, in over one third. These factors were also more frequent in the 4 largest nodes per case, than in the others.

Nodal enlargement in the presence of breast carcinoma is thus due to a proliferative reaction of follicular type that is seen in some, but far from all the nodes in a given axilla.

The nodal lymphoid tissue in the axilla can be quantitated from measurement of the area of nodal hilar sections; the latter being defined as a section passing through the hilum and the greatest nodal diameter, i.e. length. It should be noted that the plane of section determines the configuration and relative distribution of the nodal tissues measured (Fig.3). Hence the need for standardization (Hartveit, 1982). The total nodal lymphoid tissue area, that is the sum of the areas recorded from a hilar section from each node, varies from case to case in women without cancer (Hartveit and Samsonsen, 1985), and in breast cancer patients (Hartveit et al., 1985). There is however a marked difference (Fig.4). In node-negative breast cancer patients, in contrast to women without breast cancer, the total nodal lymphoid tissue in the axilla was seldom over 2 cm^2 in specimens received in the first half of the year, and rarely under this in those from the second half.

The configuration of the nodes in the first six months is like that in the non-cancer patients throughout the year (Hartveit et al., 1985) (Fig.5). In contrast the nodes in the second half are plump. On histology these nodes show marked proliferative changes of follicular type with germinal centres. In 17 node-negative cases examined between January and June a mean of 3.8 ± 4.3 nodes with germinal centres was recorded per case. In 20 cases examined between July and December over twice as many were present (8.1 ± 6.4). The reaction was more marked with tumours over 2.5 cm in diameter (p<0.02).

Thus the proliferative reaction in lymphoid tissue that accompanies progressive tumour growth is more marked in the second half of the year. These nodal reactions also vary with tumour size, but although the two may be interrelated, the influence of period of presentation appears to be stronger than that of size alone (Hartveit et al., 1983b).

Tumour size, in itself, also varies in this district with the time of year (Hartveit, 1983). The mean diameter of breast cancers removed in the first half of the year is significantly lower than that of those from the second half (Fig.6). The diameter of benign tumours does not show this

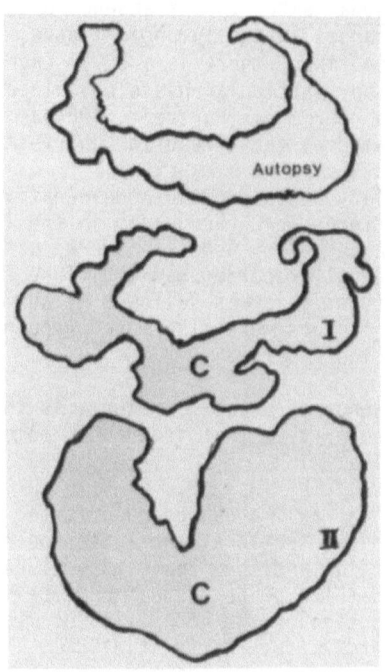

Fig. 5.
The nodal lymphoid tissue area
illustrated from charts of
hilar sections of 3 axillary
nodes. The top one shows the
configuration of nodes from the
autopsy material. This is
similar to the middle node
removed from a node-negative
breast cancer (C) patient in
the first part of the year (I),
and contrasts with the bottom
node removed from a similar
patient later in the year (II)
(Hartveit et al., 1985).

difference. The carcinomas presenting in the second half of the year are
of higher histological grade and in oestrogen receptor positive cases, the
receptor values are higher (Hartveit et al., 1983d). Further, in the zone
of host-tumour interaction the metachromatic stromal reaction, that is
related to mast cell changes in this area (Hartveit et al., 1984d), and
associated with growth of infiltrative as opposed to expansive type, is
more common in tumours removed between January and June (Hartveit et al.,
1984a).

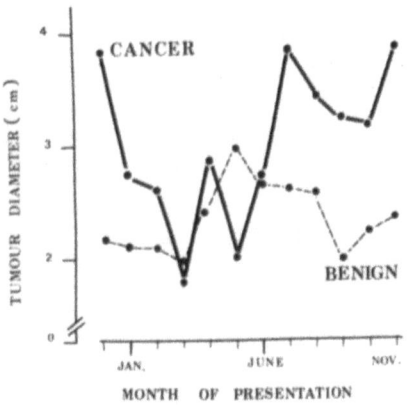

Fig. 6.
The mean (SE) diameter of the
carcinomas (—) related to the
month of presentation, compared
to that of benign lesions (---)
presenting over the same time
interval.
Note: The lack of cancers under
2 cm in diameter in the
second 6 months of the year
(Hartveit, 1983).

These findings strengthen the hypothesis that tumour growth may be synchronized to season in breast carcinoma. At the same time they serve to underline the close relationship between growth of the primary tumour and changes in the lymphatic tissue in the axillary nodes, an association that has received little previous attention.

The sinus reaction.

The nodal sinus reactions, in contrast, have long been imputed a part in the host defense against cancer (Black et al., 1953). This applies to sinus histiocytosis which has been termed an active defense mechanism (Friedel et al., 1974) and an immunity response (Anastassiades and Pryce, 1966), in keeping with its association with tumours of favourable prognosis (Black and Speer, 1958; Halsted, 1898). A different type of reaction, degenerative sinus histiocytosis (Cutler et al., 1969), was later described in advanced disease, and failure to differentiate between these two forms held to explain divergent findings on the prognostic significance of the condition.

The sinus reactions were also studied in the nodes described above in which the lymphoid tissue reactions were detailed. Three distinct patterns were recognized in the internal sinus network (Hartveit, 1982).

In some the sinuses were dilated but filled from wall to wall with a population of uniform cells, each with an oval nucleus. These cells have pale eosinophilic cytoplasm and are often fusiform. Their long axes tend to run parallel to the sinus wall. This reaction is here termed sinus histiocytosis and corresponds to the pure or syncytial form described previously (Fig. 7a) (Cutler et al., 1969).

In contrast the internal sinuses in other nodes were also dilated, often greatly so, but instead of being filled with histiocytes, contained mainly lymphocytes and other round cells. This reaction is termed sinus catarrh, to signify a condition suggesting free flow of cells and lymph through the sinuses (Fig.7c).

Many of the sinuses showed a reaction mid-way between these two extremes. They were dilated, and contained many histiocytes, but the uniform pattern of the latter seen in sinus histiocytosis was broken up by groups of lymphocytes and other round cells (Fig.7b). Their orientation parallel to the sinus walls was lost, and many were rounded and/or vacuolated. This is termed a "mixed sinus reaction". It approaches the degenerative type (Cutler et al., 1969) described previously. It should be noted that these reactions were seen in some, but not all nodes in any particular case (Hartveit, 1982). The reaction type tends to be constant in a given sinus from cortex to medulla, but different parts of the same node may show different patterns.

The distribution of nodes with these reactions varies (Fig.8) with tumour size and nodal tumour status (Hartveit, 1982). Sinus histiocytosis was present in about 30% of nodes from node-negative patients with tumours of 2 cm and under. It was virtually absent from node-positive cases. The number of nodes showing sinus catarrh increased with tumour size in node-negative cases, about one node in five showing this change. Similar

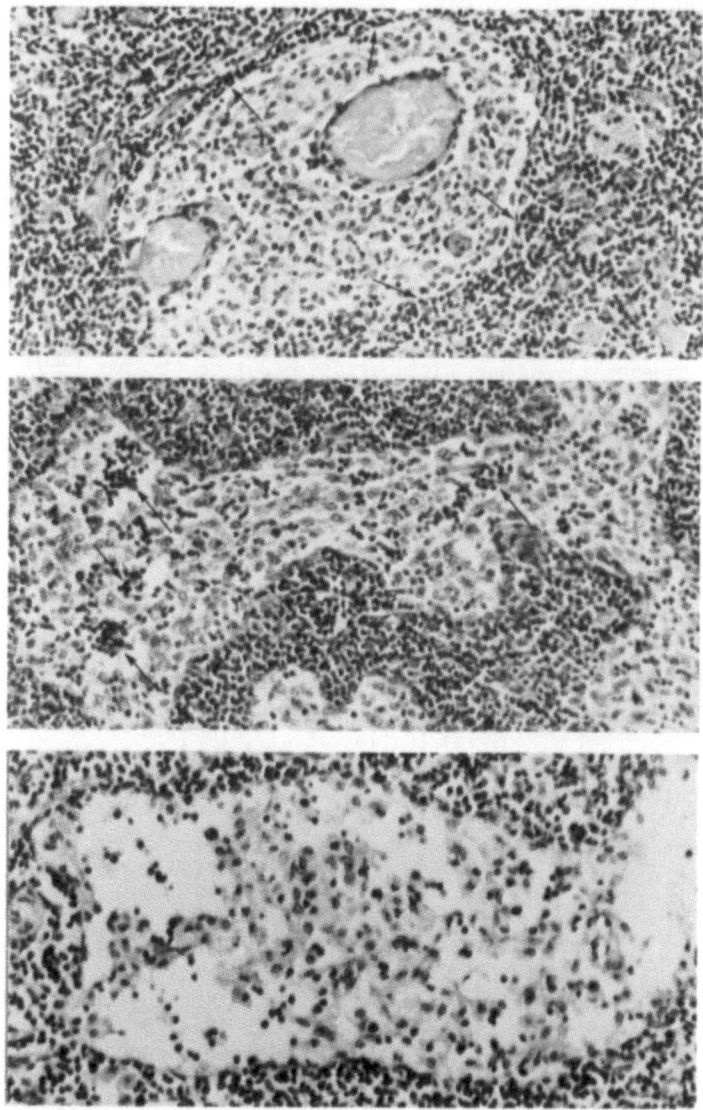

Fig. 7: Sections from lymph nodes from patients with node-negative breast
carcinoma (H&E x 300), from above down.
    a.) Sinus histiocytosis. Note: the sinus is filled with uniform
        histiocytes with oval nuclei and its edge is clearly defined
        (arrow).
    b.) Mixed sinus reaction. Note: the mass of histiocytes is broken
        up by groups of round cells (arrowed).
    c.) Sinus catarrh. Note: the lack of histiocytes in the dilated
        sinus containing scattered round cells.

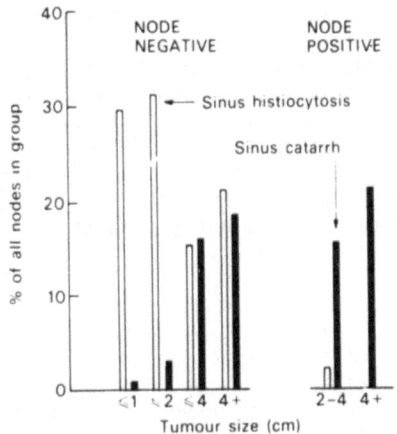

Fig. 8 The sinus reactions in the axillary lymph nodes in 59 breast
cancer patients related to tumour size and nodal state.
Note: Sinus histiocytosis is virtually confined to node-negative
    cases, while sinus catarrh increases with tumour size,
    irrespective of nodal state (Hartveit, 1982).

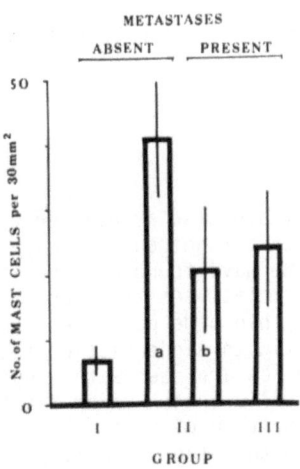

Fig. 9 The mean mast cell counts, $\pm$ SE (per 30 mm^2) in axillary lymph
nodes from patients with breast cancer, related to the absence
or presence of tumour metastases in the nodes.
Note: The highest counts were obtained from tumour-free nodes
    from patients with tumour-bearing nodes in the same axilla
    (Thoresen et al., 1982).

levels were found in all 22 node-positive cases. The mixed reaction was most common, present in over one third of the nodes in all cases, irrespective of tumour size or nodal status.

Tumours with nodes showing sinus histiocytosis tend thus to be small and without nodal metastases, in keeping with its reputed good prognosis (Black et al., 1953). However, sinus histiocytosis, in contrast to the lymphoid tissue reactions, was not significantly increased in frequency in the four largest nodes in the axilla; indicating that it is not associated with the lymphoproliferative response (Hartveit, 1981b). Recent investigations from Edinburgh suggest that the reaction is a passive one (Black et al., 1982).

The histological picture in the sinuses suggests progression from sinus histiocytosis, through the mixed reaction to sinus catarrh. The change in frequency of these reactions with progressive tumour growth supports this interaction. Sinus catarrh is also associated with tumours of high histological grade (Thoresen, 1983) which tend to show aggressive growth. These changes seem to condition the nodes for metastatic tumour growth, or indicate that they are ready to accept it.

We cannot at present distinguish between an "early" tumour confined to the breast, and a potential treatment failure in which tumour cells may have passed the nodes without colonizing them. In such cases sinus catarrh is common (Hartveit, 1980). Sinus catarrh, and the sequence of changes in the sinuses leading up to it, may thus not only precede the establishment of nodal metastases, but pose the question as to whether they may also pave the way for distant metastases. Its action may be purely mechanical; embolic tumour cells being carried on past the nodes with the free flow of lymph. That tumour cells pass through the nodes without stopping up in them has often been demonstrated experimentally (Grundmann and Vollmer, 1985).

Mast cells

These sinus reactions are also associated with changes in the nodal mast cell population, which strengthens the case for distinguishing between them. In general we have found mast cells (Fig. 9) are more frequent in nodes without metastases from node-positive cases, and less frequent in node-negative than node-positive cases (Thoresen et al., 1982). Few mast cells are present with sinus histiocytosis, most are found with the mixed reaction, while few are seen with sinus catarrh. The appearance of large numbers of mast cells in the mixed reaction and their subsequent disappearance raise the question of mast cell transport. On leaving the nodes they will empty into the blood stream, but what happens next is an open question.

The mixed sinus reaction and germinal centre proliferation both reach their peak before the establishment of nodal tumour growth, and fall off later (Hartveit et al., 1983b). Previously in the literature, germinal centre proliferation has been related to node-positive cases (Fisher et al. 1978), and attributed to tissue necrosis (Hunter et al., 1975). The nodal reactions have thus been considered secondary to establish tumour growth.

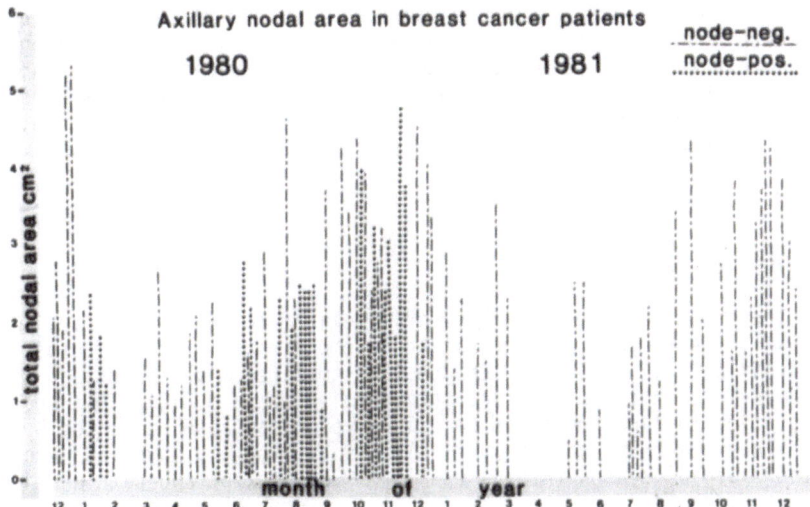

Fig. 10 The nodal lymphoid tissue area in axillary dissection specimens
from 95 breast cancer patients related to their time of operation.
Note: the increase in nodal area in the second part of the year
is not accompanied by an increase in nodal number (Hartveit
et al., 1985).

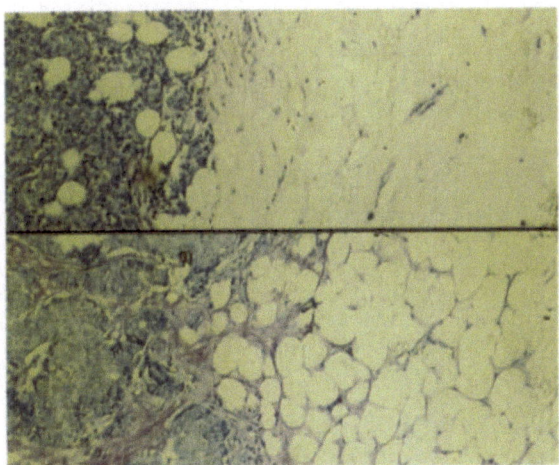

Fig. 11 Sections from the edge of 2 breast carcinomas (toluidine blue
x 125)
a.) Well-defined edge of tumour lacking stromal metachromasia
b.) Ill-defined edge of tumour with metachromasia extending into
the zone of host-tumour interaction.
Note: Stromal metachromasia beyond the tumour edge is more common
in the first part of the year (Hartveit et al., 1984d).

This view must now be questioned. The possibility that the marked germinal centre reaction seen in the nodes is reflected in the parallel presentation of poorly differentiated primary tumours must be given due consideration (Hartveit et al., 1983d). The situation may be analogous to that in experimental tumour enhancement which has long been recognized (Snell, 1970), also in connection with the occurrence of metastases (Carter and Gershon, 1966). We have thus to face a second question; "Do the nodal changes condition the nodes for metastatic growth?"

The time of year.

These nodal reactions are clearly related to the time of year in our material. Their cyclic nature has been demonstrated over 25 months (Hartveit et al., 1985). The change from proliferative to resting stage and back follows the winter and summer solstice (Fig. 10). This suggests correlation to light-mediated reactions, such as those regulated by the pineal hormone melatonin (Lewy et al., 1982), that is involved in control of the breeding season (Arendt et al., 1983; Stetson and Watson-Whitmyre, 1984) in mammals. Here there is a hint of a possible connection to the mast cells in the mixed sinus reaction that later leave the nodes. The pineal hormones are chemically related to 5-hydroxytryptamine (Namboodiri et al., 1983), a product of mast cell degranulation, and are also vasoactive (Reiter, 1980).

Mast cell degranulation in the zone of host-tumour interaction, with stromal metachromasia, is more common in the first six months of the year (Hartveit et al., 1984a). This reaction (Fig. 11) is associated with infiltrative, as opposed to proliferative tumour growth (Hartveit, 1981b). Infiltrative growth is thus linked to the action of vasoactive substances in the zone of host-tumour interaction. Thus the well-known anti-tumour effect of Tamoxifen may well, in part, be related to its anti-histamine effect (Brendes, 1985).

We have at present no knowledge of the mechanism(s) that controls the physiological distribution and/or transport of mast cells in the body. Their role in the acute inflammatory response is well established. Their vasoactive effect in the zone of host-tumour interaction, a pathological situation, initiates the production of a stroma that is receptive to the infiltrating tumour cells, and at the same time the heparin released provides them with mitogenic factors (Roche, 1985).

Tumour growth in the nodes

The establishment of nodal tumour growth has been cited as evidence of breakdown in the host's immunological defence (Devitt, 1965; 1976). The nodal changes described above indicate that it may rather be that certain changes must occur in the nodes before tumour growth can become established in them. Potential "conditioning" of nodes for metastatic growth needs experimental confirmation. There is clear evidence that tumour cells may pass right through nodes that have not been preconditioned

(Grundmann and Vollmer, 1985).

The distribution of tumour deposits in the nodes is not a random process as is often assumed (Wilkinson and Hause, 1974), but one closely related to nodal anatomy. As the afferent/efferent vessels enter/leave the node in the same plane of section, a hilar section (Hartveit, 1984a) will identify tumour cells on the way in. It is thus the section of choice for the identification of micrometastases, that is to say small groups of cells entering the nodes and settling down in them. The use of hilar sections in routine diagnostic work adds reliability to the pathologist's report at the cost of attention to detail, but little extra time or laboratory work. In contrast, if a random section is used, a 30% false negative result can be expected (Saphir and Amromin, 1948).

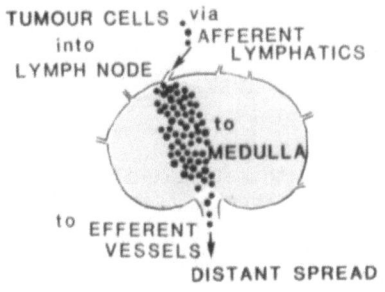

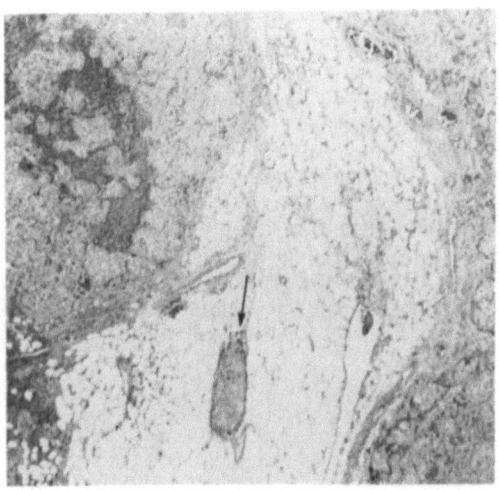

Fig. 12   Diagram showing the progressive growth of tumour cells in a lymph node. They enter via the afferent lymphatics, growing to fill the cortex and medulla. They then spread to the efferent vessels and pass on into the blood stream. Below the diagram is a section (H&E x 70) from a hilar area of a lymph node showing tumour cells (arrow) in the efferent vessels (efferent vascular invasion). Note: This is a late stage in tumour growth with correspondingly poor prognosis.

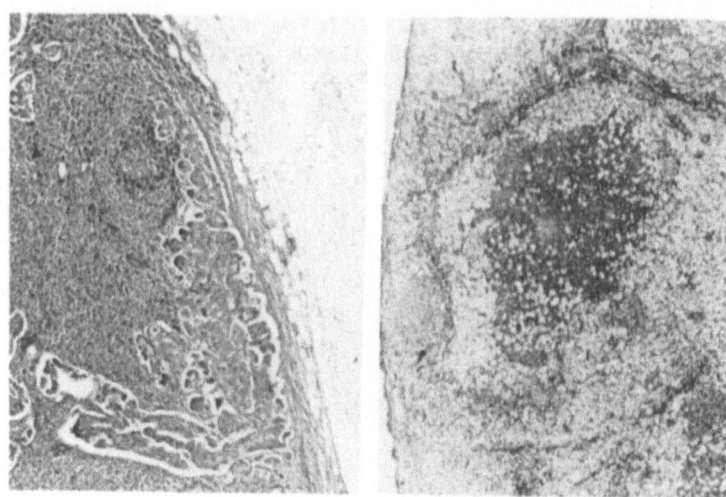

Fig. 13 Section from lymph nodes with metastatic breast carcinoma
showing sinophilic (a) and sinophobic (b) growth (H&E x 35).
Note: The former is associated with oestrogen receptor positive
    tumours, the latter with oestrogen receptor negative (Hartveit
    et al., 1983f).

     Once established within the node tumour growth is not haphazard
(Hartveit et al., 1983c). It spreads from the cortex into the medulla,
finally filling the node and extending into the efferent vessels (Fig. 12).
In the nodes tumour cells usually reflect the morphological
characteristics of the primary. They may even mimic this to the extent of
producing a basement membrane (Goldenberg et al., 1969). Irrespective of
their growth pattern their mode of growth may take two forms. Growth
within the node may be sinophilic (Hartveit et al., 1983f), the tumour
cells showing a tendency to syncytial growth, advancing through the nodes
by filling the sinuses (Fig. 13). Such tumour cells tend to be oestrogen
receptor (ER) positive. In contrast the ER negative show sinophobic growth,
with a tendency to grow in small units or as individual cells. Mixed
patterns are however common.

Efferent vascular invasion.

     Tumour growth is almost always present in both cortex and medulla if
it is found in the efferent vessels (Hartveit et al., 1983c). The
exception is cases with retrograde spread (Hartveit, 1979a). The presence
of tumour cells in the efferent nodal vessels (efferent vascular invasion,
EVI), is thus a late stage in nodal tumour growth. This is reflected in
the short survival time in such patients. It was first reported in 1979
(Hartveit, 1979b) that in a series of 98 cases only 20% with tumour cells
in the efferent vessels survived 5 years after mastectomy. They thus form

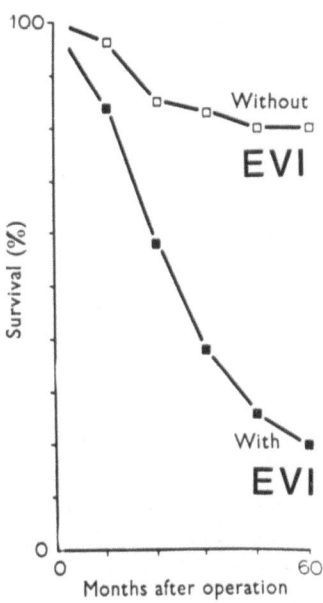

Fig. 14 Post-operative survival (percentage) in 54 patients in whom
tumour cells were found in the efferent vessels (EVI) of the
axillary lymph nodes (with), and in 47 patients without tumour
cells there (Hartveit, 1979b).

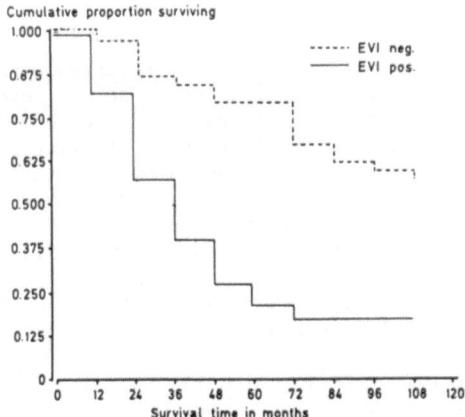

Fig. 15 The cumulative proportions surviving up to the 10th post-
operative year (same patients as in Fig. 14) related to the
presence/absence of tumour cells in the efferent nodal vessels
(Hartveit et al., 1983a).

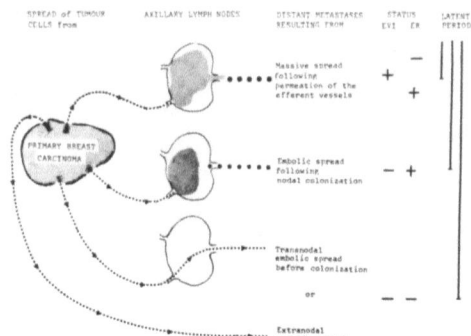

Fig. 16   Proposed system to explain the differences in time of recurrence
          in relation to efferent vascular invasion (EVI) and oestrogen
          receptor (ER) status in 50 cases of node-positive breast
          carcinoma, see text (Hartveit et al, 1983c).

a high risk group within a group, the node-positive, that is in itself of
poor prognosis (Fig. 14). The few EVI positive cases surviving 5 years
are at less risk (Hartveit et al., 1983a), while the risk of dying within
a 10 year follow-up increases in EVI negative cases (Fig. 15). A later
prospective study of 50 node-positive cases showed 11 deaths in 26 EVI
positive cases within 3 years, compared to 1 of 24 in the EVI negative
(Hartveit et al., 1983e). This criterion has not yet been taken up by
other, laboratories, and thus needs confirmation.

     The latter series also showed that while early recurrence was more
common in the first year in ER negative cases, the trend was reversed in
the third. This was in keeping with a report that the recurrence rates
tended to converge between 30 and 40 weeks (Furmanski et al., 1980). It
was suggested that this convergence would be consistent with progression
of breast cancer cells from ER positivity to negativity. In our material
the histological grade tended to be higher in the ER negative that the ER
positive, providing an alternative explanation (Hartveit et al., 1981b)

     There were also differences in time of recurrence in relation to EVI
and ER status (Fig. 16). These can be explained as follows (Hartveit
et al., 1983e):
     In the EVI positive the tumour cells colonizing the nodes have
extended into the efferent vessels. From here they may leave the nodes in
large numbers. Distant metastases formed subsequent to the establishment
of these cell groups will soon become apparent. This would explain the
rapid recurrence in EVI positive cases, their intrinsic growth rate
giving the sequence ER negative, ER positive.

In EVI negative cases growth has not yet reached the efferent vessels, but this would not exclude smaller emboli breaking away from the nodal tumour. At the time this scheme was proposed we did not know that the cell groups in ER positive cases tended to be larger than in ER negative (Hartveit et al., 1983f). While the idea that small cell groups from the nodal deposits fitted the observed time sequence for the EVI negative/ER positive, the slower development of recurrence in the ER negative did not. It was therefore proposed that such cases might be due to still smaller emboli that were the result of either transnodal or extra-nodal spread. On hindsight the difference could be explained simply on the basis of still smaller embolic cell groups being derived from nodal deposits in the ER negative.

This of course does not exclude that spread may also occur by other routes (Hartveit et al., 1983e), or to other groups of nodes (Handley and Thackray, 1949). Successful assessment of prognosis on the basis of axillary nodal findings does however demonstrate that the stage of nodal growth in them reflects the total tumour load elsewhere in the body.

It is therefore essential to know not only the extent of the tumour load, but also its potential growth rate (Hartveit et al., 1984c). These two factors will together determine the time that is to elapse before these latent metastases become clinically evident and later kill the patient.

Multiple prognostic factors

Multivariance analysis of a series of prognostic factors from our node-positive 1970-71 material (98 cases) (Mæhle and Skjærven, 1983) showed that the strongest factor in the prediction of both 5 and 10 year prognosis was EVI status, the stage of nodal growth thus reflecting the latent tumour load. The addition of a measurement of tumour growth rate increased the strength of the model, the best being the mean nuclear area (MNA) of the tumour cells. Tumour diameter, over/under 3 cm, a measure of tumour stage, gave a further increase, comparable with that obtained from the number of tumour-bearing nodes. These findings stress the need for multifactorial assessment (Haybittle et al., 1982), and more importantly that the choice of factor should be given careful consideration. Some merely reflect information given by others, while yet others may add to it.

The distinction between node-negative and node-positive cases is classically the most important prognostic indicator known. It is this that has made histological examination of the axillary nodes standard practice throughout the world. The further information gained in node-positive cases was previously confined to assessment of the tumour load on the basis of the number of nodes involved. Determination of EVI status adds a new dimension to this investigation.

Extension of tumour cell growth beyond the nodal capsule has long been considered an indicator of poor prognosis (Fisher et al., 1976). This has not been confirmed in our material, in which the presence of tumour cells in the efferent vessels was the only marker of poor prognosis found in the paranodal tissues (Hartveit, 1984b).

290

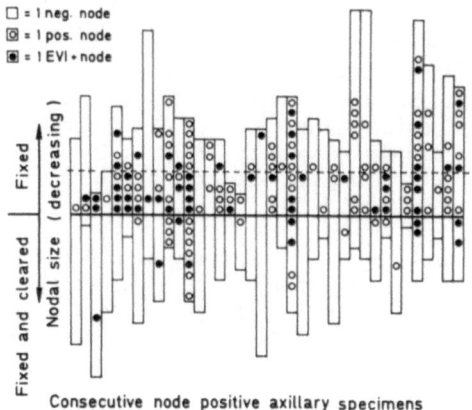

□ = 1 neg. node
◙ = 1 pos. node
◉ = 1 EVI + node

Fixed

Nodal size (decreasing)

Fixed and cleared

Consecutive node positive axillary specimens

Fig. 17   The tumour status of nodes recovered before and after clearing
of the axillary specimens related to nodal size in 37 node-
positive breast cancer patients. (The broken line marks the 4
largest nodes recovered before clearing. The largest node in each
case is placed on the base line, the others in decreasing order
of size up and down).
Note: Little information of prognostic interest is gained by
clearing the specimen (Hartveit et al., 1982b).

Axillary dissection with removal of the axillary fat up to the level
of the axillary vein is necessary to obtain a specimen that contains
sufficient nodes for prognostic assessment. The nodes of interest will be
found on palpation of the specimen provided it has been fixed in formalin
for 48 hours. By this time the nodes are markedly harder than the
surrounding fat. Little information of prognostic interest is gained
from clearing the specimen (Hartveit et al., 1982b).

Tumour, if present, is usually found in the largest nodes (Fig. 17).
These too are the nodes that show EVI. They are regularly recovered on
palpation of the formalin fixed specimen.So are 4 tumour-bearing nodes,
if so many are present in the axilla. At least one node with EVI will
also be found if such a node is present in the axilla. Prognosis in
cases with one node showing EVI is similar to that in cases with 4 or
more tumour-bearing nodes (Hartveit et al., 1983e). The recognition of
EVI as a prognostic factor has thus simplified the assessment of nodal
involvement.

At the same time a complicating factor has arisen in the assessment
of prognosis in this district. It seems that the women are becoming
progressively better at finding tumours, but that improvement is confined
to tumours in the left breast. These now present at an earlier stage
than tumours in the right breast (Hartveit et al., 1981a). The trend

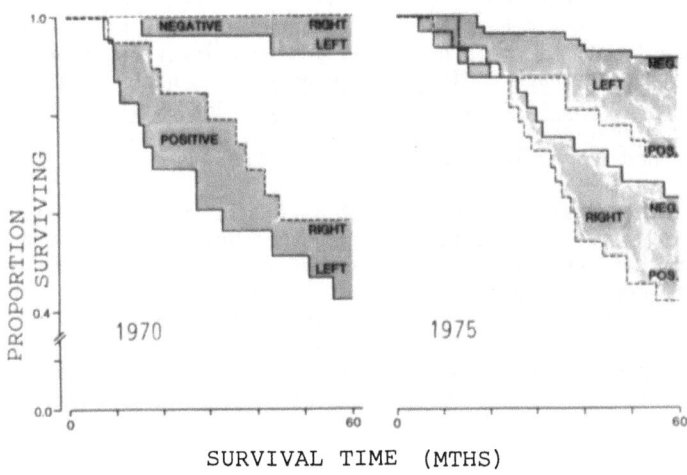

SURVIVAL TIME (MTHS)

Fig. 18   Survival curves for 87 breast cancer patients (the 1970 group)
and 163 patients (the 1975 group) both treated by modified
radical mastectomy.
Note: prognosis in 1979 was strongly related to nodal status.
   In 1975 the side involved was of greater prognostic importance
   (Hartveit et al., 1984b).

is so pronounced that the classical picture (Fig. 18) of better survival
after mastectomy in node-negative patients demonstrated in our material
from 1970, was so modified by 1974-77 that tumours in the left,
irrespective of their nodal status, showed better results than those on
the right (Hartveit et al., 1984b). It is to be hoped that this trend
continues, and spreads to the right breast.

Theoretical considerations

   The cyclical change in the amount of lymphoid tissue in the axilla
of breast cancer patients in this district calls for comment. It is
dependent on a difference in nodal size, but not in number, in the
second half of the year. The nodes are larger and show cortical
proliferation with germinal centre formation. Nodes from the first half
of the year show little evidence of proliferative change and are of
similar configuration to those from women without cancer. The difference
is present, but less marked, in cases with nodal metastases.

292

It is difficult to believe that cases coming to operation in the
first half of the year should be basically different from those presenting
later; that they should have smaller tumours, of lower histological
grade, prone to stromal metachromasia, and show lower ER values. The
alternative is that each individual cancer and its nodes go through two
different growth phases in the course of each year, that these are
repeated from year to year, as the primary increases in size, but are less
marked once nodal metastases become established.

This interpretation is perhaps as difficult to accept, but it seems
to fit facts at present available. Acceptance brings with it the
realization that the histological grade of a tumour, a measure of growth
rate, is not constant, neither is its receptor content, nor the reaction
it calls forth in the zone of host-tumour interaction. These
"characteristics" are not directly tumour related, but to some extent
under host control; albeit control that does not necessarily function to
the host's advantage. Serial biopsies would help here, but are not
available.

HOST-TUMOUR INTERACTION IN BREAST CARCINOMA

Host-tumour interaction in breast carcinoma, on the basis of the
findings described here, takes place at two levels; in the axillary nodes
and at the edge of the primary.

THE NODAL SPIRAL

Lymph draining from the primary contains a stimulus(i) that leads to
a series of reactions in the nodes (Fig. 19). Sinus histiocytosis is
followed by a mixed sinus reaction and later by sinus catarrh. Nodes with
sinus catarrh are common between July and December. The reaction is
accompanied by a proliferative follicular response with plasma cell
formation. The nodes at this stage are on the node-negative spiral. They
do not contain tumour deposits, but tumour cells may pass through them,
to give subsequent distant metastases. From January to June these same
nodes go through a non-proliferative (resting) phase. Their size decreases
and their follicular reaction regresses. Come July the follicular reaction
recurs and the nodes may enter the node-positive part of the spiral.
Tumour emboli may become established in them and grow progressively.
Regression of the proliferative reactions is now less marked between
January and June. It is also less marked as tumour growth progresses,
spreading through the node to the efferent vessels and thence to the
blood stream.

THE GROWTH CYCLE OF THE PRIMARY

Host-tumour interaction starts here with mast cell degranulation at
the tumour edge (Fig. 20). This leads to increased capillary permeability
and the formation of a metachromatic stroma. Tumour cells emigrate into
this stroma, infiltrate the tissue spaces and spread into the lymphatics

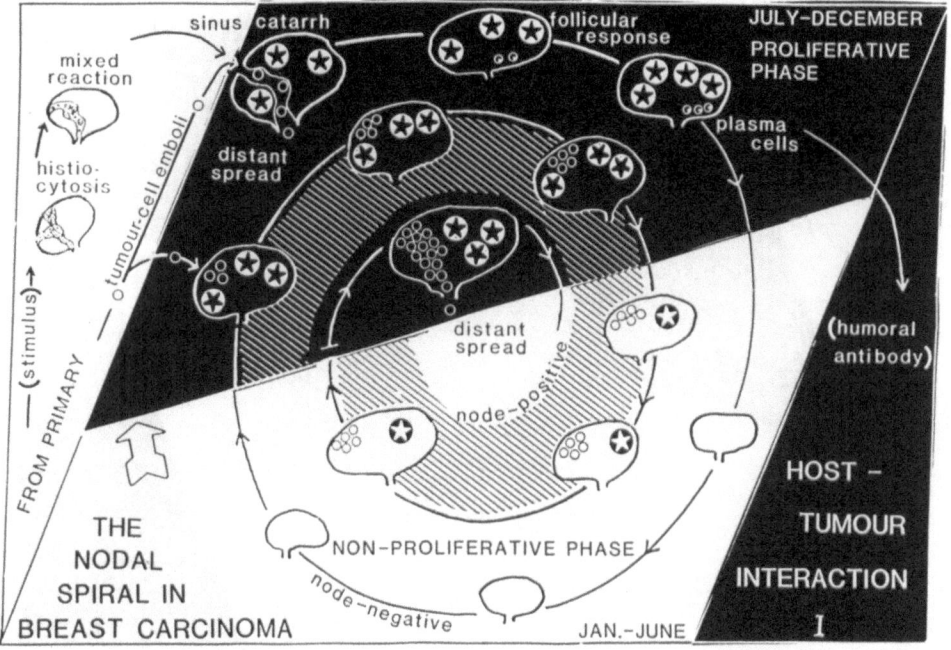

Fig. 19 The nodal spiral in breast carcinoma: A diagram relating the
        sequence of events in the axillary nodes of patients with breast
        cancer to the time of year, see text.
        Note: sinus catarrh is accompanied by a follicular response in
        the nodes. This combination may lead to distant spread in the
        absence of nodal growth (Hartveit, 1980).

that drain to the axillary nodes. These processes are marked between
January and June. Come July the tumour cells go over into a proliferative
phase, dividing to populate the new stroma. They complete the cycle by
re-establishing the tumour edge beyond that established in the preceding
year.

   The links between these two levels of reaction are not all clear. The
stimulus that leads to the sinus reactions is as yet unidentified.
Similarly the production of humoral antibody by the plasma cells in these
nodes has not been demonstrated, and the trigger that causes mast cell
degranulation in the primary is unknown.

   The mechanisms involved have yet to be unravelled. There are
indications that tumour enhancement may be involved. This was first
described in connection with experimental tumours. Treatment with dead
tumour cells enhanced the growth of existing tumours (Haaland, 1910;
Snell, 1959). This was later shown to be due to the production of humoral
antibody. Hence its relevance here, as the proliferative phase of tumour

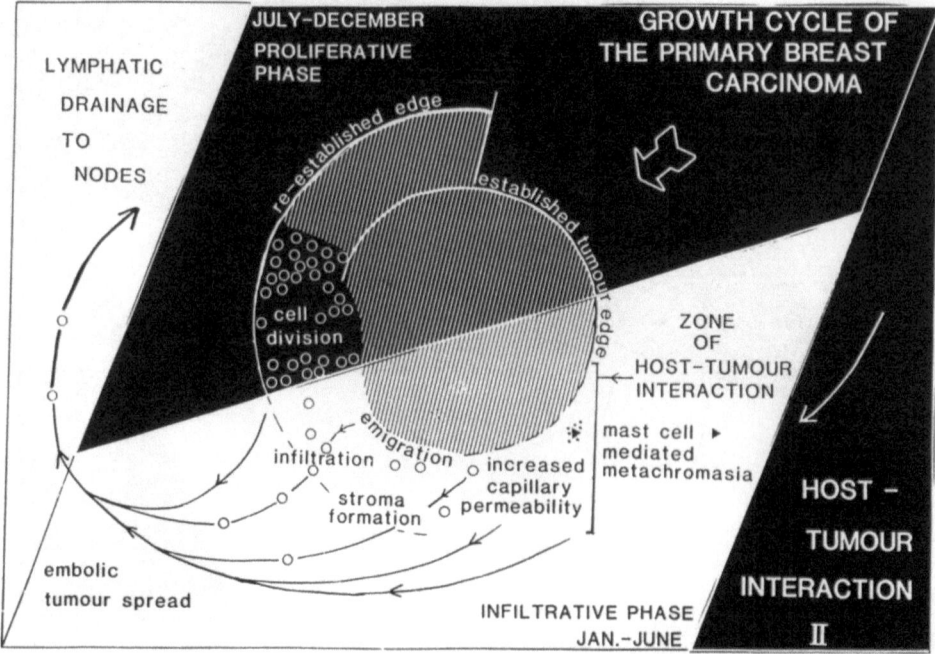

Fig. 20   The growth cycle of primary breast carcinoma: A diagram relating
           the sequence of events in the zone of host-tumour interaction to
           the time of year, see text.
           Note: The proliferative growth phase in the second part of the
              year is accompanied by higher oestrogen receptor values in
              oestrogen receptor positive cases (Hartveit et al., 1983d).
              Cyclic variation (with the seasons reversed) in the time of
              presentation of progesterone receptor positive tumours has
              been recorded in New Zealand, with a peak in late Spring
              (Meson et al., 1985), and in the mitotic activity in
              junctional naevi in Western Australia, which, from their
              figure, was highest in the first part of the year (Armstrong
              et al., 1984).

growth coincides with the follicular and germinal centre reaction in the
nodes (Carter and Gershon, 1966). Many mechanisms have been advanced that
can explain tumour enhancement by humoral antibody in the experimental
situation (Sjøgren et al., 1971; Snell, 1970). They may, or may not, be
relevant here.

    It is generally accepted that malignant tumour cells are antigenic
(Zilber, 1958), also in man. This has led to a steady stream of
publications on a cellular response, consistent with immunological
activity, at the edge of malignant tumours. It is often considered a

favourable prognostic sign, (Moore
differs on this (Gorski et al., 19
tumour growth can be expected.

A blocking effect of humoral
experimentally (Sjøgren et al., 19
consistent with a germinal centre
keeping with the idea of tumour en
being free to live undetected and

On the basis of the above int
in spite of the host immune respon
cellular immunity is concerned. Th
not conclusive.

Even so it is not the whole s
oncogenes has greatly added to our
that must occur in a cell to enabl
living organism, a transformed cel
change, that brings with it the po
synonymous with actual infiltratio
More is needed. The nodal findings
and their close relationship to pa
primary take us a step further. The
malignant tumour grows in spite of
1963), but whether it grows because
in the zone of host-tumour interact
via the draining lymph nodes. Inter
mechanisms for both the survival ar
the transformed cells might well re
body.

Changes in the zone of host-tu
to mast cell activity. This is more
tumours in the first half of the ye
consistent with increased permeabil
response (Hartveit et al., 1984d).
response results in a change in tum
an expansive pattern (Halleraker an
inflammatory reaction is self-limit
the exudate produced is anti-comple
prompted the formulation of the hyp
infiltration" (Hartveit and Hallera
uterine cervix mast cell changes ar
growth, but are seen with infiltrat
1982). It has however recently been
stromal metachromasia may precede du
situ" growth (Sandstad and Hartveit
cancer described here the factors le
and resultant infiltrative growth, s
when the proliferative phase superve
Sequential treatment with anti-infla
year by cytotoxic drugs would thus b

oote, 1949), although opinion
lowever, in general, progressive

)dy, as has been demonstrated
:an be postulated. This would be
ise in the draining nodes, and in
ient; the "masked" antigenic cells
unhindered.

ation a malignant tumour grows
is may well be so as far as
lence is highly suggestive but

The advent of the concept of
standing of the basic changes
o function on its own as a free-
ever, it is now clear that this
l ability to wander, is not
he surrounding normal tissues.
east carcinoma, detailed here,
changes in the growth of the
ing question now is not whether a
ost's immune response (Hartveit,
he response of the normal tissues
This too appears to be mediated
n is the keyword. In it lie the
ead of tumour cells. Without it
isolated from the rest of the

interaction are closely linked
ed at the growing edge of these
id leads to vascular changes,
is seen in the acute inflammatory
imentally, reduction of such a
owth from an infiltrative to
veit, 1971) (Fig. 21). This
; it is complement dependent and
y (Hartveit, 1966). This
s, "no inflammation, no
970). In carcinoma of the
nt from cases of "in situ"
owth (Hartveit and Sandstad,
, in breast carcinoma, that
infiltration from areas of "in
blished). In the cases of breast
to the inflammatory response,
o be "turned off" or "used up"
n the second half of the year.
ry agents followed later in the
ogical choice.

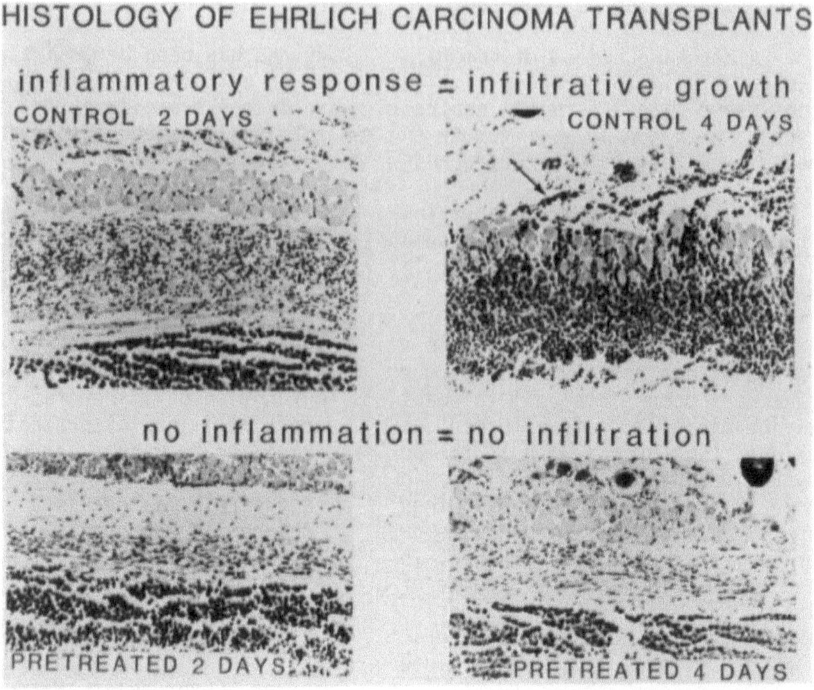

HISTOLOGY OF EHRLICH CARCINOMA TRANSPLANTS

inflammatory response = infiltrative growth
CONTROL 2 DAYS   CONTROL 4 DAYS

no inflammation = no infiltration

PRETREATED 2 DAYS   PRETREATED 4 DAYS

Fig. 21 The histology of subcutaneous transplants of the Ehrlich
         carcinoma (H&E x 150).
         Control mice: upper left: 2 day transplant with a wide band of
         loose connective tissue showing an acute inflammatory cell
         infiltrate. Upper right: 4 day transplant showing infiltrative
         tumour growth (arrow).
         Compare to lower pictures from mice that failed to produce an
         acute inflammatory reaction at 2 days. In them infiltrative
         growth was not established at 4 days (Halleraker and Hartveit,
         1971).

     In addition to inflammatory mediators mast cells also release
heparin, which is a mitogenic factor that has been shown to stimulate the
proliferation of epithelial cells. This action on tumour growth has also
been termed tumour "enhancement", but obviously different mechanisms are
involved (Roche, 1985). Heparin has also been shown to stimulate fibroblasts "in vitro" (Norrby et al., 1976). Interest in the stromal reaction,
active in the 1940's (Sylvén, 1945), is again growing. The interaction
and probable interdependence of mesenchymal and epithelial elements have
been stressed (Dürnberger et al., 1978). Similarly the mechanism(s) by
which tumour cells acquire a blood supply "in vivo" is once again open
for discussion (Folkman and Cotran, 1976; Hartveit et al., 1984d;

Shiach et al., 1985). The postulation of tumour specific angiogenic
factors "in vivo" may well be unnecessary.

These processes may well be under mast cell control, and this again
may be dependent on changes in the axillary nodes. It could be of note
that BCG stimulated T-lymphocytes are said to give rise to a mast cell
generating factor (Parwaresch et al., 1985). A similar reaction may be
operating here. All these issues are at the rapidly advancing edge of our
understanding. As they are at present they could herald the debut of
breast cancer as an auto-immune disease, one in which the price paid for
host-tumour interaction is the survival, growth and spread of its
neoplastic cells.

PRACTICAL RECOMMENDATIONS

1.) Histological examination of the axillary nodes in breast cancer is
    necessary to stage the patient's disease.
2.) A sufficient sample must be available for investigation. Removal of
    the axillary fat up to the level of the axillary vein has proved
    satisfactory.
3.) The nodes should be removed from the specimen by palpation following
    formalin fixation for 48 hours. Clearing is not necessary for routine
    tumour diagnostic work.
4.) Confirmation of the absence of metastatic deposits may be given with
    confidence when hilar sections are used. These too will show up
    tumour cells in the efferent nodal vessels. This finding, efferent
    vascular invasion (EVI), should be reported as the presence of even
    one node with EVI indicates that the patient has a high risk of early
    recurrence. The number of tumour-bearing nodes is of less interest.
5.) The presence of tumour infiltration in the paranodal tissues is of no
    prognostic significance.
6.) In the evaluation of prognosis from the axillary specimen a system
    should be used that includes the presence/absence of nodal tumour,
    the presence/absence of EVI, and a factor related to tumour growth
    rate. Here histological grade or the MNA of the nodal tumour cells
    may be used, as the results obtained are similar to those obtained on
    the primary. The ER status of the tumour should also be checked as it
    is both of therapeutic interest, and a measure of the risk of early
    recurrence. Thus it too gives a measure of tumour growth rate. If the
    ER status is not available from the primary, nodal tumour can be
    sampled at the time of surgery. Care should be taken that the hilar
    area, where the efferent vessels can be seen with the naked eye, is
    left for histology.
7.) Prognostic evaluation of the lymphoid and sinus reactions in the nodes
    in individual cases is considered premature.

SUMMARY

The lymph nodes in the axilla, their vessels, and their histology
are presented and discussed in relation to the growth of the primary
breast carcinoma.

The path of embolic tumour cells via the afferent lymphatics, through
the nodal substance, and on via the efferent vessels is illustrated. The
presence of tumour cells in the latter pin-points a high-risk group within
node-positive cases. This diagnosis can only be reached if hilar sections
of the nodes are used. These are also the sections of choice for the
identification of micro-metastases. The importance of concurrent
evaluation of the stage and rate of tumour growth is stressed.

The number of nodes found in the axilla increases with the diameter
of the primary tumour. The proliferative changes that occur in them are
of follicular type, with germinal centre formation. They reach a peak
before the establishment of nodal tumour growth. The sequence of these
changes, and those in the nodal sinuses, suggests that a certain stage of
development must be reached within the nodes before tumour cells can grow
in them. This may differ from the stage at which tumour cells can pass
through the nodes.

Synchronization between nodal changes and the growth pattern in the
primary is illustrated. These are again synchronized to the time of year;
proliferative reactions being marked in the second six months.

On this basis it is suggested that a breast carcinoma goes through a
regular cycle of changes from year to year, as it grows and metastasizes.
These changes run parallel to those in the nodes. The two sets of
reactions appear to be clearly interrelated and to have an immunological
basis. They are linked to mast cell activity, and subsequent stroma
formation.

This model implies that interaction between the primary and its nodes
facilitates progressive growth and spread of the tumour; both being
governed by the host response. In the absence of such interaction tumour
cells would remain "in situ", and thus isolated from the rest of the body.

ACKNOWLEDGEMENT.

This work has been supported by the Norwegian Cancer Society.

REFERENCES

1. Anastassiades, OT and Pryce, DM. Immunological significance of the morphological changes in lymph nodes draining breast cancer. Brit J Cancer, 20: 239-249, 1966.
2. Arendt, J, Symons, AM, Laud, CA and Pryde SJ. Melatonin can induce early onset of the breeding season in ewes. J Endocrine, 97: 395-400, 1983.
3. Armstrong, BK, Heenan, PJ, Caruso, V, Glancy, RJ and Holman, CD'AJ. Seasonal variation in the junctional component of pigmented naevi. Int J Cancer, 34: 441-442, 1984.
4. Arno, J. Atlas of lymph node pathology. Current histopathology series, vol.1, MTP Press Ltd., Lancaster, England, 1980, p.16.
5. Black, MM and Speer, FD. Sinus histiocytosis of lymph nodes in cancer. Surg Gynec Obstet. 196: 157-163, 1958.
6. Black, M, Kerpe, S and Speer, F. Lymph node structure in patients with cancer of the breast. Am J Pathol., 29: 505-522, 1953.
7. Black, RB, Steele, RJC, Collins, WCJ and Forrest, APM. Site, size and significance of palpable metastatic and "reactive" nodes in operable breast cancer. Clin Oncol., 8: 127-135, 1982.
8. Brandes, LJ. Evidence that the antiestrogen binding site is a histamine or histamine-like receptor. (abstract). Biennial International breast cancer research conference. Proceedings. 2-12. London 1985.
9. Carter, RL and Gershon, RK. Studies on homo-transplantable lymphomas in hamsters I. Histologic response in lymphoid tissues and their relationship to metastasis. Brit J Cancer, 49: 637-655, 1966.
10. Cutler, SJ, Black, MM, Mork, T, Harvei, S and Freeman, C. Further observations on prognostic factors in cancer of the female breast. Cancer, 24: 653-667, 1969.
11. Devitt, JE. The significance of regional node metastases in breast carcinoma. Canad med Ass J., 93: 289-293, 1965.
12. Devitt, JE. Clinical prediction of growth behaviour. In: Stoll BA (Ed.): Risk factors in Breast Cancer, London, W.Dienermann Medical Books Ltd., p.121, 1976.
13. Durkin, K and Haagensen, CD. An improved technique for the study of lymph nodes in surgical specimens. Ann Surg., 191: 419-429, 1980.
14. Dürnberger, H, Heuberger, B, Schwartz, P, Wasner, G and Kratchwil, K. Mesenchyme-mediated effect of testosterone on embryonic mammary epithelium. Cancer Res., 38: 4066-4070, 1978.
15. Fisher, B and Slack, NH. Number of lymph nodes examined and the prognosis of breast carcinoma. Surg Gynec Obstet., 131:79-88,1970.
16. Fisher, ER, Gregorio, RM, Redmond, C, Kim, WS and Fisher, B. Pathological findings from the National Surgical Breast Project (Protocol No.4) III. The significance of extra-nodal extension of axillary metastases. Am J Clin Pathol., 65: 439-444, 1976.
17. Fisher, ER, Palekar, A, Rockette, H, Redmond, C and Fisher, B. Pathologic findings from the national surgical adjuvant breast project (protocol no.4). Significance of axillary nodal micro-and macrometastases. Cancer 42: 2032-2038, 1978.
18. Folkman, J and Cotran, R. Relation of vascular proliferation to tumour growth. Int Rev Exp Path., 16: 207-248, 1976.
19. Friedell, GH, Soto, EA, Kumaoka, S, Abe, O, Hayward, JL and Balbrook, RD. Sinus histiocytosis in British and Japanese patients with breast cancer. Lancet, ii, 1228-1229, 1974.

20. Furmanski, P, Saunders, DE, Brooks, SC and Rich, MA. The breast cancer prognostic study clinical and pathology associates. The prognostic value of estrogen receptor determinations in patients with primary breast cancer. Cancer, 46: 2794-2796, 1980.

21. Goldenberg, WE, Goldenberg, NS and Sommers, SC. Comparative ultra-structure of atypical ductal hyperplasia, intraductal carcinoma, and infiltrating ductal carcinoma of the breast. Cancer, 24: 1152-1169, 1969.

22. Gorski, CM, Niepolamska, W, Nowak, K, Gebel, B, Plewa, I, Pysz, H and Adamus, J. Clinical evaluation and pathological grading in relation to other prognostic factors. In: Forrest APM and Kunkler PB (Eds.): Prognostic factors in breast cancer. Proceeding of the 1st Tenovus Symposium, Cardiff 1967, pp. 309-318.

23. Grundmann, E and Vollmer, E. Early local reaction and lymph node permeation of rat carcinoma HH9-d14 cells. An immunohistological approach. Path Res Pract., 178: 304-309, 1985.

24. Haaland, M. The contrast in the reactions to the implantation of cancer after the inoculation of living and mechanically disinte-grated cells. Lancet, 1: 787-789, 1910.

25. Halleraker, B and Hartveit, F. Interaction between subcutaneous and intraperitoneal transplants of the Ehrlich carcinoma; the possible role of anti-tumour antibody. J Path, 105: 95-103, 1971.

26. Halsted, W. A clinical and histological study of certain adeno-carcinomata of the breast. J Am Surg Ass., 15: 114-181, 1898.

27. Handley, RS and Thackray, AC. Internal mammary lymph chain in carcinoma of the breast; study of 50 cases. Lancet, 2: 276-278, 1949.

28. Hartveit, F. Experimental studies on the immune response to Ehrlich's ascites carcinoma. Thesis. University of Bergen, Norway,p.X, 1963.

29. Hartveit, F. In vitro abrogation of the inhibitory action of tumour ascitic fluid on the oncolytic reaction. Acta Path Microbiol Scand., 66: 55-61, 1966.

30. Hartveit, F. Tumour cells and the axillary nodes in breast cancer. Invest Cell Pathol., 2: 123-129, 1979a.

31. Hartveit, F. Paranodal vascular spread in breast cancer with axillary node involvement. J Path., 127: 111-114, 1979b.

32. Hartveit, F. Axillary node histology in cases of infiltrating breast cancer without nodal metastases dying later of disseminated disease. Invest Cell Pathol., 3: 311-314, 1980.

33. Hartveit, F. How representative is a lymph node biopsy from the axilla in a node-negative breast cancer patient? Clin Oncol. 7: 303-309, 1981a.

34. Hartveit, F. Mast cells and metachromasia in human breast cancer: their occurrence, significance and consequence: a preliminary report. J Path., 134: 7-11, 1981b

35. Hartveit, F. The sinus reaction in the axillary nodes in breast cancer related to tumour size and nodal state. Histopathology, 6: 753-764, 1982.

36. Hartveit, F. The side and size of breast tumours. Clin Oncol., 9: 135-142, 1983.

37. Hartveit, F. The routine histological investigation of axillary lymph nodes for metastatic breast cancer. J Path., 143:187-191, 1984a.

38. Hartveit, F. Paranodal tumour in breast cancer: extranodal extension versus vascular spread. J Path., 144: 253-256, 1984b.

39. Hartveit, F and Halleraker, B. Changes in the connective tissue and inflammatory response to Ehrlich's carcinoma following treatment of the host mice with butazolidine. Acta Path Microbiol Scand A, 78: 516-524, 1970.

40. Hartveit, F and Sandstad, E. Stromal metachromasia: a marker for areas of infiltrating tumour growth? Histopathology, 6: 423-428, 1982.

41. Hartveit, F. and Samsonsen, G. Quantitation of the axillary lymphoid tissue in women without cancer. J Path, 146: 95-98, 1985.

42. Hartveit, F, Skjærven, R and Mæhle, BO. Prognosis in breast cancer patients with tumour cells in the efferent vessels of their axillary nodes. J Path., 139: 379-382, 1983a.

43. Hartveit, F, Tangen, M and Halvorsen, JF. The axillary nodes and tumour size in breast cancer. Breast Cancer Research and Treatment 2: 105-109, 1982a.

44. Hartveit, F, Tangen, M, Halvorsen, JF. Is the growth of breast carcinoma regulated by the axillary nodes? Clin Oncol., 9: 239-244, 1983b.

45. Hartveit, F, Tangen, M and Halvorsen, JF. Do infiltrative and anaplastic growth patterns alternate with season in human breast cancer? Invasion and Metastasis, 4: 156-159, 1984a.

46. Hartveit, F, Tangen, M and Hartveit, E. Side and survival in breast cancer. Oncology, 41: 149-154, 1984b.

47. Hartveit, F, Thoresen, S and Mæhle, BO. Prognostic evaluation in node-positive breast carcinoma: stage versus growth rate. Brit J Surg., 71: 463-465, 1984c.

48. Hartveit, F, Mæhle, BO, Halvorsen, JF and Tangen, M. On the progressive nature of tumour growth in the axillary nodes in breast cancer. Oncology, 40: 309-314, 1983c.

49. Hartveit, F, Samsonsen, G, Tangen, M and Halvorsen, JF. Routine histological investigation of the axillary nodes in breast cancer. Clin Oncol, 8: 121-126, 1982b

50. Hartveit, F, Tangen, M, Halvorsen, JF and Samsonsen, G. Time-dependent changes in the axillary nodes in breast cancer: Nodal area. Oncology, 42: 210-216, 1985.

51. Hartveit, F, Tangen, M, Småland, R and Varhaug, JE. Side and stage in breast cancer. Clin Oncol, 7: 221-225, 1981a.

52. Hartveit, F, Thoresen, S, Tangen, M and Halvorsen, JF. Variation in histology and oestrogen receptor content in breast carcinoma related to tumour size and time of presentation. Clin Oncol, 9: 233-238, 1983d.

53. Hartveit, F, Thoresen, S, Tangen, M and Maartmann-Moe, H. Mast cell changes and tumour dissemination in human breast carcinoma. Invasion and Metastasis, 4: 146-155, 1984d.

54. Hartveit, F, Thoresen, S, Thorsen, T and Tangen, M. Histological grade and efferent vascular invasion in human breast carcinoma. Brit J Cancer, 44: 81-84, 1981b.

55. Hartveit, F, Dobbe, G, Thoresen, S, Dahl, O, Tangen M and Thorsen, T. The changing pattern of recurrence in oestrogen positive and negative breast cancer with nodal spread related to efferent vascular invasion. Oncology, 40: 81-84, 1983e.

56. Hartveit, F, Thorsen, T, Tangen, M, Mæhle, BO, Thoresen, S and Halvorsen, JF. Sinophobic growth in oestrogen receptor negative metastatic breast cancer. Oncology, 40: 241-243, 1983f.

57. Haybittle, JL, Blamey, WL, Elston, CW, Johnson, J, Doyle, DJ, Campbell, FC, Nicholson, RJ and Griffiths, K. A prognostic index in primary breast cancer. Brit J Cancer, 45: 361-366, 1982.
58. Hultborn, KA, Larsson, LG and Ragnhult, I. The lymph drainage from the breast to the axillary and parasternal lymph nodes, studied with the aid of colloidal AU[198]. Acta radiol., 43: 52-64, 1955.
59. Hunter, RL, Ferguson, DJ and Coppelson, LW. Survival with mammary cancer related to the interaction of germinal centre hyperplasia and sinus histiocytosis in axillary and internal mammary lymph nodes. Cancer, 36, 528-539, 1975.
60. Lewy, AJ, Wehr, TA, Rosenthal, NE, Nurnberger, JI, Slever, LJ, Uhde, TW, Newsome, DA, Becker, LE, Markey, SP, Kopin, IJ and Goodwin, FK. Melatonin secretion as a neurobiological "marker" and effect of light in humans. Psychopharmacology bulletin, 18: 127-128, 1982.
61. Mæhle, BO and Skjærven, R. A prognostic index based on the mean nuclear area of breast cancer cells and efferent vascular invasion in the axillary nodes. Diagn Histopathology, 6: 221-228, 1983.
62. Meson, BH, Holdaway, IH, Mullins, PR, Kay, RG and Gillmann, JC. Seasonal variation in breast cancer detection: correlation with tumour progesterone receptor status (abstract). Biannial International breast cancer research Conference. Proceedings, 3-7, London 1985.
63. Moore, O and Foote, F. The relatively favourable prognosis of medullary carcinoma of the breast. Cancer, 2: 635-642, 1949.
64. Namboodiri, MAA, Sugden, D, Klein DC and Mefford, N, 5-hydroxytryptophan elevates serum melatonin. Science, 221: 659-661, 1983.
65. Norrby, K. Enerbäck, L and Franzén, L. Mast cell activation and tissue cell proliferation. Cell Tiss Res, 170: 289-303, 1976.
66. Parwaresch, MR, Horny, H-P and Lennert, K. Tissue mast cells in health and disease. Pat Res Pract, 179: 439-461, 1985.
67. Reiter, R. The pineal and its hormones in the control of reproduction in mammals. Endocrine Rev, 1: 109-131, 1980.
68. Roche, WR. Mast cells and tumors. The specific enhancement of tumour proliferation. Am J Path, 119: 57-64, 1985.
69. Sandstad, E and Hartveit, F. (Work in progress)
70. Saphir, O and Amromin, GD. Obscure axillary lymph node metastases in carcinoma of breast. Cancer, 1: 238-241, 1948.
71. Shiach, KJ, Simpson, JG and Thompson, WD. Tumours acquire their vasculative by vessel incorporation not vessel ingrowth. (synopses) J Path, 146: 282ª, 1985.
72. Sjøgren, HO, Hellstrøm, I, Bansal, SC and Hellstrøm, KE. Suggestive evidence that the "blocking antibodies" of tumour-bearing individuals may be antigen-antibody complexes. Proc Nat Acad Sci, 68: 1372-1375, 1971.
73. Snell, GD. Transplantable tumors. In: The physiopathology of cancer, p.293, Ed.Homburger, 2nd ed. New York, Paul B. Hoeber Inc, 1959.
74. Snell, GD. Immunologic enhancement. Collective review. Surg Gynec Obstet, 130: 1109-1119, 1970.
75. Stetson, MH and Watson-Whitmyre, M. Physiology of the pineal and its hormone melatonin in annual reproduction in rodents. In: The pineal gland (Ed.R.J. Reiter), pp. 109-153, Raven Press, New York, 1984.

76. Sylvén, B. Ester sulpharic acids of high molecular weight and mast cells in mesenchymal tumours. Acta Radiol, (Stockholm) suppl. 59, 1945.

77. Thoresen, S, Tangen, M and Hartveit, F. Mast cells in the axillary nodes of breast cancer patients. Diagn Histopathology, 5: 65-67, 1982.

78. Thoresen, S, Hartveit, F, Tangen, M and Halvorsen, JF. Sinus catarrh and histological grade in breast cancer. Histopathology, 7: 753-757, 1983.

79. Wilkinson, EJ and Hause, L. Probability in lymph node sectioning. Cancer, 33: 1269-1274, 1974.

80. Zilber, LA. Specific tumor antigens. In: Advances in Cancer Research 5, p.291, New York, Academic Press Inc, 1958.

USE OF IMMUNOCYTOCHEMICAL MARKERS IN THE EVALUATION OF

BREAST CANCER INVASION AND METASTATIC SPREAD.

G. BUSSOLATI[1], P. GUGLIOTTA[1], I. MORRA[1], F. PIETRIBIASI[1], AND E. BERARDENGO[2]

1. Dipartimento di Scienze Biomediche e Oncologia Umana dell'Università,
2. Servizio di Anatomia et Istologia Patologica, Ospedale Maggiore di S. Giovanni Battista, 10.126 Torino, Italy.

INTRODUCTION

Cell markers identifiable with specific antibodies can supplement classical morphological parameters giving evidence of stromal or vascular invasion and of the metastatic spread in lymph nodes, bone marrow, and serous effusions. Such data allow a better staging and therefore a more precise prognosis and therapeutic approach.

Different markers of breast cancer cells have been described in recent years (Hageman and Peterse, 1985). The use of such markers in following the various steps involved in the breast cancer metastatic process will be analysed here, taking into consideration the value and clinical interest of the immunocytochemical data and focusing on the present status and future prospects.

Transition from in situ to invasive primary cancer

Classical light and electron microscopical studies showing breaches in the basement membrane in areas of in situ ductal carcinoma (Ozzello and Sanpitak, 1970) have been extended by investigations with antibodies against collagen IV, fibronectin and laminin. Studies by Liotta et al. (1979) with antibodies against basement membrane collagen gave evidence of focal disruption of such membranes as a possible area of micro-invasion. Further investigations on fibronectin (Labat-Robert et al., 1980; Natali et al., 1984; Birembaut et al., 1985), and on laminin (Albrechtsen et al.,

1981; Nielsen et al., 1983) indicate, however, a rather heterogeneous expression of basement membrane antigens by invasive breast cancer cells. Some invasive breast cancers, namely medullary carcinomas, seem, in fact, able to produce fibronectin. Albrechtsen et al. (1981), on the basis of staining for laminin, have suggested that the more differentiated carcinomas, even when metastatic in lymph nodes, should be able to produce basement membranes, but thinner and discontinuous.

The lack in in situ carcinoma of the myoepithelial cell layer normally present in the mammary ducts and ductules has long been regarded as a histopathologic character of diagnostic significance (W.H.O., 1982). The behaviour of the myoepithelial cells in areas of in situ carcinoma has been investigated with immunocytochemical markers typical, if not specific, of these cells. To trace the myoepithelial cells, we have been employing rabbit antiactin sera, which allow detection of this contractile protein in formalin-fixed paraffin embedded tissues, thus allowing retrospective and prospective studies (Bussolati et al., 1984). Mono-clonal antibodies (Dairkee et al., 1985) and conventional sera (Gusterson et al., 1982) against keratin and antibodies against myosin have also been empoyed to detect the myoepi-thelial cells. They give, however, better results on frozen section than on paraffin-embedded tissues.

There is now consensus by different groups of workers on the presence of only focal remnants of flattened myoepi-thelial cells in ductal in situ carcinomas, while most lesions and areas of lobular cancerization are deprived of these cells (Ozzello and Sanpitak, 1970; Bussolati et al., 1980; Gusterson et al., 1982). Since one of the functions of myoepithelial cells seems to be that of the production of the basement membrane, it appears that the lack of these cells in focal areas might indirectly allow micro-invasion. Accordingly, in a preliminary study of three cases of in situ ductal carcinoma (as diagnosed on the basis of sub-serial sections of the breast lesion), but accompanied by metastatic spread in lymph nodes, we noticed (Eusebi et al., 1985, unpublished observation) a lack of the actin-rich myoepithelial cell layer in most (about 90%) of the carcin-omatous areas.

In lobular (as opposed to ductal) in situ carcinomas, the myoepithelial cell layer is often present, as we have shown by immunohistochemical and parallel electron micro-scopical investigations (Bussolati, 1980; Bussolati et al.,

1981). In some of the lesions, the myoepithelial cell layer is disarranged, and cancer cells seem to reach the basement membrane. This might be the precursor stage to stromal invasion.

The immunocytochemical detection of the myoepithelial cell layer is of diagnostic interest in the differential diagnosis between florid adenosis and well differentiated invasive carcinomas, a single epithelial cell type being regarded as typical of the latter. An exception to this well recognized principle is the absence of myoepithelial cells in focal areas of microglandular adenosis, a rare hyperplastic lesion apparently devoid of malignant potential and behaviour (Clement and Azzopardi, 1983).

The presence, and most probably the progression, of breast cancer cells along the ducts (s.c. pagetoid spread) and into the epidermis can be followed by means of epithelial cell markers. Although there is presently no univocal interpretation of the nature of Paget cells, a strong evidence in favour of the invasive nature of Paget cells is the identification, among the epidermal cells of the nipple, of cells positive for the same markers found positive in the breast cancer cells in the underlying ducts (Bussolati and Pich, 1975; Kirkham et al., 1985).

In seven cases of Paget disease of the nipple associated with carcinoma in the ducts, we have conducted an immunocytochemical investigation both on the epidermal and the ductal lesions, which were stained for callous keratin, epithelial membrane antigen (EMA), carcinoembryonic antigen (CEA), and the apocrine marker 15,000 M.W. glycoprotein of cystic diease fluid (GCDFP-15). The high degree of correlation (Table 1) of the reactions in the Paget cells and the cancer cells in the ducts is in agreement with the hypothesis that Paget cells are not of epidermal origin, but originate from cancer cells migrating along the ducts. The positivity of Paget cells with mono- or polyclonal antibodies against EMA and against tumor-associated antigens (such as Ca 1), as well as their negativity with antibodies against callous keratin (which stain instead the epidermal cells) are in agreement with the carcinomatous and infiltrative nature of the Paget cells.

In a recent investigation of a large series of breast carcinomas (Eusebi et al., submitted for publication), we found only 14% of carcinomas to be positive for a 15,000 dalton M.W. glycoprotein of the cystic disease fluid, a

TABLE 1

PAGET DISEASE OF THE NIPPLE
(7 cases)

Immunocytochemical reactivity of epidermal Paget cells (A)
and of intra-ductal carcinoma cells (B)

	Keratin	GCDFP-15	EMA	CEA	Cal
A+ B+	/	4	7	7	6
A+ B-	/	/	/	/	/
A- B+	/	1	/	/	/
A- B-	7	2	/	/	1

Cases regarded as positive (+) when more than 20% of cells were stained.
Keratin: Rabbit anti-callous human keratin (Dako, Denmark).
GCDFP-15: Rabbit anti-Gross Cystic Disease Fluid Protein 15,000 dalton M.W.
EMA: Rabbit anti-human milk fat globule membrane antigen.
CEA: Rabbit anti-human CEA (Dako, Denmark).
Cal: Mouse anti-human tumor-associated antigen (Wellcome, U.K.).

marker of apocrine metaplasia. In five of our seven cases of Paget disease, we found that the intraductal carcinoma cells, as well as the Paget cells, were positive for the apocrine marker. This might be interpreted as evidence in favour of the hypothesis that apocrine carcinomas of the

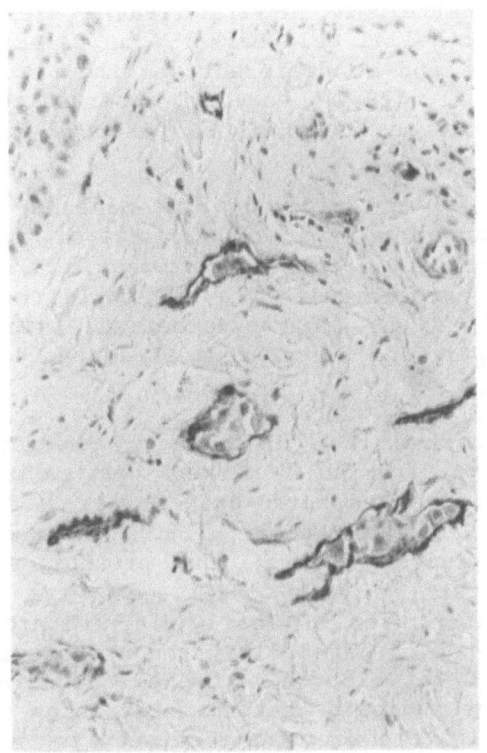

Fig. 1.   Human breast cancer. In areas peripheral to the main tumoral node, cancer cells are present in irregularly shaped spaces. The positivity of the endothelial cells for Factor VIII (immunoperoxy-dase procedure) demonstrates that such spaces are likely correspond to blood capillaries. Nuclei counterstained with Haemalun, x 200.

breast constitute a subgroup of tumor with a high tendency to epidermal invasion. Accordingly, and in agreement with the results of Mazoujian et al. (1984), we found positivity for the apocrine marker in four cases of extramammary (vulvar) Paget disease.

Markers of vascular endothelium can be employed in the identification of areas of vascular invasion in primary breast cancer, a topic of high prognostic significance (Fig. 1). According to Bettelheim et al. (1984), staining for Factor VIII, an endothelial cell marker, can be employed to detect blood vessels and to differentiate them from lymphatics. Svanholm et al. (1984), however, observed that lymph vessels also can on some occasions be positive for Factor VIII.

We have recently investigated intra-vascular invasion in a series of signet ring and/or squamous carcinomas of the breast (Bussolati et al., 1985). Comparing electron microscopical and immunocytochemical data, we could not confirm the absolute value of the immunocytochemical staining for Factor VIII in identifying cancer-permeated spaces as blood vessels.

It is not clear whether presence or absence of any immunocytochemically detectable marker has a predictory value on the recurrence and metastatic behaviour of breast cancer. While some authors (Walker, 1980) observed a worse prognosis in CEA-positive cases, the present status of experience (Gilchrist et al., 1985) does not seem to indicate immunostaining for CEA as a discriminatory value for early recurrence. Similarly, recent studies with monoclonal anti-milk fat globule membrane antibodies (Berry et al., 1985) do not indicate that immunostaining with such antibodies might help to discriminate between the metastatic potential of different primary breast cancers.

Lymph node metastases

The involvement of axillary lymph nodes by breast cancer has an important bearing on prognosis and therapeutic treatment. While generally the detection of metastatic foci in lymph nodes offers no difficult diagnostic problem, the detection of micrometastatic foci is indeed a more difficult task. Wells et al. (1984) have recently shown, in an extensive investigation of cases of breast cancer reported to be lymph node negative, the presence of immunocytochemically detectable micrometastatic foci of ductal or lobular cancer in about 20% of the cases. The authors employed three monoclonals, two raised against human milk fat globule membrane antigens and one against cytokeratin, and it is interesting to note that their results differ from those previously reported by Sloane et al. (1980), who made a similar study but using a polyclonal antiserum against human milk fat globule membrane antigen. These authors were not able to reveal, by immunohistochemistry, metastases which had not been observed by conventional histopathological examination.

These studies raise a series of important points of diagnostic and clinical significance:
1. The relative value of monoclonal antibodies and conventional sera.

Theoretically, the latter, if specific for cancerous or epithelial cells, should be more apt to detect all meta-static cells in lymph nodes, being able to detect a higher number of antigenic determinants, due to the well recognized heterogeneous population of breast cancer cells.

2. The real advantages of immunocytochemistry over classical morphological criteria of diagnosis.

Special staining procedures have to be performed on new, serially cut, histological sections, different from those employed for routine examination. It might well be that the new sections reveal micrometastatic foci not present in the conventionally stained sections. In the experience of Fisher et al. (1978), serial sectioning of lymph nodes can reveal micrometastases in up to 24% of the cases. In addition, the histological type of breast cancer has also to be considered. Metastases of ductal carcinomas are characterized by highly atypical and/or gland forming cells, easily differentiable from the reactive lymph nodular tissue. Cells of infiltrating lobular carcinoma have instead a more benign aspect (Ashton et al., 1975), are isolated or diffuse in the lymph node in a lymphoma-like pattern, as originally described by McDivitt et al. (1968) and tend to fill up the sinuses in a way which can mimic sinus histiocytosis (Rossi, 1981).

Consistent with the above considerations, Wells et al. (1984) detected immunocytochemically micrometastatic involvement in lymph nodes previously considered as negative, in 33% of lobular carcinomas and in 9% of ductal carcinomas. However, it should be assumed that the mere presence of cells reactive with mono- or polyclonal anti-bodies against tumor associated antigens is not an absolute proof of their malignant nature, since such tumor-derived antigens might have been taken up from macrophages.

3. The clinical significance of micrometastases has been discussed by several authors.

According to Huvos et al., 1971; Attiyeh et al., 1977; Fisher et al., 1978a and b, the prognosis of breast cancer should be related to the macrometastatic rather than to the micrometastatic spread. Rosen et al. (1981) showed that in patients with a single node metastasis, the presence of micrometastases might indicate a tendency to later diffusion of the disease.

In view of the above considerations, we have set up an extensive study of 50 cases of breast cancer in order to investigate the real value of an immunocytochemical detection of micrometastatic spread in lymph nodes. Only cases of lobular carcinoma with negative axillary lymph nodes and a minimum follow-up of two years were retained. Cases were considered eligible when at least ten negative lymph nodes had been examined. Formalin-fixed paraffin embedded tissue blocks were recut, and serial sections were stained with: (1) Haematoxyline-Eosin; (2) Goat anti-Epithelial Membrane Antigen (EMA) (Sera Lab., U.K.); (3) Monoclonal antibody HMFG-2 (kindly supplied by Dr. J. Taylor-Papadimitriou, ICRF, London); (4) Monoclonal antibody anti-54 kd cytokeratin (ENZO Biochem., USA). Sections serial to those found positive in the immunocytochemical staining for cancer associated antigens were stained with rabbit sera against chymotrypsin, a macrophage marker.

Micrometastatic foci were found in twelve cases in which one or more lymph nodes were affected. No special advantage was found with the use of monoclonal antibodies versus conventional antiserum; on the contrary, the number of positive cells was generally higher with anti-EMA serum, and in at least one case, a group of EMA-positive cells appeared completely negative with monoclonal HMFG-2 anti-body. In agreement with Delsol et al. (1984), we observed that anti-EMA serum and, to a minor extent, a monoclonal HMFG-2, occasionally stained lymphoid cells, mainly plasma cells; the non-epithelial nature of these cells was, however, easily interpreted by morphological criteria.

Anti-keratin monoclonal antibody gave rather weak staining in most cases of metastatic epithelial cells (as identified on parallel sections by conventional stains and immunocytochemical reactions with anti-EMA and HMFG-2 antibodies). We interpreted such weak reaction as related to the fact that the lymph nodes had been fixed in formalin, while alcohol fixation is regarded as ideal for keratin staining (Altmannsberger et al., 1981).

More difficult was the interpreation of macrophage-like cells in lymph sinuses showing small cytoplasmic vacuoles positive for HMFG-2 and EMA, but not for keratin. These cells were found positive for chymotrypsin and accordingly interpreted as macrophages engulfed with antigens derived from the primary tumor. To rule out the occurrence of an histiocytoid variety of lobular carcinoma, which has been recently identified by Eusebi et al. (1984) and characterized by apocrine features, we have stained sections with rabbit anti-GCDFP-15 serum, a marker of apocrine metaplasia (Mazoujian et al., 1983).

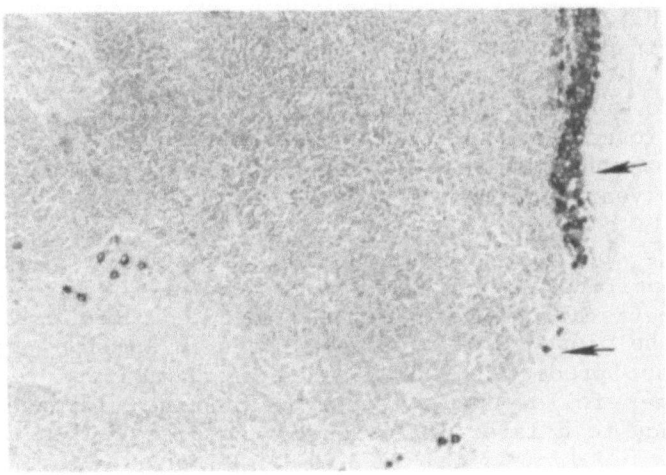

Fig. 2.   Axillary lymph node from a patient with infiltrat-
          ing lobular carcinoma of the breast. Immunoper-
          oxidase staining with rabbit anti-EMA serum. Most
          of the lymph node is negative, but isolated EMA-
          positive cancers (arrows) are scattered in the
          marginal sinus. X 80.

In most of the positive cases, the neoplastic cells were found in the sinuses, mainly in the marginal one (Fig. 2). In some cases, however, the cancer cells were diffusely present in the lymph-reticular tissue. On some occasions, the typical intra-cytoplasmic vacuoles were observed, with most of the neoplastic cells showing a diffuse staining in the cytoplasm and/or of the cell membrane with anti-EMA or HMFG-2 antibodies. Anti-keratin staining resulted in a diffuse cytoplasmic staining.

To answer the question whether the immunocytochemical detection of micrometastases was only related to the fact that the staining had been performed on new sections, we examined the serial sections after conventional staining. Out of the 12 positive cases, an independent examination could detect micrometastatic foci in 5 cases. It can therefore be concluded that in some cases, micrometastatic foci from lobular breast carcinoma were not morphologically recognizable because of the lack of cellular atypia and of structural disarrangement of lymph nodes. This was also confirmed in selected cases in which sections were stained with H. and E., photographed, and then unmounted and re-stained for EMA.

To answer questions on the clinical and prognostic significance of micrometastatic spread, we have obtained data on the follow-up of all the 50 patients for a minimum of two years and on the average for 3.5 years.

We observed relapse or death from tumor in two of the 12 "positive" cases and in seven of the 38 cases when micrometastatic spread was not found. These data indicate that the presence of micrometastases in axillary lymph nodes does not predict the occurrence of short term recurrences. A longer follow-up is needed to obtain information on the tendency to a later diffusion of the disease.

Bone metastases

Metastases in the bone marrow have been described as an early and frequent occurrence in breast cancer patients, resulting in early recurrence and poor prognosis (Ingle, 1978; Riddel and Landys, 1979). The identification of single neoplastic cells within bone marrow haematopoietic cells is difficult on a morphological basis, and immunocytochemical procedures have been proposed to detect breast cancer cells. In a previous investigation (Gugliotta et al., 1981), we tested antisera against seven different tumor associated markers and found, in agreement with the results of Dearnaley et al. (1981, 1983), that an antiserum against milk fat globule membrane revealed metastatic breast cancer cells in all the ten cases of bone metastases examined. An antiserum against CEA was also found highly sensitive, i.e., able to recognize cancer cells in nine out of ten cases examined. It was not specific, however, since conventional sera as well as most anti-CEA monoclonals also recognize an antigen expressed by myeloid cells (Navone et al., 1985).

According to the hypothesis that a small number of cancer cells might already be metastatic in bone marrow when the patients first present with breast cancer and that such currently undetectable cancer cells might be the source of relapse, Redding et al. (1983) conducted an immunocytochemical investigation in 110 breast cancer patients at the time of the primary surgery.

Samples of bone marrow were aspirated from eight sites, and smears were tested in an immuno-phosphatase procedure with an anti-milk fat globule membrane (anti-EMA) rabbit serum. Tumor cells were detected in the bone marrow of 28% of the patients, and it was suggested that these patients without lymph node involvement and thus "at low risk" should be treated like those with a diffuse diseaes. The prognostic significance of these observations has still to be evaluated after a long follow-up. There are indeed some doubts concerning the specificity of the method. Recently, Delsol et al. (1984) have shown that lymphoid cells can react with poly- or monoclonal antibodies against epithelial membrane antigen. Thus, the identification of metastatic cells in bone marrow cannot be based only on its reactivity with presently available immunological probes, but also on its morphology.

We have conducted an investigation similar to that of Redding et al. (1983), but on histological sections of needle biopsies taken at the moment of mastectomy from 112 patients without clinical or radiological evidence of diffuse disease. The biopsies were taken from the iliac crest, monolaterally in 63 cases and bilaterally in 49 cases, fixed-decalcified in Bouin fluid (Bussolati, 1978), and tested on sections with rabbit anti-EMA serum and on immunoperoxidase procedure. Positive cases were tested on serial sections with monoclonal antibodies HMFG-2 and Ca 1.

In this study, only two cases came as positive: one patient, where the metastatic diffusion was rather extensive and already appreciable with conventional histology, died within one year after the operation; the other patient showed only sparse neoplastic cells, positive with all the markers employed but not identifiable with conventional cytology (Fig. 3). This patient shows no evidence of disease four years after surgery. In our opinion, this indicates that the presence of micrometastases of breast cancer cells in bone marrow does not necessarily mean an early recurrence.

Of interest is the application of immunocytochemical markers for the detection of metastatic breast cancer cells in cases of clinical or radiological suspicion of bone metastases. In five out of seventeen cases of bone biopsies from such patients, we were able to detect EMA-positive cells. In at least one of these cases, the cancer cells were not appreciable with conventional staining procedures. All five patients died from tumor within two years after biopsy.

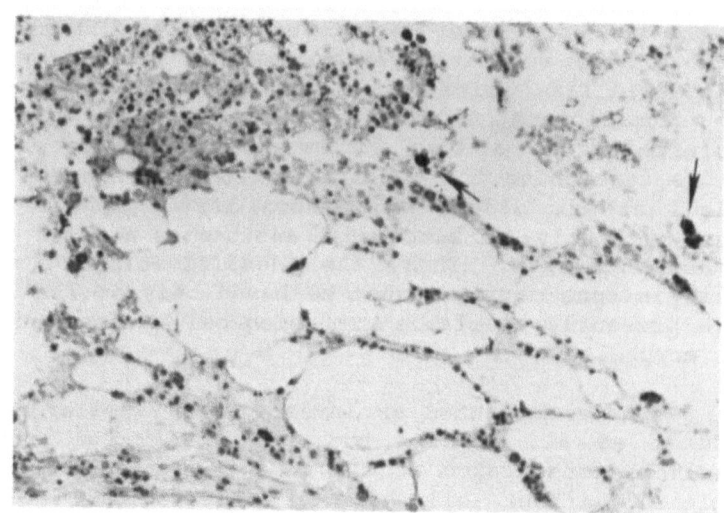

Fig. 3. Bone marrow biopsy obtained during mastectomy from a patient with infiltrating lobular carcinoma. A few scattered EMA-positive cells are present (arrows). Four years after mastectomy, the patient is still alive, without evidence of disease. X 200.

Serous effusions

Difficulties in recognizing cancer cells in serous effusions and their correct differentiation from reactive mesothelial cells is a well-known diagnostic problem. The use of conventional antisera and of monoclonal antibodies against tumor-associated antigens has been proposed by various authors to detect breast cancer cells in pleural and peritoneal effusions as an adjunct to cytomorphological procedures. The percentage of immunocytochemically positive cases varies from 50 to 100% according to the criteria of evaluation of the different authors and to the antibodies employed. Some of these antibodies, such as HMFG-2, Ca 1, and B 72.3, were originally regarded as cancer- or at least epithelium-specific, but recent evidences have been presented against such assumption (Ghosh et al., 1983; Delsol et al., 1984). The highest percentage of positive cases has been reported by Johnston et al. (1985), who investigated 21 patients with metastatic breast cancer in effusions as diagnosed by conventional cytomorphology; in all cases, tumor cells were recognized by antibody B 72.3 while mesothelium was always negative. However, the authors did not study the usefulness of MAB B 72.3 in the detection of sparse cancer cells which escaped from conventional histology.

We have employed conventional antisera against EMA and CEA and monoclonal antibodies HMFG-2, Ca 1, B 72.3, and against 54 kd cytokeratin (ENZO Bioch., USA) on a series of pleural effusions. The immunperoxidase (ABC) procedure was applied on serial sections of the alcohol-fixed sediment embedded in paraffin according to the cell-bag procedure (Bussolati, 1982).

Poly- or monoclonal antibodies against CEA were often positive in cancer cells, as already observed by Sehested et al. (1983) and Szpak et al. (1984). We also observed a positive staining of granulocytes and of macrophages having ingested heterogeneous material, a finding which makes anti-CEA antibodies not specific and not very reliable in the immunocytochemical detection of cancer cells in serous effusions. The Ca 1 antibody, in our experience, gave positive results in ten cases of pleural effusions from breast cancer patients (Gugliotta et al., 1983). Contrary to the findings of Ghosh et al. (1983), we did not observe staining of mesothelial cells, possibly since we employed the antibody at a very low concentration (0.2 µg/ml). The monoclonal antibody against 54 kd cytokeratin (ENZO Biochem., USA) was highly selective but not specific since there was a positive staining in the reactive mesothelial cells, as already described by Gown and Vogel (1984).

In a series of fifty cases of patients mastectomized for breast cancer and presenting with serous effusions, we conducted a parallel cytomorphological and immunocytochemical investigation. The results were evaluated on the base of follow-up and clinical outcome, since all patients were dead from tumor after two years. Serial sections of the paraffin-embedded sediment were stained with Haematoxylin-Eosin and with the immunoperoxidase reactions for EMA (goat serum), with monoclonals HMFG-2 and B 72.3 (Fig. 4a and b). Papanicolaou-stained smears of the same cases were also examined. The results are summarized in Table 2. Cytomorphology was positive in 25, suspicious in ten, and negative in fifteen cases. EMA staining revealed positive cells in all morphologically positive cases, in eight of the suspicious, and in eight of the false-negative cases. In

TABLE 2

IMMUNOCYTOCHEMICAL DETECTION OF CANCER CELLS IN SEROUS EFFUSIONS
from
50 breast cancer patients with relapse or death from tumor and 10 patients without evidence of tumor (controls)

		Cytology	EMA+	HMFG-2	B 72.3
Breast- cancer- patients	Positive	25	25	23	21
	Suspicious	10	8	9	7
	Negative	15	8	6	6
	TOTAL	50	41	38	34
Controls	Negative	10	3	0	0

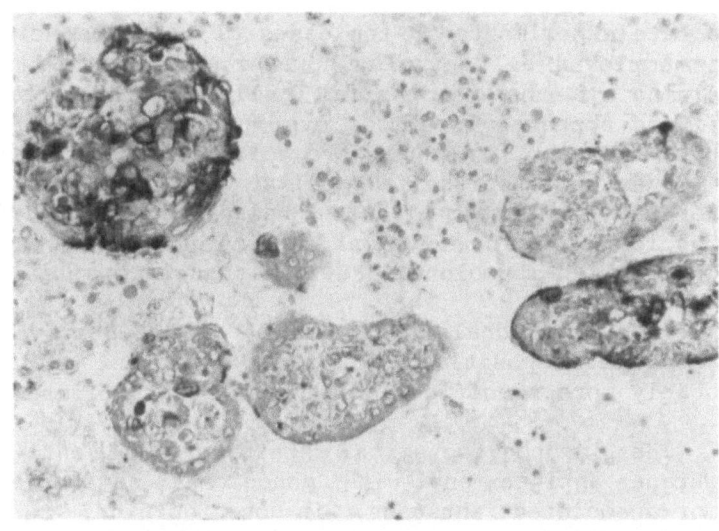

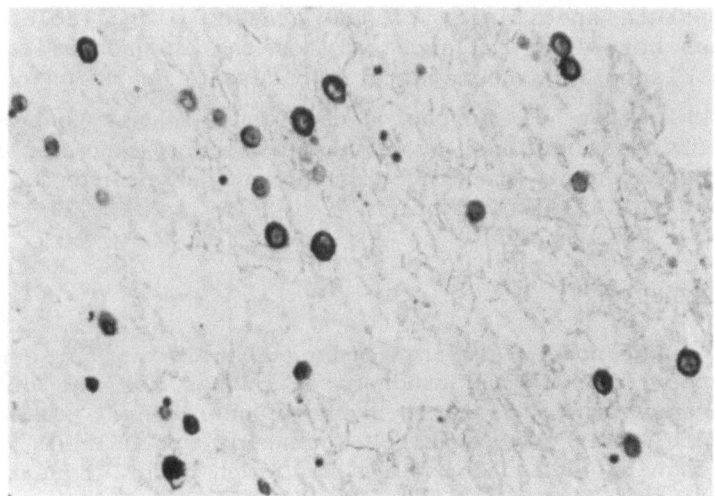

Fig. 4 a and b. Paraffin-embedded sediments of pleural
effusions from breast cancer patients.
(a) Immunocytochemical staining with B 72.3
monoclonal antibody. The cancer cells are
arranged in clumps and some, but not all, of them
are positive with the marker. Mesothelial and
reactive cells are negative. (b) Isolated metastatic cancer cells are revealed by a peripheral
immunoperoxidase staining with antibody HMFG-2.
X 320.

separate experiments in ten cases of reactive serous effusions employed as controls, however, we observed a positive staining of the mesothelial cells in three cases; such staining appeared localized over part of the cell membrane, with a distribution, therefore, different form that observed in metastatic epithelial cells. In addition, we also observed, in agreement with Delsol et al. (1984), that lymphoid cells in effusions can be positive with anti-EMA and even with monoclonal HFG-2, although to a lesser extent.

The monoclonals HMFG-2 and B 72.3 gave a lower percentage of positive cases in the present series but are probably more specific than the anti-EMA antiserum.

The immunocytochemical staining with anti-epithelial membrane antigen and with monoclonal antibodies against tumor-associated antigens, in our opinion, represents a useful adjunct to conventional cytomorphological criteria, especially in detecting sparse cancer cells intermingled with reactive mesothelial cells and in providing additional differentiation criteria in suspicious cases. The lack of absolute specificity of the presently available antibodies does not allow reliance only on the immunochemical reaction in diagnosing the metastatic nature of an effusion. The combination of morphological and immunocytochemical criteria, as obtained by immunoperoxidase (and not by immunofluorescence) staining procedures can presently allow the most reliable information.

CONCLUSION

Antibodies against tumor-associated antigens can be employed as immunocytochemical probes for the detection of invasive and metastatic breast cancer cells. Among the most useful markers, anti-EMA mono-or polyclonal antibodies recognize metastatic cells in lymph nodes, bone marrow, and serous effusions. Other antibodies, such as anticytokeratin, Ca 1, and B 72.3, also present a high prospect of application to specific problems.

Monoclonal antibodies HMFG-2 and B 72.3, employed either alone or in parallel, present a great diagnostic interest in recognizing sparse breast cancer cells in serous effusions and have a great clinical application. The use of these antibodies can solve doubtful cases, particularly those cases originallly diagnosed as negative by classical cytological means.

The immunological probes detect micrometastatic spreads
in lymph nodes and bone marrow, especially from infiltrating
lobular carcinoma, which would be difficult or even impossible to recognize by conventional histology. The clinical
significance of such findings in terms of prognosis, however, appears uncertain at the present time.

ACKNOWLEDGEMENTS

Work supported by grants from the A.I.R.C. (Milan), the
M.P.I. (Rome and the Italian CNR (Finalized Project
"Oncologia") grant n° 85.02058.44.

Dr. Joyce Taylor-Papadimitriou, Imperial Cancer
Research Fund, London, and Dr. Jeffrey Schlom, National
Cancer Institute, Bethesda, kindly supplied monoclonals
HMFG-2 and B 72.3, respectively.

REFERENCES

Albrechtsen, R., Nielsen, M., Wewer, U., Engvall, E., and
Ruoslahti, E., Basement membrane changes in breast
cancer detected by immunohistochemical staining for
laminin. Cancer Res., 41, 5076-5081, 1981.

Altmannsberger, M., Osborn, M., Holscher, A., Schauer, A.,
and Weber, K., The distribution of keratin type
intermediate filaments in human breast cancer: an
immunohistological study. Virchows Arch. (Cell
Pathol.), 37, 277-284, 1981.

Ashton, P.R., Hollingsworth, A.S. Jr., and Johnston, W.W.,
The cytopathology of metastatic breast cancer, 19,
1-6, 1975.

Attiyeh, F.F., Jensen, M., Huvos, A.G., and Fracchia, A.,
Axillary micrometastases and macrometastases in
carcinoma of the breast. Surg. Gynecol. Obstet.,
144, 839-842, 1977.

322

Berry, N., Jones, D.B., Smallwood, J., Taylor, I., Kirkham, N., and Taylor-Papadimitriou, J., The prognostic value of the monoclonal antibodies HMFG1 and HMFG2 in breast cancer. Br. J. Cancer, 51, 179-186, 1985.

Bettelheim, R., Mitchell, D., and Gusterson, B.A., Immunocytochemistry in the identification of vascular invasion in breast cancer. J. Clin. Pathol., 37, 364-366, 1984.

Birembaut, P., Caron, Y., and Adnet, J.J., Usefulness of basement membrane markers in tumoural pathology. J. Pathol., 145, 283-296, 1985.

Bussolati, G., A fixation-decalcification procedure for bone biopsies. Histopathology, 2, 329-334, 1978.

Bussolati, G., Actin-rich (myoepithelial) cells in lobular carcinoma in situ of the breast. Virchows Arch. (Cell Pathol.), 32, 165-176, 1980.

Bussolati, G., A celloidin bag for the histological preparation of cytologic material. J. Clin. Pathol., 35, 574-576, 1982.

Bussolati, G., and Pich, A., Mammary and extramammary Paget's disease. Am. J. Pathol., 80, 117-124, 1975

Bussolati, G., Botta, G., and Gugliotta, P., Actin-rich (myoepithelial) cells in ductal carcinoma in situ of the breast. Virchows Arch. (Cell Pathol.), 34, 251-269, 1980.

Bussolati, G., Botto Micca, F., Eusebi, V., and Betts, C.M., Myoepithelial cells in lobular carcinoma in situ of the breast: a parallel immunocytochemical and ultrastructural study. Ultrastruct. Pathol., 2, 219-230, 1981.

Bussolati, G., Gugliotta, P., and Fulcheri, E., Immunocytochemistry of actin in normal and neoplastic tissues. In: Advances in Immunohistochemistry, R.A. De Lellis, ed., Masson, U.S.A., pp. 325-341, 1984.

Bussolati, G., Sapino, A., Morra, I., and Ghiringhello, B., Carcinoma of the breast with signet ring cell and/or squamous metaplasia. In: Progress in Surgical Pathology, C.M. Fenoglio-Preiser, ed., Field, Rich and Ass., New York, 1986, in press.

Clement, P.B., and Azzopardi, J.G., Microglandular adenosis of the breast - a lesion simulating tubular carcinoma. Histopathology, 7, 169-180, 1983.

Dairkee, S.H., Blayney, C.M., Smith, H.S., and Hackett, A.J., A monoclonal antibody that defines human myoepithelium. Biennial International Breast Cancer Research Conference, London, 1985.

Dearnaley, D.P., Sloane, J.P., Ormerod, M.G., Steele, K., Coombes, R.C., Clink H. McD., Powles, T.J., Ford, H.T., Gazet, J.-C., and Neville, A.M., Increased detection of mammary carcinoma cells in marrow smears using antisera to epithelial membrane antigen. Br. J. Cancer, 44, 85-90, 1981.

Dearnaley, D.P., Ormerod, M.G., Sloane, J.P., Humley, H., Imrie, S. , Jones, M., Coombes, R.C., and Neville, A. M., Detection of isolated mammary carcinoma cells in marrow of patients with primary breast cancer. J. Roy. Soc. Med., 76, 359-364, 1983.

Delsol, G., Gatter, K.C., Stein, H., Erber, W.N., Pulford., K.A.F., Zinne, K., and Meson, D.Y., Human lymphoid cells express epithelial membrane antigen. Implications for diagnosis of human neoplasms. Lancet, ii, 1124-1128, 1984.

Eusebi, V., Betts, C.M., Haagensen, D.E. Jr., Gugliotta, P., Bussolati, G., and Azzopardi, J.G., Apocrine differentiation in lobular carcinoma of the breast: a morphologic, immunologic and ultrastructural study. Hum. Path., 15 134-140, 1984.

Fisher, E.R., Palekar, A., Rockette, H.,Redmond, C. and Fisher, B., Pathologic findings from the National Surgery Adjuvant Breast Project (protocol no.4). V. Significance of axillary nodal micro- and macrometastases. Cancer, 42, 2032-2038, 1978 a.

Fisher, E.R., Swamidoss, S., Lee, C.H., Rockette,H., Redmond, C. and Fisher, B., Detection and significance of occult axillary node metastases in patients with invasive breasr cancer. Cancer, 42, 2025-2031, 1978 b.

Gosh, A.K., Spriggs, A.I., Taylor-Papadimitriou, J., and Mason, D.Y., Immunocytochemical staining of cells in pleural and peritoneal effusions with a panel of monoclonal antibodies. J. Clin. Pathol., 36, 1154-1164, 1983.

Gilchrist, K.W., Kalish, L., Could, V.E., Hirschl, S., Imbriglia, J.E., Levy, W.M., Patchefsky, A.S., Pickren, J., Roth, J.A., Schinella, R.A., Schwartz, I.S., Wheeler, J.E., and Tormey, D.C., Immuno-staining for carcinoembryonic antigen does not discriminate for early recurrence in breast cancer. The ECOG experience. Cancer, 56, 351-355, 1985.

Gown, A.M., and Vogel, A.M., Monoclonal antibodies to human intermediate filament proteins. II.Distribution of filament proteins in normal human tissues. Am. J. Path., 114, 309-321, 1984.

Gugliatta, P., Botta, G., and Bussolati, G., Immunocyto-chemical detection of tumour markers in bone metastases from carcinoma of the breast. Histochem. J., 13, 953-959, 1981.

Gugliatta, P., Papotti, M., Varalli, M., and Bussolati, G., Carcino-embryonic antigen (CEA) localisation in primary and metastatic breast cancer: a methodo-logical approach. International Association for Breast Cancer Research. Breast Cancer Research Conference. Denver, Colorado, 1983.

Gusterson, B.A., Warburton, M.J., Mitchell, D., Ellison, M., Neville, A.M., and Rudland, P.S., Distribution of myoepithelial cells and basement membrane proteins in the normal breast and in benign and malignant breast diseases. Cancer Res., 42, 4763-4770, 1972.

Hageman, P.H., and Peterse, J.L., New approaches to the pathology of breast cancer: can immunohistochemistry add new information? Biennial International Breast Cancer Research Conference, London, 1985.

Huvos, A.G., Hutter, R.V.P., and Berg, J.W., Significance of axillary macrometastases and micrometastases in mammary cancer. Ann. Surg., 173, 44-46, 1971.

Ingle, J.N., Tormey, D.C., and Tan, H.K., The bone marrow examination in breast cancer. Cancer, 41, 670-674, 1978.

Johnston, W.W., Szpak, C.A., Lottich, S.C. Thor, A., and Schlom,J., Use of monoclonal antibody (B 72.3) as an immunocytochemical adjunct to diagnosis of adeno-carcinoma in human effusions. Cancer Res., 45, 1894-1900, 1985.

Kirkham, N., Berry, N., Jones, D.B., and Taylor-Papadimitriou, J., Paget's disease of the nipple. Cancer, 55, 1510-1512, 1985.

Labat-Robert, J., Birembaut, P., Adnet, J.J., Mercantini, F., and Robert, L., Loss of fibronectin in human breast cancer. Cell Biol. Internat. Rep., 4, 609-616, 1980.

Liotta, L.A., Foidart, J.M., Gehron Robey, P., Martin, G.R., and Gullino, P.M., Identification of micrometastases of breast carcinomas by presence of basement membrane collagen. Lancet, ii, 146-147, 1979.

Mazoujian, G., Pinkus, G.S., Davis, S., and Haagensen, D.E. Jr., Immunohistochemistry of a gross cystic disease fluid protein (GCDFP-15) of the breast. A marker of apocrine epithelium and breast carcinomas with apocrine features. Am. J. Pathol., 110, 105-112, 1983.

Mazoujian, G., Pinkus, G.S., and Haagensen, D.E. Jr., Extramammary Paget's disease. Evidence for an apocrine origin. Am. J. Surg. Pathol., 8, 43-50, 1984.

McDivitt, R.W., Stewart, F.W., and Berg, J.W., Tumors of the breast. In: Atlas of tumor pathology, 2nd series, fascicle 2. Armed Forces Institute of Pathology, Washington, DC, 1968.

Natali, P.G., Giacomini, P., Bigotti, G., Nicotra, M.R., Bellocci, M., and de Martino, C., Heterogeneous distribution of actin, myosin, fibronectin and basement membrane antigens in primary and metastatic human breast cancer. Virchows Arch. (Pathol. Anat.), 405, 69-83, 1984.

Navone, R., Gugliotta, P., and Bussolati, G., Applicazione di un anticorpo monoclonale anti-CEA come marcatore del tessuto mieloide in biopsie ossee. XX Congresso Società Italiana di Istochimica, Milano, 1985.

Nielsen, M., Christensen, L., and Albrechtsen, R., The basement membrane component laminin in breast carcinomas and axillary lymph node metastases. Acta Path. Microbiol. Immunol. Scand., Sect. A., 91, 257-264, 1983.

Ozzello, L., and Sanpitak, P., Epithelial-stromal junction of intraductal carcinoma of the breast. Cancer, 26, 1186-1198, 1970.

Redding, W.H., Coombes, R.C., Monaghan, P., Clink, H.McD., Imrie, S.F., Dearnaley, D.P., Ormerod, M.G., Sloane, J.P., Gazet, J.-C., Powles, T.J., and Neville, A.M., Detection of micrometastases in patients with primary breast cancer. Lancet, ii, 1271-1273, 1983.

Ridell, B., and Landys, K., Incidence and histopathology of metastases of mammary carcinoma in biopsies from the posterior iliac crest. Cancer, 44, 1782-1788, 1979.

Rosai, J., Ackerman's Surgical Pathology. Mosby, St. Louis, Toronto, London, 1981, p.1214.

Rosen, P.P., Saigo, P.E., Braun, D.W., Weathers, E., Fracchia, A.A., and Kinne, D.W., Axillary micro- and macrometastases in breast cancer: prognostic significance of tumor size. Ann. Surg., 194, 585-591, 1981.

Sehested, M., Ralfkjaer, E., and Rasmussen, J., Immunoperoxydase demonstration of carcinoembryonic antigen in pleural and peritoneal effusions. Acta Cytol., 27, 124-127, 1983.

Sloane, J.P., Ormerod, M.G., Imrie, S.F., and Coombes, R.C., The use of antisera to epithelial membrane antigen in detecting micrometastases in histological sections. Br. J. Cancer, 42, 392-398, 1980.

Swanholm, H., Nielsen, K., and Hauge, P., Factor VIII-related antigen and lymphatic collecting vessels. Virchows Arch. (Pathol. Anat.), 404, 223-228, 1984.

Szpak, C.A., Johnston,W.W., Lottich, S.C., Kufe, D., Thor, A., and Schlom, J., Patterns of reactivity of four novel monoclonal antibodies (B 72.3, DF3, B 1.1, and B 6.2) with cells in human malignant and benign effusions. Acta Cytol., 28, 356-367, 1984.

Walker, R.A., Demonstration of carcinoembryonic antigen in human breast carcinomas by the immunoperoxydase technique. J. Clin. Pathol., 33, 356-360, 1980.

Wells,   C.A.,   Heryet, A., Brochier, J., Catter,   K.C.,   and
        Mason,   D.Y.,   The   immunocytochemical detection   of
        axillary micrometastases   in   breast cancer. Br. J.
        Cancer, 50, 193-197, 1984.

W.H.O., The World Health Organization histological typing of
        breast tumors. Second edition, Am. J. Clin. Pathol.,
        78, 806-816, 1982.

TUMOUR-HOST INTERACTIONS IN BREAST CANCER METASTASIS

DAVID TARIN

University of Oxford, Nuffield Department of Pathology,
John Radcliffe Hospital, Oxford OX3 9DU, England

INTRINSIC PROPERTIES OF TUMOUR CELLS AND METASTASIS

Tumour metastasis is a property separate and additional to tumourigenicity, as demonstrated by the fact that several undeniably tumourigenic cell lines are incapable of forming metastatic colonies in distant sites even if deliberately disseminated by inoculation into the bloodstream. Evidence confirming this comes from studies on animals with malignant mammary neoplasms, as well as on patients with inoperable malignancy.

Observations on animal tumours

Our studies on spontaneous murine mammary tumours showed that the cells from some could heavily colonise the lungs after intravenous inoculation in mice, whereas those from others did so weakly or not at all, and the results in autologous animals were similar to those in syngeneic recipients. The tumours were all adenocarcinomas, and there were no features which correlated with this behavioural variation. However, the high reproducibility of the findings in each batch of animals inoculated with a given tumour indicated that the differences between individual tumours were due to intrinsic differences in their constituent cells (Tarin and Price, 1979; Tarin and Price, 1980; Price et al., 1982). Similarly, numerous investigations (Fidler, 1978; Kripke et al., 1978; Fidler et al., 1981; Poste et al., 1982) have now shown convincingly that there is considerable diversity in experimental metastatic capability among different cloned tumour cell populations even within a single neoplasm, some clones being totally ineffective in lung colonisation but still tumourigenic on subcutaneous inoculation. There is, therefore, little room for doubt that metastatic capability is determined by intrinsic properties of the tumour cell, separate and additional to those responsible for its tumourigenicity. However, non-neoplastic cells do not make progressively growing colonies after subcutaneous or intravenous inoculation (Price et al., 1982), so the process of metastasis requires an initial tumourigenic capability. This is not to say that non-neoplastic cells cannot, in some circumstances, disseminate and survive in ectopic sites. Lymphocytes, polymorphs, and monocytes/macrophages, for instance, after dispersal in the blood, enter or travel through many tissues. Endometriosis, a condition in which endometrium seeds the pelvic cavity (Blaustein, 1982), and the presence of trophoblastic cells in the blood in pregnancy (Covone et al., 1984) are other possible examples, but in metastasis the end result is unlimited growth and destruction of adjacent normal tissue by multiple colonies of disorganised cells. Thus, some cell traffic may occur in normal subjects, but go largely unrecognised because the elements concerned do not multiplty to form focal aggregates where they come to rest (see Tarin, 1976, for further discussion).

As the process of metastasis consists of the relentless growth of tumour deposits in distant sites after dissemination from the primary, it must by definition take place on a background of tumourigenicity and is, therefore, de facto evidence of progression in the behaviour of the tumour.

Observations on human tumours

Five years ago, a new opportunity for studying some aspects of tumour metastasis in living humans became available as a result of the introduction of recently developed techniques for the treatment of intractable malignant ascites due to inoperable abdominal cancer. In these patients, recurrent accumulation of fluid causes pain and distress, and the traditional means of removing it by paracentesis (aspiration of ascites through the abdominal wall) results in loss of salts and proteins and severe metabolic imbalance. Such patients subjectively fare much better if the fluid is shunted into the jugular vein via a plastic tube; but, of course, the malignant cells are thus infused directly into the circulation, there being no possibility of interposing a filter because it would rapidly block with cells and debris. Autopsy studies on 19 such patients (Tarin et al., 1986) [now updated to 22 patients] showed that half the patients had small seedling metastases and the remainder had none, although the median survival time of the second group was not strikingly different. It was also observed that among patients with histologically identical tumours of the same organ, some had metastases at the time of death whereas others did not, although they had survived much longer. It would seem, therefore, that individual tumours differ from each other in their capability to establish metastatic colonies, or that host mechanisms are more effective in some patients than in others; but we could find no pathological evidence of cellular immune attack on tumour emboli or small colonies in any of the patients in this series. Differences in therapy did not account for the differences in metastatic behaviour among tumours because all patients were considered terminal, and shunting was used as a palliative measure when all other treatment had failed and had been discontinued.

The sample of patients in this study is not large, and interpretation should be guarded. However, the mode of infusion of tumour cells was directly homologous to that used in our earlier studies on murine mammary tumours, and the findings indicate the underlying mechanisms involved in tumour metastasis are similar in these two species.

STEPWISE NATURE OF METASTASIS

Metastasis, being a kinetic event in a living organism, must involve interplay between the tumour cells and the anatomical and physiological constitution of the host. The pathological sequence of events involves local invasion and destruction of intercellular matrix including collagen, intravasation into blood vessels, lymphatics, or other channels of transport (for example, the subarachnoid space), survival in the jetstream of the blood and of impaction in the next capillary network, extravasation out of the vessel, growth in the new location, and destruction of indigenous cells, as well as coercion of the local tissues to provide a fibro-vascular stroma. Ability to survive in the alien metabolic environment of a different organ is also an essential requirement. Success in the metastatic process requires tumour cells to be able to accomplish all these steps in the right sequence and, as cellular behaviour is governed by the prevailing pattern of gene expression, the coordinate or at least the concomitant malfunction of genes giving a selective advantage in each step of the metastatic process is required. Failure to achieve any of these steps renders the cells generally unfit to metastasise and aborts the whole sequence.

ORGAN MICROENVIRONMENT AND METASTASIS DISTRIBUTION

The process of metastasis is not random because even when ubiquitous vascular dissemination of tumour cells can be demonstrated, metastases only grow in certain sites, and the preferential patterns of organ colonisation bear a relationship to the sites and types of the primary tumours. Therefore, even cells known to be capable of forming metastatic colonies in some sites cannot do so in others, and it follows that their growth is suppressed or at least not encouraged in the organs where metastases fail to grow. Evidence demonstrating this both in patients treated with peritoneovenous shunts for malignant ascites and in animals bearing mammary tumours is also available.

By labelling disaggregated murine mammary tumour cells with fluorescein isothiocyanate before injecting them intravascularly and subsequently examining frozen sections of several organs of the recipients with an ultraviolet microscope, it was demonstrated that viable tumour cells arrive in all organs examined within 15 min of inoculation either intravenously or arterially (Potter et al., 1983) and are still detectable in various organs 30 days later. Although the method is not quantitatively accurate, its advantages are that the cells can be directly visualised, and it can be confirmed that the label is attached to whole viable cells and not to cellular fragments. The findings effectively disposed of the possibility that the consistent absence of deposits in certain sites in animals inoculated with cells from spontaneous murine mammary tumours is due to failure of the cells to reach them. It was also confirmed that FITC-labelled cells were still capable of forming deposits, and occasional fluorescent cells were detected in these secondary neoplasms.

As mentioned above, we had demonstrated earlier that cells from some spontaneous murine mammary tumours heavily colonised the lungs of every inoculated animal when injected intravenously, whereas those from others did so weakly or not at all. Extrapulmonary deposits were rare when cells are inoculated by this route. In further experiments (Juacaba et al., 1983), we found that if the cells were inoculated retrograde along the subclavian artery into the arch of the aorta, or directly into the abdominal aorta, they were capable of colonising organs other than the lungs and that individual tumours had reproducible preferences for establishing colonies in certain sites. The combinations of organs favoured varied from tumour to tumour, but most still showed a predilection for forming pulmonary deposits. Several organs were not colonised by any tumour in any recipient. It was concluded that the distribution of metastatic colonies formed by these spontaneous mammary tumours was influenced by interplay between intrinsic properties of tumour cells and microenvironmental influences in the organs in which the cells arrest as well as rheological considerations.

In patients with malignant ascites treated by P-V shunting, who subsequently had evidence of haematogenous metastasis, it was found that metastases were forming in some organs but not in others. Indeed, in some the lungs were not colonised, even though they are the first site where sieving effects due to capillary beds are encountered by tumour cells released intravascularly, and it can there-fore be concluded that tumours cannot colonise all sites in which substantial numbers of viable tumour cells lodge. This experimentally confirms, in living human subjects, Paget's deduction, based on autopsy data, and the findings demolish the contention of Ewing (Ewing, 1928) and others, that the distribution of metastases is solely determined by the anatomy of vascular and lymphatic drainage from the site of the primary tumour. Even so, it remains necessary to realise that the sieving effects of capillary beds can reduce the tumour cell burden entering the arterial circula-tion and thus have some influence on whether metastases form downstream. Among patients with shunts, some had no pulmo-nary deposits (Tarin et al., 1984a,b, 1986) yet still demonstrated preferential colonisation of other (downstream) organs via the systemic arterial pathway and hence failure to colonise others. These patterns of metastasis were not relatable to blood flow through the organs concerned nor to proportions of tumour cells arriving in various sites (which can be deduced from the proportion of cardiac output distri-bution to each organ). They also varied with different tumour types and between different individuals with the same types of tumours.

The collective evidence from these patients, therefore, provides direct experimental support for Paget's (Paget, 1889) "seed and soil" hypothesis, which was based on a study of over 700 autopsies on patients dying with mammary cancer. In this study, he observed that metastatic breast tumour deposits were found much more frequently in the bones than in any other organ and then most often in the lungs and liver. The presence of tumour deposits in these organs was clearly due to haematogenous spread via the systemic circulation, and yet tumour deposits clearly did not form equally readily in all organs. Paget therefore proposed that tumour cells ("seeds") randomly scattered by vascular routes could only form metastatic deposits if they had appropriate intrinsic properties and also landed in congenial territory ("soil"). The molecular mechanisms by which the microenvironment affects the growth rate of tumour cells are presently unknown but, clearly, such evidence suggesting epigenetic suppression of the metastatic phenotype by normal tissues has profound implications reaching beyond explanation of patterns of metastatic dissemination. Once it is accepted that populations of heterogenous tumour cells are scattered more or less representatively throughout the body after mixing in the vortex of the blood, and that they reproducibly grow in some sites and not others, it follows that individual organs can permit or inhibit secondary tumour formation by metastasis-competent cells, and hence that cells of normal organs can, on occasion, suppress or at least fail to support, malignant growth. Verification of this interpretation requires demonstration of the mechanisms of the microenvironmental effects deduced to be operative in vivo, and recent work in this laboratory has been directed towards analysis of how the microenvironment in individual organs may affect full expression of metastatic tumour growth. Using naturally-occurring murine mammary tumours, which preferentially metastasise to the lungs, it was found (Horak et al., 1985a,b; Horak et al., 1986) that the tissues of many organs produce soluble components which can affect the survival of the tumour cells in vitro. Culture medium conditioned by fragments of normal lung was either neutral or actually facilitatory to tumour cell survival but that from most other organs was inhibitory or lethal. Of further interest was the observation that survival of non-neoplastic proliferating mammary epithelium from pregnant animals was diminished by conditioned medium from all organs tested. As normal cells are known not to flourish in alien organs even after deliberate vascular inoculation (Price et al., 1982), the findings would be compatible with the hypothesis that homeostasis of cellular composition in various organs, which presumably is essential in complex multicellular animals, is achieved by killing or inhibiting intruding cells accidentally released from other sites (Horak et al., 1986, for further discussion). In this scheme, successfully metastatic cells would be the ones which had evolved ways of circumventing these regulatory controls.

INSTABILITY OF THE PROCESS

By transplantation of pulmonary metastases back into the mammary fatpads of fresh recipients, it has been found that the constituent cells were nearly always tumourigenic (95%) but not necessarily able to recapitulate the metastatic process (35%) (Price et al., 1984). This suggests that the progeny of cells which have already shown their fitness for the metastatic process do not necessarily all inherit or retain this capability, although repeated selection of metastases and reinoculation of their cells (Fidler, 1973) can eventually lead to the development of cell lines which have high metastatic potency.

Recent observations on serially passaged cloned cell lines from transplantable tumours also indicate that metastatic capability is inherently unstable and that the instability is greater in populations of high metastatic capability than in those with low metastatic performance (Cifone and Fidler, 1981). Currently available evidence therefore suggests that the pathway to metastatic behaviour is a "two-way street," some cells becoming more potent and others less so.

Evidence obtained by Poste and colleagues (Poste et al., 1981; Poste et al., 1982) working with the B16 melanoma indicates that this instability in metastatic potency increases if individual cells are cloned and isolated from others within the same tumour and is stabilised by recombination of isolated clones. This suggests that short-range cell interactions in the original tumour limit the generation of new phenotypes.

SUMMARY

The findings collectively indicate that metastasis is a phenomenon in which select populations of tumour cells with inherent capability for dissemination shower out of the primary tumour to lodge in innumerable inappropriate sites where the microenvironment supports or curtails their proliferative capability. Superimposed on this interaction are systemic effects exerted by the host immune and endocrine systems, the magnitude of which depend on the nature and quantity of exposed receptors and antigens.

Therapeutic attack on the problems of metastasis therefore needs to be focussed on three main areas:

1.   analysis of the intrinsic properties of the
      spreading tumour cells;

2.   understanding why some microenvironments are
      inhospitable to metastatic cells and mobilising
      such inhibitory effects in as many organs as
      possible; and

3.   stimulating systemic factors which handicap the
      growth of tumour cells.

Tumours of the breast, because of their clinical importance and ready availability, are particularly appropriate for investigation of these issues.

ACKNOWLEDGEMENTS

The financial support of the Cancer Research Campaign of Great Britain is gratefully acknowledged. I wish to thank Mrs. P. Messer for typing the manuscript and for help in coordinating the work.

REFERENCES

Blaustein, A. Pathology of the Female Genital Tract, Springer Verlag, New York, 1982, pp. 464-479.

Cifone, M.A., and Fidler, I.J. Increasing metastatic potential is associated with increasing genetic instability of clones isolated from murine neoplasms. Proc. Natl. Acad. Sci. USA 78, 6949-6952, 1981.

Covone, A.E., Johnson, P.M., Mutton, D., and Adinolfi, M. Trophoblast cells in peripheral blood from pregnant women. Lancet ii, 841-843, 1984.

Ewing, J. Neoplastic Diseases, 3rd Edn., W.B. Saunders Co., Philadelphia, 1928.

Fidler, I.J. Selection of successive tumour lines for metastasis. Nature New Biol. 242, 148-149, 1973.

Fidler, I.J. Tumour heterogeneity and the biology of cancer invasion and metastasis. Cancer Res. 38, 2651-2660, 1978.

Fidler, I.J., Gruys, E., Cifone, M.A., Barnes, Z., and Bucana, C. Demonstration of multiple phenotypic diversity in murine melanoma of recent origin. J. Natl. Cancer Inst. 67, 947-956, 1981.

Horak, E., Darling, D.L., and Tarin, D. Organ-specific effects on metastatic tumour growth: studies involving

transplantation techniques. In: Treatment of
Metastasis: Problems and Prospects, K. Hellmann and
S.A. Eccles, eds., Taylor and Francis, London, 1985a,
pp. 307-310.

Horak, E., Darling, D.L., and Tarin, D. Organ-specific
effects on metastatic tumour growth studied in vitro.
In: Treatment of Metastasis: Problems and Prospects,
K. Hellmann and S.A. Eccles, eds., Taylor and Francis,
London, 1985b, pp. 369-372.

Horak, E., Darling, D.L., and Tarin D. Analysis of
organ-specific effects on metastatic tumour formation
by studies in vitro. J. Natl. Cancer Inst. 1986 (in
press).

Juacaba, S.F., Jones, L.D., and Tarin D. Organ preferences
in metastatic colony formation by spontaneous mammary
carcinomas after intra-arterial inoculation. Invasion
Metastasis 3, 208-220, 1983.

Kripke, M.L., Gruys, E., and Fidler, I.J. Metastatic
heterogeneity of cells from an ultraviolet
light-induced murine fibrosarcoma of recent origin.
Cancer Res. 38, 2962-2967, 1978.

Paget, S. The distribution of secondary growths in cancer
of the breast. Lancet 1, 571-573, 1889.

Poste, G., Doll, J., and Fidler, I.J. Interactions among
clonal subpopulations affect stability of the
metastatic phenotype in polyclonal populations of B16
melanoma cells. Proc. Natl. Acad. Sci. USA 78,
6226-6230, 1981.

Poste, G., Doll, J., Brown, A.E., Tzeng, J., and Zeidman, I.
Comparison of the metastatic properties of B16 melanoma
clones isolated from cultured cell lines, subcutaneous
tumours, and individual lung metastases. Cancer Res.
42, 2770-2778, 1982.

Potter, K.M., Juacaba, S.F., Price, J.E., and Tarin, D.
Observations on organ distribution of fluorescein
labelled tumour cells released intravascularly.
Invasion Metastasis 3, 221-233, 1983.

Price, J.E., Carr, D., Jones, L.D., Messer, P., and Tarin,
D. Experimental analysis of factors affecting
metastatic spread using naturally occurring tumours.
Invasion Metastasis 2, 77-112, 1982.

Price, J.E., Carr, D., and Tarin, D. Spontaneous and
induced metastasis of naturally-occurring tumours in
mice: Analysis of cell shedding into the blood. J.
Natl. Cancer Inst. 73, 1319-1326, 1984.

Tarin, D. Cellular interactions in neoplasia. In:
Fundamental Aspects of Metastasis, L. Weiss, ed.
North-Holland Publishing Co., Amsterdam, 1976, pp.
151-187.

Tarin, D. Clinicopathologic studies on mechanisms of
     metastasis in man and other vertebrates. In: Biology
     and Treatment of Colorectal Cancer Metastasis, A.J.
     Mastromarino, ed. Martinus Nijhoff Publishing, Boston,
     1986, pp. 41-52.
Tarin, D. and Price, J.E. Metastatic colonization potential
     of primary tumour cells in mice. Br. J. Cancer 39,
     740-754, 1979.
Tarin, D. and Price, J.E. Studies on the metastatic
     colonisation potential of cells from primary tumours.
     In: Metastatic Tumor Growth, Cancer Campaign Series,
     Vol. 4, E. Grundmann, ed. G. Fischer Press, Stuttgart,
     1980, pp. 65-70.
Tarin, D., Price, J.E., Kettlewell, M.G.W., Souter, R.G.,
     Vass, A.C.R., and Crossley, B. Clinicopathological
     observations on metastasis in man studied in patients
     treated with peritoneovenous shunts. Br. Med. J. 288,
     749-751, 1984a.
Tarin, D., Price, J.E., Kettlewell, M.G.W., Souter, R.G.,
     Vass, A.C.R., and Crossley, B., Mechanisms of human
     tumor metastasis studied in patients with
     peritoneovenous shunts. Cancer Res. 44, 3584-3592,
     1984b.

MALIGNANCY- AND METASTASIS-RELATED CELL PROPERTIES

B. HAGMAR, L.-J. ERKELL, and W. RYD

1. Department of Pathology, Faculty of Medicine, Kuwait University,
2. Deutsches Krebsforschungszentrum, Heidelberg, FRG.
3. Sahlgrenska Hospital, Göteborg, Sweden.

In the 1960ies Sumner Wood became famous when he made microcinemato-graphic recordings from rabbit ear chambers and decided that thrombus formation was very important, if not necessary, for the entrapment of tumor cells in capillaries and for the establishment of metastases (Wood 1964). The theory was well presented and to this day it is sort of a dogma in certain quarters that thrombi promote metastasis. The experimental support for this theory is very weak, however, except under rare experimental conditions.

We do not want to minimize the importance of serious studies of blood coagulation and cancer. Certainly, the platelets may have an important function in the retention and growth control of disseminated cancer cells. But the theory that thrombus formation is necessary for metastasis establ-ishement is unfounded. Yet, it was so simple and attractive, that many workers were carried away and did not evaluate their data critically any longer. One of us (BH) reviewed the subject 15 years ago (Hagmar 1970) and Peter Hilgard has since presented several balanced overviews, which show the complexity of the topic (Hilgard and Thornes 1976, Hilgard and Maat 1979). In such studies, it is necessary to use an appropriate system; in this case one where extra-pulmonary tumors develop, as well as pulmonary ones. Otherwise, the shunting of metastases past the lung will falsely be interpreted as a metastasis reduction (Hagmar and Boeryd, 1969).

The next major vogue in metastasis research, as for cancer as whole, was related to the Tumor Specific Transplantation Antigens (TSTAs). McFarlane Burnet´s theory on immunesurveillance was related to cancerogenesis, but it could also be applied to other aspects of malignancies, such as their spread. Briefly, the appearance of a cancer, or a metastasis, was regarded as a deficiency in the body´s surveillance of aberrant, neoplastic cells. Innumerable articles described the impact of immune-modulation on tumor growth and dissemination.

It was not until the end of 1970ies that the weakness of the theory was clearly pointed out by Hewitt (1979), among others: the antigenicity of cancers is to a large extent a laboratory artefact. Naturally occurring, spontaneous tumors have a negligible antigenicity. Except for the rare cases of choriocarcinoma and other strongly antigenic tumours, the concept of immunesurveillance does not seem valid.

We must recall here that already in 1970, Dr. Richmond Prehn, one of the pioneers in detecting TSTAs, warned at the Cancer Congress in Houston that immune reactions towards tumours may equally well favour their growth as prevent it. Prehn has since (1977) given many examples of the trophic effect of a weak immune reaction on cancers. He has compared the situation with the growth of the placenta, for which immune-stimulation is a prerequisite.

We must also stress the point that, of course, host factors may modify tumor growth and spread. Lately, natural killer (NK) cells (Hanna 1985) and macrophages (Fidler and Poste 1982) have been particularly studied in this respect. Unfortunately, the purpose seems very often to be the search for one single cause of cancer dissemination. Such a simple state of affairs would permit one single modality for prevention or cure, like for instance the injection of interferon or "armed macrophages". The design of the experiment is less often to prove that this or that studied parameter is part of a complex chain of events, where is addition, the relative importance of each factor may vary considerably, depending on the circumstances.

Parallels can again be drawn to hopeful thinking about coagulation factors, fibrinolysis and other enzyme activities of tumor cells. If someone is interested in, say fibrinolysis, it is not appropriate to interprete all data in terms of this one, selected parameter. As one example, we could show that the action of fibrinolytic inhibitors could be mimicked by antihypertensive treatment of mice (Boeryd et al. 1974). The reason was, aparently, that the anti-fibrinolytic drug we used, EACA, also has a antihypertensive action. The effect of EACA on experimental metastases could, at least in part, be imitated by another anti-hypertensive drug, guanethidine, which has no antifibrinolytic action.

The next major issue, related to metastasis, was Fidler´s Clonal Selection Theory. It is also a simple and attractive hypothesis: the survival of only the fittest cancer cell in a hostile environment. By mutation there would be stable sublines in tumors with a particular potential for metastasis. The theory offers a comparable situation to that of bacteria, which mutate for virulence and chemoresistance.

Fidler has rightly been honoured for this theory, where the initial experiments were based on a Luria-Delbruck´s fluctuation analysis of Melanoma B16´s i.v. transplantation potential (Fidler and Kripke 1977). But this theory predicted that cells from metastases would metastasize more than unselected cells. We and others could show, however, that selection of metastatic cells by in vivo procedures failed to give rise to a more metastatic tumour (Ryd et al. 1986). Poste and co-workers (1981) subsequently could show that isolated tumour cell clones were unstable. Genetic stability was achieved only in heterogenous tumours. Examples of this will be given later : we have developed ascites tumors which are stable in terms of transplantability. Then the matter started to become really complicated, for the changes seen in metastasizibility by in vitro selection procedures were too quick to occur by a mutation-selection process (Ling et al. 1984). Various genetic and epigenetic mechanisms have henceforth been discussed in this context (Schirrmacher 1980, Kerbel et al. 1983, Chambers et al. 1984). We will return to this subject of clonal stability later. But our main conclusion now, from all the various experiments performed, is that metastasis is not a clonal selection phenomenon. It is reflecting the heterogeneity of the primary tumour, however, where some cells may be permanently or transiently able to metastasize, others are not. And this heterogeneity is a very important fact to keep in mind when one tries to kill all the cancer cells in a patient with immuno- or chemo-therapy for instance.

A parenthetic comment on genetic stability - instability may be warranted: maybe the genetic instability of a cancer is the clue to both its heterogeneity and adaptability ? Cifone and Fidler (1981) even suggested it is the basis of metastasis. Auer and co-workers (1980) have made cytophotometric DNA measurements on breast carcinomas and their results seem to contradict such a conclusion. They found that aneuploid tumours were significantly more frequent among patients dying from their tumour, than among survivors. The survivors had largely euploid tumours. But interestingly, the metastases showed the same DNA distribution pattern as the primary tumor (Auer et al. 1979). This would not indicate a genetic instability, rather the opposite, in the metastatic cell. The authors conclude "progression in breast cancer is more likely to be due to a net increase and/or dissemination of tumour cells exhibiting similar genetic properties, than to a progressive dedifferentiation and increase of malignancy of tumour cells" (Auer et al. 1984).

This rather lengthy introduction will serve as a background for the main topic of our presentation: the importance of tumour cell properties for metastasis. The purpose of our introduction was mainly to show that there is not likely to be one single cell characteristic of overriding importance, but several factors acting together.

In Göteborg, in the 1960ies, we studied the effect of anticoagulation on experimental metastases in mice. Heparin had a different action on metastases that other anticoagulants, and we could ascribe this to absorption onto the tumor cell surfaces (Hagmar, 1970). From this observation originated the hypothesis that the pattern of spread of a cancer is in part governed by surface properties of the tumour cells. This theory would serve as a complement, rather than an alternative to pre-existing theories on the location of metastases, i.e., the mechanical theory (Ewing 1928) or the seed-soil theory (Paget 1889). The means we had to investigate this matter was by modifying tumor cells in a reproducible manner and monitor changes in their spontaneous or experimental dissemination patterns (Hagmar and Ryd 1981).

The cells were modified

i. by coating with polar substances, polyanions and polycations and also with neutrally charged molecules such as dextran;

ii. by treating the cells with enzymes prior to injection;

iii. by paralysing the cells (Hagmar and Ryd 1977, Ryd and Hagmar 1977);

iv. by cloning ascites tumors from solid tumors. The cloning achieves, by mutation-selection, different subpopulations of cells with new surface properties. The tumors remain equally malignant, but change their dissemination pattern.

Nicholson (1984) has extended such studies greatly, and added another method of cell surface modification: v/the fusion of surface vesicles from more metastasiogenic cells onto less metastatic ones and thereby increasing their metastatic potential.

All these procedures have demonstrated that chemical changes in the surface coat of tumor cells affect the distribution of experimental metastases. The distribution of radiolabelled cells have not been significantly changed on such experimental occasions, however (Ryd and Hagmar 1984). This either depends on:

i. the fact that our methods monitoring the radio-distribution of tumor cells are too insensitive to detect small but functionally important shifts of tumor cells from one organ to another; or,

ii. the changed distribution of metastses is in greater part due to changes in growth conditions than to a changed initial distribution of tumor cells.

The first alternative would add increased weight to the cell surface governed spread hypothesis. The latter alternative would further the seed-soil hypothesis, i.e., that certain organs offer a better soil than others for growth of disseminated cells.

Our more recent approach to these questions is to use a panel of 12 ascites-transformed tumors, epithelial as well as mesenchymal. The tumors represent various combinations of malignancy - and metastasis-related behaviours (Hagmar et al. 1985). There are quickly growing tumors, which metastasize or do not metastasize, and slowly growing tumours with or without the potential for spread. First we assess the malignancy and the metastasis-forming capacity as 2 independent properties. Then we determine a number of cell factors, which we think are related to either malignancy and/or metastasis:

endothelial adhesivity
tumor cell deformability
growth factor dependency and production
enzyme production
cell surface carbohydrate groups with quantitative lectin
    determination.

I shall first present the tumors and then disclose some of the experimental data. It must be pointed out that the results are still preliminary.

The tumours are, with 2 exceptions, methylcholanthrene-induced. This procedure of induction includes the artifact that the tumours may be antigenic. This has not proved to be the case, however, when we have tested it, probably because the tumors were arising late after MC-treatment. The first arising tumours generally are the more antigenic ones (Old et al.1962).

<u>TABLE 1</u>

Tumor-host systems used for
malignancy and metastasis grading.

MCG 1   MC-induced rhabdomyosarcoma (CBA mice)
Mellgren, J. et. al: Acta Path Microbiol Scand 68 (1966) 535
Hagmar, B.: Acta Path Microbiol Scand Sect A, Suppl. 211 (1970)

MCG 101 MC-induced fibrosarcoma (C57Bl/6J mice)
Hagmar, B.: Acta Path Microbiol Scand Sect A 82 (1974) 358; 369; 379
Hagmar, B., Ryd, W.: Acta Path Microbiol Scand Sect A 83 (1975) 328

MCB 21   MC-induced fibrosarcoma (CBA mice)
Hagmar, B., Ryd, W.: Acta Path Microbiol Scand Sect A 86 (1978) 231
Ryd, W., Hagmar, B.: Acta Path Microbiol Scand Sect A 87 (1979) 97
Ryd, W., Hagmar, B.: J Cancer Res Clin Oncol 94 (1979) 185

MCB 31   MC-induced squamous cell carcinoma (CBA mice)
For references, see MCB 21

Sq 1   MC-induced squamous cell carcinoma (CBA mice)
Hagmar, B., Ryd, W.: Invasion and Metastasis 5 (1985) 31

MCB 28   MC-induced squamous cell carcinoma (CBA mice)
Hagmar, B., Ryd, W.: "MCB 28, an ascites converted carcinoma in inbred CBA mice" (manuscript)

B 16   Melanoma (C57Bl/6J mice)

TA3Ha   Ascites-transformed mammary carcinoma (A/SN mice)
Hauschka, T.S. et. al: J.Natl. Cancer Inst. 47 (1971) 343

The criterion of selection for these tumours, among hundreds induced, is that they metastasize spontaneously and they let themselves be transformed into ascites form. The ascites transformation is important, from at least 2 points of view:

i.   The transformation is a true mutation-selection phenomenon, which in our hands has changed the metastasis pattern of the respective tumour each time it has succeeded. There is sometimes, but not always, a change for greater metastasizibility. More often there is a change in metastasis pattern, i.e. the organs where the resulting spontaneous metastases are located. So it is not a finding which supports the Mutation Selection Theory of Metastasis. But it shows that stable mutational changes can affect not only the primary growth of a tumour, but also the metastasis pattern.

ii.   Ascites tumours give us the advantage of a practically unlimited supply of native tumour cells for characterization. They need not be treated by any of the mechanical or enzymatical procedures, which are required to bring solid tumours into suspension. The fact that the tumours are stable means that we have been able to establish how they differ in malignancy, i.e. in growth rate and transplantability, and also in terms of spontaneous and i.v. induced so-called experimental metastasis formation.

We consider this a satisfactory, but not ideal, model. Autochtonous tumours would be preferable, but unfortunately it is not experimentally possible. In particular, we have been keen not to use in vitro cultivated cell lines. We know from the work of others (Stackpole 1983, Weiss et al. 1983) that such lines offer experimental artifacts due to selection and adaptation to in vitro conditions.

The Melanoma B16 is included in our panel of tumours as an international "standard", and in some respects the different B16 sublines may be used for comparison. For instance, it has been found that Melanoma B16 produces an insulin-like growth factor (Bajzer et al. 1984). We have found that B16 also produces PDGF-like activity in higher amounts than any of our other tumours (Nistér et al., unpublished data).

The ascites-transformed mammary carcinoma TA3Ha is included as a non-MC-induced, spontaneous epithelial tumour. It is interesting from many points of view, not least because it has a strong colony growth promoting effect on haematopoetic cells. But it is too old to offer a good model of breast cancer. Dr. Tarin´s breast cancers (Tarin and Price 1979), always used in early generations, certainly are preferable.

Our characterization program, apart from the malignancy and metastasis assessment, is just started and we have made no break-through disclosures yet.

The endothelial adhesivity is reflecting a necessary step in metastasis: the contact between a circulating cancer cell and the endothelium in a distant part of the body. A perfect model of this is difficult to achieve in vitro, because it requires the confluent growth in monolayer of endothelial cells. In addition, the cells should grow on an intact basement membrane, to simulate the in vivo situation.

We have data from a more primitive model in vitro, where we coated microwells with collagen IV, with and without fibronectin or laminin. They show that the highly metastatic tumor MCG1-SS adheres significanlty better to laminin than to either fibronectin or collagen IV. For other tumours the data are still incomplete.

TABLE 2

Adhesion tests performed in microwells coated with
different proteins. The results are given as an index
with the actual no. of adherent cells as numerator and cells
adherent to plastic (controls) as denominator.

Tumor (Temp., No. of Exper.)	Collagen	Fibronectin	Laminin
MCG1-SS			
37 (6)	0.79	0.87	1.04
0 (5)	0.90	1.02	1.05
MCG1-AA			
37 (4)	0.62	0.85	(0.76)*
0 (5)	0.98	1.25	(1.14)*
Sq1-AA			
37 (2)	0.89	0.94	–
0 (2)	1.0	0.91	–
TA3Ha			
37 (1)	0.87	1.16	
0 (1)	0.45	0.49	

*Figures in brackets based on 2 experiments only

The flexibility (deformability) as opposed to rigidity of the cell
wall is potentially a decisive factor for metastasis.   The same is true
for mechanical strength of the cell membrane. Weiss and Dimitrov (1984)
have   calculated the stress forces encountered by circulating cancer cells
and found them to be in an order of magnitude that they can be a major
cause of "metastatic inefficiency", which Weiss (1982) has called the
phenomenon that most cancer cells succumb in the circulation. Our
deformability data are preliminary, but they do not entirely support a
contention by Sato and Suzuki (1976), that tumours giving rise to
extrapulmonary metastases are made up by more deformable cells than those
giving rise to lung metastases.

TABLE 3

Filtration time and survival of tumor cells in
Nucleopore deformability tests.
The average cell size is also given ($\pm$ SD)

Tumour	Filtration time (sec)	Survival (%)	Diameter (μ)
MCG1-SS	92 (6)	45 (4)	12.9 (0.3)
1-AA	365 (68)	35 (3)	13.4 (0.1)
MCG101-SS	977 (16)	45 (7)	11.4 (0.3)
101-AA	758 (11)	51 (5)	11.4 (0.3)
MCB21-SS	90	44 (8)	-
21-AA	298 (43)	13 (3)	11.4 (0.3)
MCB31-SC	-	-	-
31-AA	190	20 (3)	14.0 (0.3)
Sq1-SC	-	-	-
1-AA	326	45 (7)	13.7 (0.7)
MCB28-SS	-	-	-
28-AA	273 (57)	-	-
Mel.B16	27 (4.2)	15 (2)	12.9 (0.3)
TA3Ha	141 (27)	27 (4)	11.4 (0.2)

The growth factor production and dependency studies are also still in
a preliminary stage.   Such factors have to be studied, not only in terms
of growth stimulation on other cells such as fibroblasts, but also
immunologically for growth factor typing.   In addition, the relationship
to known oncogenes and their products has to be defined.   The theoretical
interest for growth factor determination is related to the question of
independence and autocrine stimulation of cancer cells.   This may be a
major determinant in the survival of dissociated tumor cells, lacking the
protective and presumably stimulatory surrounding of homologous cells.

Lately, a peculiar family of growth factors, TAF (Tumour Angiogenic
Growth Factor) in crude tumour extracts, has regained interest.   Its
discoverer, Judah Folkman, has found out that TAF acts synergistically
with heparin and that it can be counteracted by basic polypeptides like
protamine.   From a theoretical point of view, TAF may be a limiting
factor, not only for the growth of a primary tumour, but also for
metastases, albeit in a later stage when tumour cells have started
multiplying in a new site and established a gross metastatic colony.   The
practical consequences of growth factor inhibition, as in this case with
protamine, may open up new therapeutic avenues. Our tumours do show TAF
activity in a chorio-allantois-membrane assay.   There are quantitative

differences, but as yet there is no clear-cut relationship to metastasis formation. Yet it can be noted that the highest percentual activity is shown by the most actively metastasizing tumour, MCG1-SS. The ascites transformed counterpart, MCG1-AA, shows less than half of MCG1-SS's activity.

TABLE 4

Angiogenic activity of 4 experimental mouse
tumors transplanted into hen chorioallantois membranes

Tumor	No. of Exper.	No. of eggs	Implant loss No.	Angiogenic No.	Activity %
MCG1-SS	5	57	14	29	67
MCG1-AS	4	49	13	10	28
MCG101-AS	4	46	15	18	58
MCG101-AS	5	51	16	14	33

The quantitative determination of cell surface carbohydrates is also a tedious work. It requires radio-labelled lectins and very much standardized conditions to give reproducible results.

We have used 5 lectins, detecting

    galactose (Gal)
    fucose (F)
    N-acetyl-D-galactoseamine (GalNac)
    N-acetyl-D-glucoseamine (GluNac)
    x-methyl-mannoside (Man)

So far, we have not found any significant quantitative difference between our tested tumour lines. We have concentrated our efforts on the pair of tumours MCG-SS - MCG1-AA. The first one, as mentioned, is an early and avid metastasizer. The latter is equally malignant, but does not metastasize. They share, as it turns out, similar amounts of Man and GluNac on their surfaces. What remains to be determined is whether part of their surface sugars are covered with sialic acid, or not (Fogel et al. 1983). In addition, the spatial configuration of surface sugars is being studied with electron microscopy.

We want to characterize the cells not only in terms of the amount of surface sugars, but also in terms of their heterogeneity in this respect. For this purpose we use cell column affinity chromatography with immobilized lectins.

The stated evidence may be sufficient examples of ongoing work. Other groups are attacking the same problems from different angels. What we all have to deal with in metastasis research is the dichotomy between specialization and generalization. By specialization we restrict ourselves to the study of one or a few factors in a very complex multifactorial process. We may very well end up misinterpreting (usually exaggerating) the importance of the factor(s) under study. On the other hand, broad attacks on the metastatic process have the tendency to become superficial. The resources are not sufficient to create in depth studies, except for restricted fields.

The problem is that we attack a complex multi-step process, where practically everything in biology may be involved. There is probably not one solution to the problem of metastasis, but very many important aspects. Let us help in the future to avoid unnecessary generalizations and one-eyedness. Let us also help to develop appropriate experimental models.

In summary, we think

i)   in metastasis, the major cause is to be sought for in the cancer cell, not in any defect in the host defence;

ii) most cancer cells die in the circulation or after being trapped in tissues;

iii) the main problem now is to define the metastatic cancer cell as distinct from the non-metastatic ones. We must define its pheno-type in order to draw conclusions about its genotype.

This is the background, against which our experiments are performed.

ACKNOWLEDGEMENTS

On-going studies in Kuwait are supported by grant No. MG 004, which is gratefully acknowledged.

We thank Mr. James Luke for his skillful secreterial help in preparing the manuscript.

REFERENCES

1. Auer GU, Caspersoon TO, and Wallgren AS: DNA content and survival in mammary carcinoma. Analytical and Quantitative Cytol. J. 2: 161-165, 1980.
2. Auer GU, Arrhenius E, Granberg PO, and Fox C: Comparison of DNA distributions in primary human breast cancers and their metastases. Europ. J. Cancer 16 : 273-278, 1979.
3. Auer GU, Fallenius AG, Erhardt KY and Sundelin SB: Progression of mammary adencarcinomas as reflected by nuclear DNA content. Cytometry 5: 420-425, 1984.
4. Boeryd B, Hagmar B, Johnsson G, and Ryd W: Effects of EACA, AMCHA and guanethidine on metastases induced by intravenously injected tumour cells. Path. Europ.9 : 119-123, 1974.
5. Bajzer Z, Parelic K, and Vuk-Pavlovic, S: Growth self-incitement in murine melanoma B 16 : A phenomenological model. Science 225 : 930-932, 1984.
6. Cifone MA, and Fidler IJ: Increasing metastatic potential is associated with increasing instability of clones isolated from murine neoplasms. Proc. Nat. Acad. Sci. USA.78 : 6949-6952 1981.
7. Chambers AF, Harris JF, Sing V, and Hill RP: Rapid phenotype variation in cells derived from lung metastases of KHT fibrosarcoma. Invasion and Metastasis 4: 225-237, 1984.
8. Ewing J(ed): Neoplastic Diseases, Saunders,Philadelphia, 1928.
9. Fidler IJ, and Kripke ML: Metastasis results from pre-existing variant cells within a malignant tumor. Science 197: 893-895, 1977.
10. Fidler IJ, and Poste G: Macrophage-mediated destruction of malignant tumor cells and new strategies for the therapy of metastatic disease. Springer Semin. Immunopath. 5: 161-174, 1982.
11. Fogel, M., Altevogt, P. and Schirrmacher, V.: Metastatic potential severely altered by changes in tumor cell adhesiveness and cell surface sialylation. J. Exp. Med. 157: 371-376, 1983.
12. Hagmar, B: Experimental tumor metastases and blood coagulability. Acta Path. Microbiol. Scandinav. suppl., No. 211, 1970.
13. Hagmar B, and Boeryd B: Action of heparin and coumarin on the distribution of experimental metastases. Acta Path. Microbiol. Scand. 76: 651-656, 1969.
14. Hagmar B, and Ryd W: Tumor cell locomotion - a factor in metastasis formation. Influence of Cytochalasin B on a tumor dissemination pattern. Int. J. Cancer 19: 576-580, 1977.
15. Hagmar B, and Ryd W: Cancer cell properties in relation to metastases. Proc. of the 6th Meeting of the European Association for Cancer Research. Kugler, Amsterdam, 1981 pp 123-129 .
16. Hagmar B, Erkell LJ, and Ryd W: Malignancy and metastasis grading of experimental tumors. Manuscript 1985.
17. Hanna N: The role of natural killer cells in the control of tumor growth and metastasis. Biochim. Biophys. Acta 780: 213-226, 1985.
18. Hewitt HB: A critical examination of the foundations of immunotherapy for cancer. Clin. Radiol 31: 361-369, 1979.
19. Hilgard P, and Thornes RD: Anticoagulants in the treatment of cancer. Europ. J. Cancer 12: 755-762, 1976.
20. Hilgard P, and Maat B: Mechanism of lung tumour colony reduction caused by coumarin anticoagulation. Europ. J. Cancer 15: 183-187, 1979.

350

21. Kerbel RS, Frost P, and Liteplo RG: Genetic and epigenetic regulations of the metastatic phenotype : a basis for resolving the controversy regarding its selective or random nature and variable phenotypic stability. In "Biochemistry and Molecular Genetics of Metastasis" Liotta et al(ed), Martinus Nijhoff, Amsterdam, 1983.
22. Ling V, Chambers AF, Harris JF, and Hill RP: Dynamic heterogeneity and metastasis. J. Cell Physiol. Suppl. 3: 99-103, 1984.
23. Nicolson GL: Cell surface molecules and tumor metastasis. Regulation of metastatic diversity. Exp. Cell. Res. 150: 3-22, 1984.
24. Old LJ, Boyse EA, Clarke DA, and Carswell EA: Antigenic properties of chemically induced tumors. Ann. N.Y. Acad. Sci. 101: 80-106, 1962.
25. Paget S: The distribution of secondary growths in cancer of the breast. Lancet 1: 571-573, 1889.
26. Poste G, Doll J, and Fidler IJ: Interaction between clonal subpopulations affect the stability of the metastatic phenotype in polyclonal populations of B 16 melanoma cells. Proc. Nat. Acad. Sci. USA 78: 6226-6230, 1981.
27. Prehn R: Immunostimulation of the lymphodependent phase of neoplastic growth. J. Nat. Cancer Inst. 59: 1043-1049, 1977.
28. Ryd W, and Hagmar B: In vitro effects of Cytochalasin B on TA3 tumor cells. Beitr. Pathol. 161: 131-141, 1977.
29. Ryd W, and Hagmar B: The elimination of i.v. injected tumor cells. Studies with IUDR labelled cells in four syngeneic murine tumor systems. Acta path. microbiol. scand. Sect. A. 92: 23-30, 1984.
30. Ryd W, Hagmar B, and Erkell LJ: Characterization of two murine tumor sublines selected strictly in vivo for specific metastasis patterns. Invasion and Metastasis, 6: 21-32, 1986.
31. Sato H, and Suzuki M: Deformability and viability of tumor cells by transcapillary passage with reference to organ affinity of metastasis in cancer. In "Fundamental Aspects of Cancer". Weiss L(ed), North-Holland, Amsterdam, 1976, pp 311-317.
32. Schirrmacher V: Shifts in tumor cell phenotypes induced by signals from the microenvironment. Immunobiol. 157: 89-98, 1980.
33. Stackpole CW: Generation of phenotypic diversity in the B 16 mouse melanoma relative to spontaneous metastasis. Cancer Res. 43: 3057-3065, 1983.
34. Tarin D, and Price JE: Metastatic colonization potential of primary tumor cells in mice. Brit. J. Cancer 39: 740-754, 1979.
35. Weiss L, Holmes JC, and Ward PM: Do metastases arise from pre-existing subpopulations of cancer cells ? Brit. J. Cancer 47: 81-89, 1983.
36. Weiss L, and Dimitrov DS: A fluid mechanical analysis of the velocity, adhesion and destruction of cancer cells in capillaries during metastasis. Cell Biophys. 6: 9-22, 1984.
37. Weiss L: Metastatic inefficiency. In "Liver Metastasis". Weiss and Gilbert (eds), Hall, Boston, 1982, pp. 126-157.
38. Wood S Jr: Experimental studies of the intravascular dissemination of ascitic V2 carcinoma cells in the rabbit, with special reference to fibrinogen and fibrinolytic agents. Bull. Swiss. Acad, Med. Sci. 20: 92-121, 1964.

EXPERIMENTAL RESULTS ON INVASIVENESS OF MOUSE MAMMARY CELLS:

CLINICAL IMPLICATIONS?

MARC M. MAREEL[1], GEORGES K. DE BRUYNE[1], ARNOUD
SONNENBERG[2], AND JO HILGERS[2]

1. Laboratory of Experimental Cancerology,
    Department of Radiotherapy and Nuclear
    Medicine, University Hospital,
    De Pintelaan, 185, 9000 Ghent, Belgium.
2. Division of Tumor Biology, The Netherlands
    Cancer Institute, Antoni van Leeuwenhoekhuis,
    Amsterdam, The Netherlands

INTRODUCTION

Multicellular organisms are characterized by the organization of their cells in domains building tissues and organs. Maintenance of the territorial integrity of these domains is under regulatory control not only during embryogenesis but also in adult life. Invasion can be defined as a loss of this territorial integrity: Invasive cells break through the boundary of their tissue of origin and penetrate into the territory of another tissue within the same or in another organ. Most invasive cells have the capacity to break through vessel walls and penetrate into the vessel lumen (intravasation). After transport by the circulation, invasive cells can leave the vessels (extravasation) and lodge at secondary sites to produce metastases. Since metastases are, like primary tumours, invasive, they put cells into a new (second, third, etc.) metastatic cascade.

Invasiveness is the hallmark of malignancy because invasiveness marks the difference between benign and malignant in surgical pathology, because levels of invasiveness are considered to have prognostic value in a number of tumours, and because invasion is a major obstacle to therapeutic success (Mareel et al., 1986). For recent reviews about tumour invasiveness, the reader is referred to "Tumor Invasion and Metastasis" edited by L.A. Liotta and I.R. Hart, Martinus Nijhoff Publishers, The Hague, Boston,

London, 1982, and to "Invasion. Experimental and Clinical Implications" edited by Marc M. Mareel and Kenneth C. Calman, Oxford University Press, Oxford, New York, Tokyo, 1984.

During the last decade, the attention of experimental oncologists has been drawn to tumour heterogeneity (Fidler and Kripke, 1977). Solid tumours have been shown to be heterogeneous for a number of characteristics: histology, cellular structure; karyotype; biochemistry; differentiation; growth patterns; receptors; hormone dependence; antigen expression; immunogenicity; sensitivity to drugs, radiotherapy, and hyperthermia; invasiveness; and metastatic capability. Cellular heterogeneity of mammary tumours has been recently reviewed (McCormack, 1984). In its most simple presentation, heterogeneity of invasiveness means that a tumour is composed of invasive and non-invasive cells. The invasive subpopulation constitutes the harmful factor for the patient and should be, therefore, the principal target for therapy. However, tumour heterogeneity does not mean that a tumour is just a bag of mixed cells. Heterogeneous tumours probably are sensitive to population equilibrium: deprivation of interactions between distinct subpopulations, e.g. by cloning, makes these subpopulations unstable so that they become polyclonal again (Poste, 1983). Further, the generation of tumour heterogeneity is constantly influenced by genetic and epigenetic factors (Kim, 1986). Finally, subpopulations probably do not evolve in a single direction, e.g. towards invasiveness, but may also revert, e.g. towards non-invasiveness (Ling et al., 1985). Including heterogeneity of tumour invasiveness into our therapeutic thinking raises several questions: What is the proportion of invasive cells in a tumour at a given moment? How do relative proportions shift during tumour progression? How is this shift influenced by therapy? Are invasive cells more sensitive to treatment than non-invasive ones or is it the other way around? These and other questions about the therapeutic implications of tumour cell heterogeneity have been discussed recently in Volume XII, No. 3, of "Seminars in Oncology," Grune and Stratton, Inc., 1985.

In human tumours, at present, these questions are hard to investigate. Therefore, experimental systems with animal tumours and with cells from these and from human tumours are utilized. Such experimental systems are more readable than the natural situation. It is, however, important to stress that the price for better readability is the risk of irrelevance. The following description of phenotypic heterogeneity in an RIII-MMTV induced Balb/c mouse mammary tumour is meant to discuss which kind of information can be gained from experimental systems.

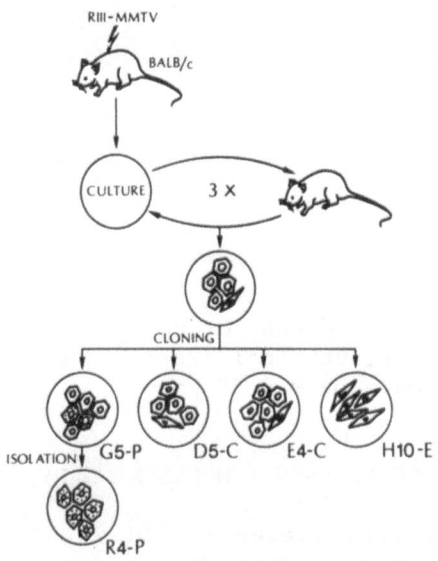

Fig. 1.   Schematic presentation of the origin and isolation of phenotypically diverse clonal cell lines from an RIII-MMTV induced Balb/c mouse mammary tumour. The last character of the code for cell lines indicates phenotypes in culture as follows: P = polygonal; C = cuboidal; E = elongated. (After data from Sonnenberg et al., 1986)

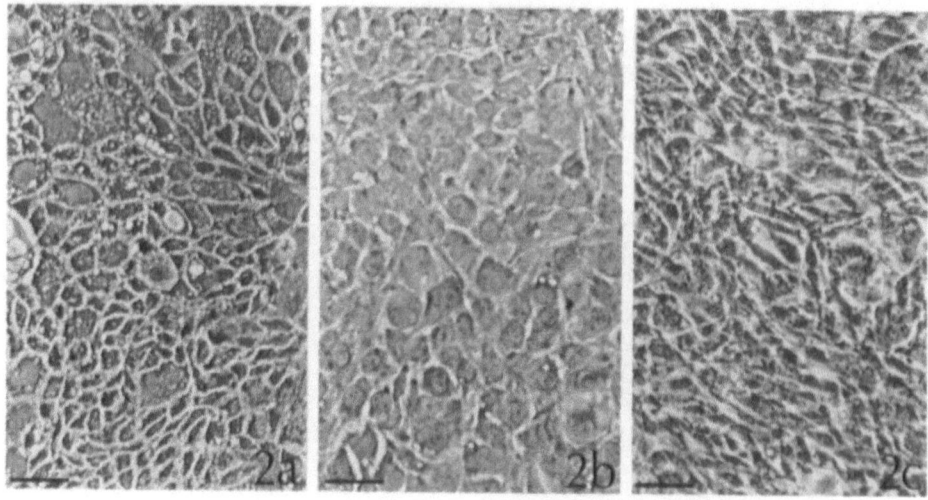

Fig. 2.   Phase contrast micrographs of confluent cultures
           of polygonal (2a), cuboidal (2b), and elongated
           (2c) cells. Scale bars = 50 μm.

PHENOTYPIC DIVERSITY IN CELLS FROM A MOUSE MAMMARY TUMOUR

     Various cell lines were prepared from a Balb/c mouse
mammary tumour induced by RIII-MMTV (mouse mammary tumour
virus). The procedures of isolation and cloning of these
cell lines are presented in Fig. 1. Analysis of the cultures by phase contrast microscopy revealed three phenotypes
designated as polygonal (P) cells, cuboidal (C) cells, and
elongated (E) cells (Fig. 2). The evolution of cloned cell
lines indicated the following sequence of transitions
between these phenotypes: P cells convert to C cells, a
process that is reversible for some time; C cells irrevers-
ibly produce E cells. The arguments in favour of this
sequence are: 1) Cell lines had a clonal origin; they were
prepared by limiting dilution 1x at 5 cells/well and 2x at
0.5 cells/well, and wells were selected for distinct
phenotypes (see Fig. 2). 2) These cell lines were characterized not only phenotypically, but also ultrastructurally,

by their growth patterns in vitro, and by unique insertions of proviruses (Sonnenberg et al., 1986). 3) P cell and C cell cultures were phenotypically unstable; E cell cultures were phenotypically stable. 4) P cell cultures regularly gave rise to C cell cultures; C cell cultures transformed into E cell cultures. 5) P cell cultures could be isolated from low passage C cell cultures.

Growth characteristics of E cell lines, such as high saturation density, and efficient colony formation in soft agar suggested that the transition from C to E cells was critical for the acquisition of malignancy. A similar transition in cell lines from mouse and rat mammary tumours has been described by others (Hager et al., 1981; Dunnington et al., 1983; Barnett and Eccles, 1984). One serious criticism concerning the relevance of all these observations for tumour cell heterogeneity in vivo is that the phenotypic diversity of the cell lines is caused by cloning in vitro (Heppner, 1984). The observation that in vivo transitions from epithelial (P and/or C cell-like) into sarcomatous (E cell-like) tumours do occur (Dunn, 1958) invalidates to some extent this criticism.

Table 1. Behaviour in vivo of cells isolated from an
RIII-MMTV induced Balb/c mouse mammary tumour

Phenotype	Tumori-genicity	Latency period (months)	Histology	Invas.	Phenotype TD-line
P	+	<3	Ca	−	P
C	±(a)	>3	CaSa	+	E
E	+	<2	CaSa	+	N.D.

Invas.: invasiveness
(a) In 20 to 50% of mice.
TD-line: cell line der_ived from a tumour; P: polygonal; C: cuboidal; E: elongated; Ca: carcinoma; CaSa: carcinosarcoma; N.D.: not done.
(Modified after Sonnenberg et al., 1986)

BEHAVIOUR OF MAMMARY CELL LINES IN VIVO

The behaviour of cells from P, C, and E cultures after injection into syngeneic mice is summarized in Table 1.

Cells from P cultures produced tumours with a glandular morphology (adenocarcinoma, type B; variable tumour; papillary cystadenocarcinoma; carcinoma simplex; intratubular carcinoma; see Dunn, 1958) which were not invasive. The latter characteristic makes P cell cultures particularly important since relatively few cell lines are known that produce non-invasive tumours after injection into an appropriate host (Mareel and Van Roy, 1986).

Cells from E cultures produced invasive sarcoma-like tumours (carcinosarcoma; carcinoma with spindle cell formation; anaplastic carcinoma; mixed tumour; see Dunn, 1958). Cells from C cultures produced sarcoma-like tumours, which were invasive. However, tumours appeared after long latency periods, and only a fraction of the injected mice developed a tumour. Theoretically, long latency periods can be interpreted in various ways: The fraction of tumorigenic cells in the inoculum might be low. Or, a subpopulation of the injected cells might acquire the tumorigenic phenotype in vivo. Or, the growth rate of the total tumour cell population might be slow. Our interpretation of the present results is that C cell tumors are, in fact, produced by a minor subpopulation of E cells which evolved during the assay for tumorigenicity or which pre-existed in the inoculum. The arguments are: 1) The histology of C cell tumours closely resembles that of E cell tumours. 2) Cell lines derived from C cell tumours displayed the E phenotype, unlike P tumour-derived cell lines (see Table 1). 3) C cell cultures are known to produce E cells. This interpretation implies that C cells per se are not tumorigenic and, hence, that the conversion from P to C cells is accompanied by a loss of tumorigenicity. The latter features remain to be verified experimentally.

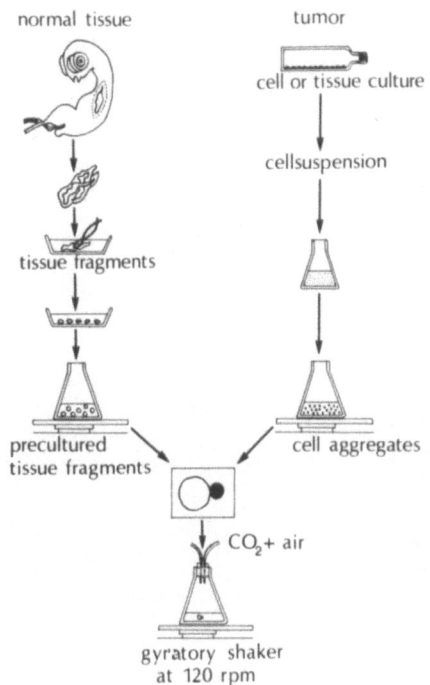

Fig. 3   Schematic presentation of the assay for invasiveness in vitro. (Modified from Mareel et al., 1980.)

Table 2.   Invasion in vitro of cells isolated from a
            RIII-MMTV induced Balb/c mouse mammary tumour

Cell type	Invasion after					
	2 days	4 days	7 days	14 days	21 days	28 days
P	-	-	-	-	-	-
C	-,±	-,±,+	-,±,+	-,±,+	-,±,+	-,±,+
E	+	+	+	+	N.D.	N.D.

-: no invasion; ±: suggestive for two populations;
+: invasive; N.D.: not done.

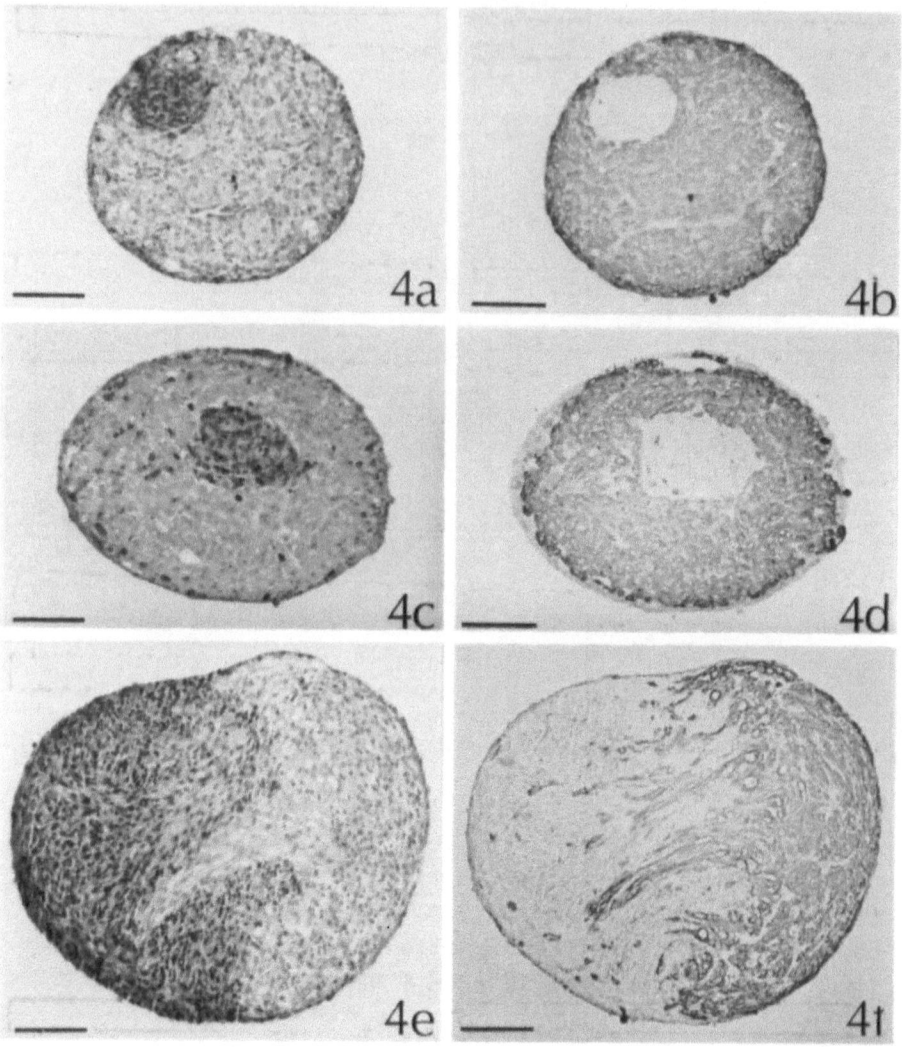

Fig. 4.   Micrographs of paraffin sections from confronting
cultures of chick heart with C2 cells (4a and 4b),
D5-AC cells (4c and 4d), and D5-C cells (4e and
4f); for codes of cell lines see Fig. 1. Cultures
were fixed after 4 days (4a and 4b), and after 7
days (4c to 4f) and stained with hematoxylin-eosin
(4a, 4c, and 4e) and with an antiserum against
chick heart (4b, 4d, 4f). Invasion was scored
(see Table 2) as follows: - (4a and 4b); ± (4c
and 4d); + (4e and 4f). Scale bars = 100 μm.

INVASIVENESS OF MAMMARY CELL LINES IN VITRO

The invasiveness of P, C, and E cells was analyzed in vitro. Cellular aggregates (diameter = 0.2 mm) or fragments of monolayers were confronted with precultured embryonic chick heart fragments (diameter - 0.4 mm) in organ culture following a method described earlier (Mareel et al., 1979). The procedure is shown in Fig. 3. After various periods of incubation, confronting cultures were analyzed histologically after staining of serial sections with hematoxylin-eosin or after immunostaining with either an antiserum against chick heart or an antiserum against mouse cells. The relevance of this method for invasion in vivo has been discussed (Mareel, 1982, 1983). The main argument in favour of this relevance is the good correlation between invasiveness or non-invasiveness of cells in the assay in vitro and invasiveness or non-invasiveness of the same cells in vivo.

Our results with the present mammary cell lines are summarized in Table 2. Clear-cut results were obtained with P cells and with E cells. P cells were not invasive. E cells were readily invasive; they progressively occupied and replaced the heart tissue. With C cells, large culture to culture variations in invasiveness were observed (Fig. 4). Nevertheless, as a rule these cells behaved differently as compared to either P or E cells. In most early cultures (day 2 to day 7) invasion was absent (Fig. 4a), or a minor population of invasive cells was seen next to a nodule of non-invasive cells (Fig. 4b). Later (day 7 to day 28) invasion became obvious in some cultures (Fig. 4c), and these cultures could no longer be distinguished from confronting cultures with E cells. With one cell line, double populations were no longer observed after the fourth day of incubation. Taken together, the results of the assay of invasiveness in vitro resemble the results of the assay for tumorigenicity in vivo. They confirmed the non-invasive and the invasive characters of P cells and E cells respectively. Further, these results suggest that C cells per se are not invasive, but that they contain or generate during the assay a minor subpopulation of invasive (presumably E) cells.

CONCLUSION

The RIII-MMTV Balb/c mouse mammary tumour contained at least three distinct cell populations as evident from isolation and cloning of phenotypically diverse cell lines.

P (polygonal) cells were not invasive in vitro and produced benign tumours in vivo. E (elongated) cells were invasive in vitro and produced invasive tumours in vivo. C (cuboidal) cells per se were not invasive in vitro and not, or poorly, tumorigenic in vivo. However, C cells regularly produced E-like cells. The proposed sequence of conversion between cell populations is:

$$P \rightleftharpoons C \longrightarrow E$$

where P to C is temporarily reversible. These observations confirmed that mouse mammary tumours are heterogeneous. They further indicated a remarkable type of shift: Non-invasive, tumorigenic cell populations (P) gave rise to invasive, tumorigenic cell populations (E), passing through an intermediate state of non-invasiveness and non-tumorigenicity (C cell populations).

There is little evidence to accept or to deny that the invasiveness of human mammary tumours resembles that of the MMTV-induced mouse mammary tumour. Our experiments indicate heterogeneity of invasiveness in mammary tumours. This heterogeneity appears to be dynamic with a tendency towards increased invasiveness. The novel finding is that the malignant (invasive) or benign (non-invasive) course of a tumour may be determined by the evolution of an intermediate subpopulation of cells which per se are neither tumorigenic nor invasive. Then, the question relevant for therapy is: How does incomplete removal, radiotherapy, hyperthermia, or chemotherapy influence the evolution of the intermediate cell population?

ACKNOWLEDGEMENTS

Research in the authors' laboratories is supported by grants from the Kankerfonds van de Algemene Spaar- en Lijfrentekas, the F.G.W.O. (No. 20.093 and 39.000.983), the Sport Vereniging tegen de Kanker and Eli Lilly, Benelux, Belgium, and by grant NKI 79-6 from the Netherlands Cancer Foundation. The authors thank J. Roels van Kerckvoorde for preparing the illustrations and G. Matthys-De Smet for typing the manuscript.

REFERENCES

Barnett, S.C., Eccles, S.A. Studies of mammary carcinoma metastasis in a mouse model system. I. Derivation and characterization of cells with different metastatic properties during tumour progression in vivo. Clin. Exp. Metastasis 2, 15-35, 1984.

Dunn, T.B. Morphology of mammary tumors in mice. In: Homburger, F. (ed) The physiopathology of cancer, 2nd ed. Hoebner Inc., New York, 1958, pp 38-84.

Dunnington, D.J., Hughes, C.M., Monaghan, P., Rudland, P.S. Phenotypic instability of rat mammary tumor epithelial cells. J. Natl. Cancer Inst. 71, 1227-1240, 1983.

Fidler, I.J., Kripke, M.L. Metastasis results from pre-existing variant cells within a malignant tumor. Science 197, 893-895, 1977.

Hager, J.C., Fligiel, S., Stanley, W., Richardson, A.M., Heppner, G.H. Characterization of a variant-producing tumor cell line from a heterogeneous strain BALB/cfC3H mouse mammary tumor. Cancer Res. 41, 1293-1300, 1981.

Heppner, G.H. Tumor heterogeneity. Cancer Res. 44, 2259-2265, 1984.

Kim, U. Factors influencing the generation of phenotypic heterogeneity in mammary tumours. In: Mihich, E. (ed) Biological responses in cancer, Vol. 3. Plenum Press, New York, 1986.

Ling, V., Chambers, A.F., Harris, J.F., Hill, R.P. Quantitative genetic analysis of tumor progression. Cancer Metastasis Rev. 4, 173-194, 1985.

Mareel, M.M.K. The use of embryo organ cultures to study invasion in vitro. In: Liotta, L.A. and Hart, I.R. (eds) Tumor invasion and metastasis. Martinus Nijhoff Publ., The Hague, Boston, London, 1982, pp 207-230.

Mareel, M.M. Invasion in vitro: methods of analysis. Cancer Metastasis Rev. 2, 201-218, 1983.

Mareel, M.M., Van Roy, F.M. Are oncogenes involved in invasion and metastasis? Anticancer Res. 1986.

Mareel, M.M., Bracke, M.E., Boghaert, E.R. Tumour invasion and metastasis: major causes of therapeutic failure. Radiotherapy and Oncology, 1986.

Mareel, M., Kint, J., Meyvisch, C. Methods of study of the invasion of malignant C3H mouse fibroblasts into embryonic chick heart in vitro. Virchows Arch. (Cell Pathol.) 30, 95-111, 1979.

Mareel, M., Bruyneel, E., De Bruyne, G., Dragonetti, C. Methods for morphological and biochemical analysis of invasion in vitro. In: De Brabander, M., Borgers, M., and De Mey, M. (eds) Cell movement and neoplasia. Pergamon Press, Oxford, New York, 1980, pp 87-95.

McCormack, S.A. Mixed cell populations in human mammary cancer. Rev. Endocrine-Related Cancer 17, 17-23, 1984.

Poste, G. Tumor cell heterogeneity and the metastatic process. In: Rich, M.A., Hager, J.C., and Furmanski, P. (eds) Understanding breast cancer. Clinical and laboratory concepts. Marcel Dekker, Inc., New York and Basel, 1983, pp 119-143.

Sonnenberg, A., Daams, J., Calafat, J., Hilgers, J. In vitro differentiation and progression of mouse mammary tumor cells. Cancer Res., 1986.

EXPERIMENTAL MODIFICATION OF METASTATIC PATTERNS

OF MAMMARY CARCINOMA CELLS

L. OZZELLO[1] AND C. LEUCHTENBERGER[2]

[1]Arthur Purdy Stout Laboratory of Surgical
Pathology, Columbia University, College of
Physicians and Surgeons, New York, NY 10032,
U.S.A. [2]Department of Cytochemistry, Swiss
Institute for Experimental Cancer Research,
Lausanne, Switzerland

INTRODUCTION

The patterns of metastatic spread of human tumors are
well known and are fairly characteristic of each tumor type.
Nevertheless, the factors that regulate the frequency and
distribution of metastases are largely unknown. Nor is it
known whether and how the metastatic behavior of malignant
cells can be modified by endogenous or exogenous agents.

The purpose of this report is to illustrate some
observations that we made in the course of experiments on
tobacco and marihuana smoke carcinogenesis, observations
suggesting that, under certain circumstances, it may be
possible to modify the metastatic potential and the way of
spreading of breast cancer cells by means of exogenous
factors. The background of this work was provided by
earlier observations indicating that L-cysteine and ascorbic
acid used to counteract the carcinogenic effects of
SH-reactive groups present in the gas vapor phase of cigarette smoke produced morphological changes in pulmonary
cells cultured in vitro (Leuchtenberger and Leuchtenberger,
1977). When these metabolites were applied to non-smoked
human breast cancer cells from the SK-Br-3 line, similar
morphological and growth alterations were seen
(Leuchtenberger and Ozzello, 1983). In a subsequent study,
we investigated how these modified SK-Br-3 cells behaved in
an in vivo system by transplanting them into nude mice, and
we found that the treated cells, as compared to control
cells, exhibited different tumorigenicity, produced tumors
of different morphology and of different degree of

differentiation, and had a different metastatic potential. Some of these findings have been reported previously (Ozzello and Leuchtenberger, 1980; Ozzello et al., 1983).

MATERIALS AND METHODS

Cell cultures

Cloned SK-Br-3 cells were kindly donated by Dr. S. Carrel of the Ludwig Institute for Cancer Research, Lausanne, Switzerland. The SK-Br-3 cell line was originally established from the pleural effusion of a 41-year-old woman with disseminated breast carcinoma (Fogh and Trempe, 1975).

Experimental cultures used for transplantation consisted of SK-Br-3 cells grown in monolayers and fed with Eagle-Dulbecco medium (ED) supplemented with either L-cysteine (0.3 g/l) for 71-1/2 to 73 weeks or with ascorbic acid (8 mg/l) for 11 to 71-1/2 weeks. SK-Br-3 cells grown in ED alone were used as controls. The media of all cultures were supplemented with 20% calf serum.

The features of these cultures were described in detail elsewhere (Leuchtenberger and Leuchtenberger, 1977). Briefly, control cultures were made up of a mixture of small and large cells growing in epithelial-like monolayers. Some of the large cells were multinucleated. SK-Br-3 cells exposed to L-cysteine exhibited a spindle, fibroblast-like appearance, while the cultures treated with ascorbic acid presented an epithelial type of growth, with cells that were uniformly small and sometimes formed rosette-like structures. No large multinucleated cells were seen in the ascorbic acid-treated cultures.

Heterotransplantation

Homozygous nude mice with BALB/c genetic background were raised and uninterruptedly maintained under pathogen-limited conditions. Virgin females were used throughout these experiments. For the original transplantations, the cells were trypsinized, resuspended in a few drops of ED, and injected subcutaneously (sc) into the lateral thoracic region of the mice. Subsequent passages were carried out by transplanting sc finely minced tissue from surgically excised tumors.

Tumors were allowed to grow until the animals showed signs of wasting and were sacrificed. To check for recurrences, some of the tumors from each passage were excised and the mice followed until death. A complete autopsy was performed on all animals.

Excised tumors and autopsy specimens were fixed in 10% buffered formalin, embedded in paraffin, and stained with hematoxylin and eosin. In addition, selected tumors were stained for epithelial mucins (PAS and Alcian blue) and for reticulin. The presence of milk proteins was checked by the immunoperoxidase technique or immunofluorescence, using antibodies to human α-lactalbumin prepared by Dr. J. Hurlimann of the Institute of Pathology, University of Lausanne (Ozzello et al., 1983).

The volumes of the tumors were calculated using the formula for a prolate ellipsoid:

$$V = \frac{\pi}{6} \ (d_1 \cdot d_2 \cdot d_3)$$

in which $d_{1,2,3}$ represent the three largest diameters. The daily growth rate of the tumors (GI) was estimated with the following formula:

$$GI = \frac{\text{tumor volume}}{\text{age of tumor in days}} \times 10$$

RESULTS AND DISCUSSION

The tumorigenicity of these cells varied greatly from one group to another. While inocula of 3×10^7 control cells were needed to obtain successful takes after latency periods of 3 months or longer, inocula of 1.5×10^6 of L-cysteine or ascorbic acid-treated cells gave rise to tumors after latent periods of 2 weeks. Likewise, in subsequent passages using approximately the same amount of transplanted tissue, the tumors of L-cysteine or ascorbic acid-treated cells grew after shorter latency periods (3-10 days) than the control tumors (14-30 days).

Morphological features

Control tumors were moderately differentiated carcinomas whose cells grew in masses and broad sheets with no particular orientation (Fig. 1). The epithelial pattern was further supported by the reticulin stain showing reticulin fibers delimiting large islands of cells.

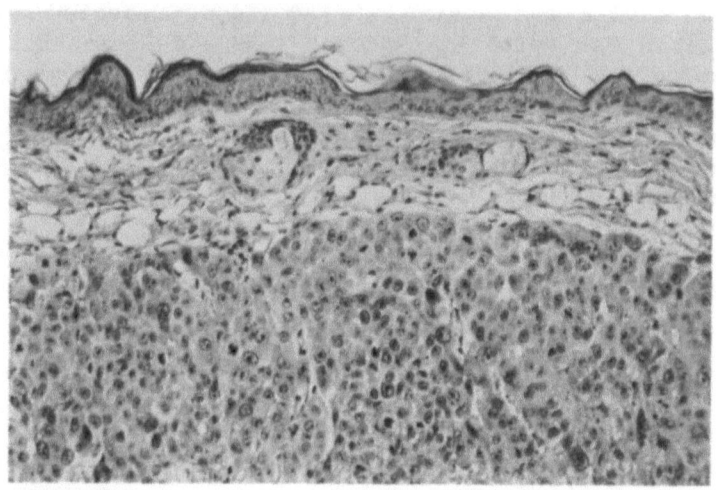

Fig. 1.   Tumor of untreated SK-Br-3 cells (42 days after the 5th passage). It is well delimited from the overlying skin and is composed of broad sheets of haphazardly oriented cells. H&E, X120.

The tumors produced by L-cysteine-treated cells (Fig. 2) were composed of poorly differentiated spindle cells arranged haphazardly or in interlacing bundles. These tumors had a tight reticulin network with fibers surrounding single cells or small groups of cells. The human mammary nature of these cells, however, could be confirmed by their karyotype and by the presence of positive immunostaining with antibodies to human α-lactalbumin in some of the tumor cells. Therefore, these tumors were human mammary carcinomas with some features reminiscent of the spindle cell carcinomas occasionally seen in the human breast.

The tumors of ascorbic acid-treated cells had an adenocarcinomatous appearance with many gland-like lumens (Fig. 3). Copious amounts of mucin and of α-lactalbumin could be demonstrated in many cells and in the intercellular lumens. In one of the experiments with ascorbic acid-treated cells, after approximately 2 months of growth

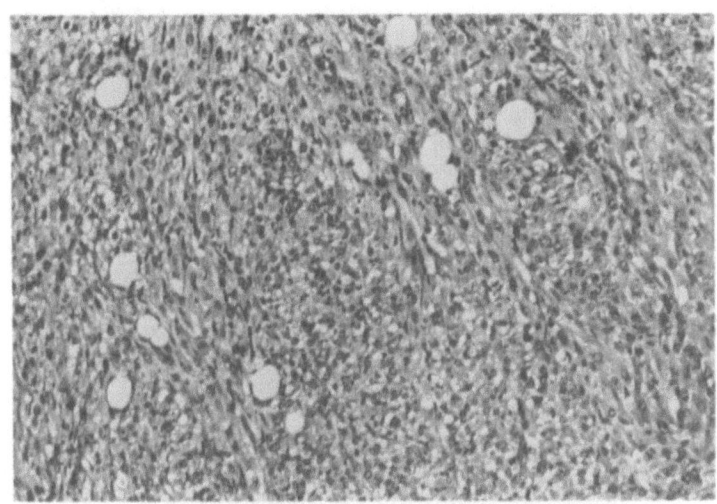

Fig. 2.   Tumor of L-cysteine-treated SK-Br-3 cells (113
           days after the 1st passage, 152 days after the
           original transplantation) invading fat. The
           malignant cells are spindle shaped and are
           arranged in interlacing bundles. H&E, X120.

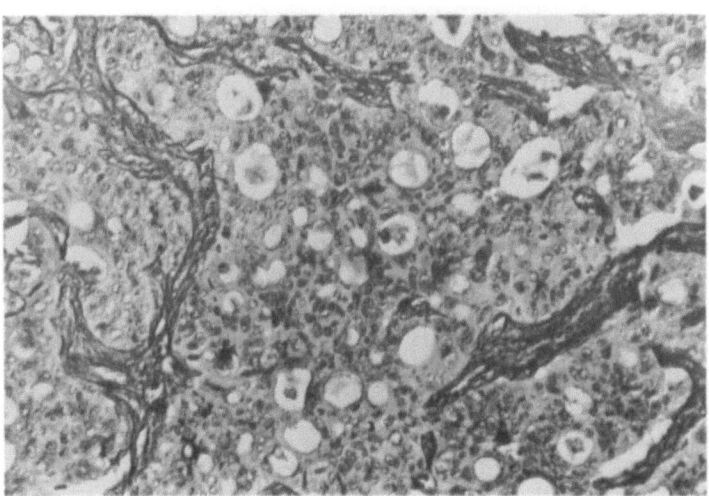

Fig. 3.   Tumor of ascorbic acid-treated SK-Br-3 cells (55
           days after the original transplantation) featuring
           an adenocarcinomatous architecture and scanty
           fibrillar stroma. H&E, X120.

in nude mice, atypical spindle cells appeared and progressively replaced the adenocarcinomatous components (Fig. 4)
until the tumors were made up entirely of spindle cells
resembling those of the L-cysteine group. Nevertheless,
when one of these spindle cell tumors was re-explanted in
vitro, it produced an outgrowth of epithelial-like cells
very similar to those of the original cultures of ascorbic
acid-treated SK-Br-3 cells.

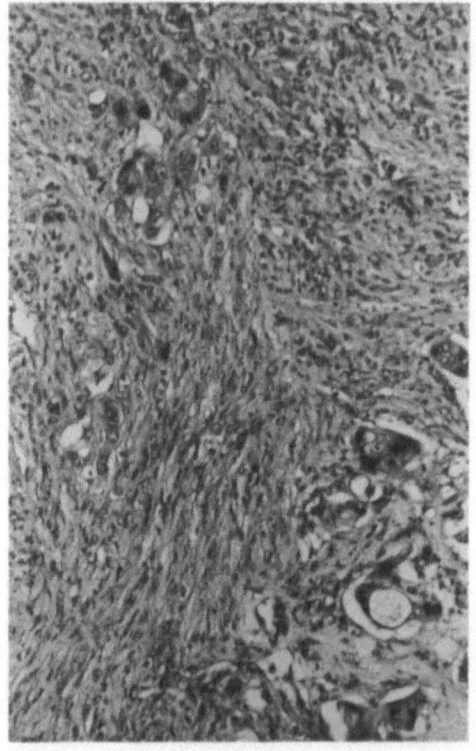

Fig. 4.   Tumor of ascorbic acid-treated SK-Br-3 cells (57
           days after the 1st passage, 96 days after the
           original transplantation). The tumor is made up
           of spindle cells surrounding a few residual
           adenocarcinomatous nests. H&E, X120.

Table 1

SK-Br-3 Tumors in BALB/c nu/nu mice

Cells	Transplants			Tumors		
	No.	Takes	Histologic type	Volume* (cm^3)	Age in days	GI*
Control	31	28	Carcinoma NST	2.0±0.3	11-145	3.4±0.4
Treated:						
L-cysteine	74	74	Spindle cell carcinoma	4.7±0.5	9-46	22.3±1.6
Ascorb. ac.	49	49	Adenocarcin.	1.7±0.3	21-70	3.8±0.5
Ascorb. ac.	31	31	Adenocarcin. with spindle metaplasia	4.7±0.7	11-42	21.5±1.8

*Mean ± S.E.

The growth features of these tumors are shown in Table 1. Control tumors had a mean volume of 2 cm^3 and a GI of 3.4. It is interesting to note that while the well differentiated adenocarcinomas produced by ascorbic acid-treated cells had growth figures comparable to those of the controls, the tumors of the L-cysteine group and the spindle cell carcinomas of the ascorbic acid-treated cells attained much larger volumes in shorter periods of time and had higher GI values. It should be pointed out that the more vigorous growth rate of these last 2 groups of tumors was paralled by a greater local aggressiveness.

Table 2

SK-Br-3 Tumors in BALB/c nu/nu mice

Follow up

Cells	Histologic type	Recurrences'	Mice with metastases"	Metastases	
				Lymph.	Hemat.
Control	Carcinoma NST	0/10	0/28	0	0
Treated:					
L-cysteine	Spindle cell carcinoma	24/34	50/74	10	78
Ascorb. ac.	Adenocarcinoma	14/26	24/49	20	20
Ascorb. ac.	Adenocarcinoma with spindle metaplasia	8/15	17/24	2	35

' Recurrences / excised tumors
'' Number of mice with metastases / number of mice followed to death with a minimum of 8 post-operative days. Most mice had multiple metastatic foci.

Tumor behavior.

As seen in Table 2, no recurrences and no metastases were observed in the control tumors. On the contrary, the tumors of treated cells had high rates of local recurrences and of metastases following surgical excision. It is important to note that most mice with metastatic involvement had multiple metastases. Of the mice with L-cysteine treated tumors 68% had metastases, while among the animals with ascorbic acid-treated tumors, metastases were found in 49% of those with adenocarcinomas and in 71% of those with carcinomas with spindle cell metaplasia. The distribution and pathway of the metastases is of particular interest. One-half of the metastases of the adenocarcinomas in the ascorbic acid group were found in regional lymph nodes and the other half in distant sites. In contrast, carcinomas with spindle cell features, from both L-cysteine and ascorbic acid groups, metastasized predominantly to distant sites. The latter included the lungs and less frequently the mediastinum, pleura, pericardium and kidneys, and were most likely the result of hematogenous spread.

It would thus appear that L-cysteine and ascorbic acid can modify the morphology and degree of differentiation of SK-Br-3 cells in vitro and that these modifications are accompanied by alterations in the growth and behavior of the tumors in vivo. The mechanisms by which these modifications take place are at the present time matter of conjecture. It is possible that differences in the biology of these cells resulted from enhancement of particular clones of cells by L-cysteine and by ascorbic acid. Or, since the cultures used in these experiments were derived from an originally cloned cell population, the two metabolites might have induced the appearance of new clones with different biological potentials. However, these observations point out the possibility that the behavior of neoplastic cells may be manipulated and altered by exogenous factors. Further experimentation is required to elucidate this phenomenon and whether it can be observed in other cell types as well.

REFERENCES

Fogh, J. and Trempe, G. New human tumor cell lines. In: Human Tumor Cells in Vitro, J. Fogh ed., Plenum Press, New York, 1975, pp 115-159.

Leuchtenberger, C. and Leuchtenberger, R. Protection of hamster lung cultures by L-cysteine or vitamin C against carcinogenic effects of fresh smoke from tobacco or marihuana cigarettes. Br. J. Exp. Path. 58, 625-634, 1977.

Leuchtenberger, C. and Ozzello, L. Morphological and behavioral modifications of human mammary carcinoma cells caused by L-cysteine and ascorbic acid. I. In vitro experiments. In: Progress in Surgical Pathology, Vol. 5, C.M. Fenoglio and M. Wolff eds., Masson Publishing U.S.A., New York, 1983, pp 243-249.

Ozzello, L. and Leuchtenberger, C. Metastatic potential of SK-Br-3 cells treated with L-cysteine or ascorbic acid.

<u>In</u>: Metastases - Clinical and Experimental Aspects, K. Hellman, P. Hilgard, and S. Eccles eds., Martinus Nijhoff, Publish., The Hague, 1980, pp 232-236.

Ozzello, L., Leuchtenberger, C., and Hurlimann, J. Morphological and behavioral modifications of human mammary carcinoma cells caused by L-cysteine and by ascorbic acid. II. Observations in xenografts. <u>In</u>: Progress in Surgical Pathology, Vol. 5, C.M. Fenoglio and M. Wolff eds., Masson Publishing U.S.A., New York, 1983, pp 251-262.

CLINICAL ASPECTS OF METASTASES IN BREAST CANCER

A. ONNIS

Institute of Gynaecology and Obstetrics,
University of Padua, 35100 Padua, Italy.

New concepts in the management of metastases from breast cancer have developed in recent years out of a better understanding of the natural history and malignant potential of the disease.

The fact that breast cancer is already a systemic disease at the time of clinical diagnosis explains the high percentage of failures with traditional regional treatments even when carried to the extreme limits of radical surgery. In a preoperative staging of 172 cases with clinically operable breast cancer, Roberts et al. (1976) found 22% positive bone scintigrams, 16% positive liver scintigrams and 29% positive blood chemistry markers, indicating early metastasis.

As a result, systemic therapy, such as hormonotherapy, chemotherapy, immunotherapy with monoclonal antibodies etc, should be planned in association with local therapy, from the beginning of the treatment.

Appropriate treatment should take into account different aspects of the disease: tumor stage and lymph node status, tumor volume, histologic and nuclear grade, steroid receptor positivity, tumor margin, lymphocytic infiltration, invasion of capillary spaces and others (Fisher et al., 1975; Maehle and Jarven, 1984; Stenkvist et al., 1982; Osborne et al., 1980).

The Cooperative Breast Cancer Group (1978) found that after extended local therapy, breast cancer metastases were regional (skin, lymph nodes, soft tissue) in 28% of the cases, visceral (lung, liver, brain) in 43% and in bone in 28%.

It is therefore important for each patient to be accurately screened for the presence and location of metastases (Galasco, 1977).

The incidence and location of regional or distant metastases depend on the type of breast cancer and the biological characteristics of the latter.

By way of example, the incidence of metastases in various organs differs with the estrogen receptor status of the tumor. The incidence of metastases in the soft tissues is significantly higher in ER-positive breast cancers, while metastases in the liver and brain are more frequent in ER-negative cancers (Samaan et al., 1981).

This explains the higher rate of success with anti-estrogen therapy in metastases involving soft tissue compared with metastases in other sites. Patterson et al., (1982) observed that the rate of response to anti-estrogen therapy was related to the site of metastasis and was noticeably higher in soft tissues (56%) than in bone (33%) and the visceral organs (35%).

In a detailed study of different locations, De Lena and Volonterio (1982) obtained results similar to those of Patterson et al. (1982) favouring the use of antiestrogenic therapy in metastases of soft tissues and the skin.

Our personal series (Nardelli et al., 1985) also showed a correlation between the presence of estrogen receptors and response to endocrine therapy in advanced and metastatic breast cancer (Table 1).

A more accurate prediction of response to endocrine therapy may be obtained by determining progesterone as well as estrogen receptor status. In our series, the rate of response to hormonal therapy reached 76% in ER+/PgR+ tumors, fell to 9% in ER-/PgR- tumors but was equal to 28% in ER-/PgR+ tumors and 27% in ER+/PgR- tumors (Table 2). Since cellular growth depends on the estrogen-progesterone balance, the response to hormonal therapy is a function of both estrogen and progesterone receptor status.

Since estrogens, after translocation to the nucleus, stimulate the production of progesterone receptors which, in turn, modulate ER production, progesterone receptors may be considered the end product of estrogen stimulation.

Unfortunately, receptor characterization which is predictive of hormone sensitivity does not offer any valid indication of tumor chemosensitivity, as shown by Umsawasdi et al., (1981) who observed that complete and partial response to chemotherapy was independent of estrogen receptors in advanced and metastatic breast cancer. They recorded response rates of 56% in ER+ and 49.5% in ER- tumors.

That the response to hormonal treatment is not always in agreement with the receptor status of the tumor may be explained by the fact that receptors are not permanent and unchanging. Primary tumors and metastases may show dissimilar receptor characteristics and also dissimilar responsiveness to therapy (Webster et al., 1978). Subsequent biopsies may show a different receptor distribution. The receptor content in multiple tumor specimens from individual patients varies more often in subsequent than in simultaneous biopsies (Rosen et al., 1977). In the course of endocrine therapy, ER+ tumors may become ER-, and under chemotherapy, ER- tumors may become ER+ (Allegra et al., 1980.

TABLE 1

RESPONSE RATE TO ENDOCRINE THERAPY
ACCORDING TO ER STATUS IN ADVANCED
AND METASTATIC BREAST CANCER

	CASES	RESPONSE RATE
ER-	8/72	11%
ER+/-	13/87	15%
ER+	29/58	50%
ER++	34/46	74%

-= 0-3 fmol   ;   +- = 3-10 fmol
+= 10-100 fmol ;   ++ > 100 fmol

TABLE 2

RESPONSE RATE TO ENDOCRINE THERAPY
ACCORDING TO ER STATUS IN ADVANCED
AND METASTATIC BREAST CANCER

	CASES	RESPONSE RATE
ER+/PgR+	62/81	76%
ER-/PgR+	11/39	28%
ER+/PgR-	7/26	27%
ER-/PgR	7/78	9%

- $<$10 fmol
+ $>$10 fmol

For this reason, several authors and Tormey (1981) in particular, have stressed the greater efficacy of combined chemohormonal treatments (Çocconi et al., 1979; Mouridsen, 1980; Tormey, 1981) (Table 3).

The antimitotic action of combined therapy is probably more complete, since it adds the action of antiblastic agents on receptor-negative cell clones to the selective effect of hormonotherapy on specific receptors. Moreover, hormonal treatment can make receptor-positive clones more sensitive to antimitotic agents. This reinforcement has a valid clinical application.

Engelsman et al., (1981) have shown the efficacy of chemotherapy (CMF) combined with hormonotherapy (Tamoxifen) particularly in visceral metastases which are notoriously the most resistant to either chemotherapy or hormonotherapy unaccompanied by other types of treatment.

The problem of combined therapy in metastatic disease is an old one, if one considers the controversy over ovariectomy in premenopausal women in the context of endocrine surgery (hypophysectomy, adrenalectomy, etc.) (Table 4).

On the basis of the receptor status of the neoplasm, modern hormonotherapy combines compounds such as dexametason or aminoglutetamid in premenopause or Tamoxifen and ciproterone acetate in postmenopause.

Our clinical experience has revealed that about one-third of patients with metastatic breast cancer in premenopause show an objective improvement after ovariectomy. Furthermore, in patients responsive to ovariectomy, the clinical course has a better outcome than in non-responsive patients irrespective of subsequent medical treatment. This indicates that hormone sensitivity, defined by steroid receptor determinations constitutes a favourable prognostic index which is corroborated by the remission rate of responsive patients following hormonal therapy (Table 5).

In spite of the percentage of favourable responses to the new combined chemo-hormonal therapy, the survival rate of patients with disseminated disease is still deemed unsatisfactory today.

This means that a very close follow-up of metastatic breast cancer is necessary for the early detection of relapse by means of sensitive markers such as monoclonal antibodies (Croghan et al., 1983; Ciocca et al., 1983; Rasmussen et al., 1982).

The clinical problems connected with metastatic breast cancer remain numerous and are still extremely complex but we have gained and continue to gain greater insight as a result of significant progress in the understanding of tumor biology and its influence on the clinical course of the disease.

TABLE 3

CONTROLLED TRIALS OF HORMONOTHERAPY COMBINED WITH
CHEMOTHERAPY IN ADVANCED ANS METASTATIC BREAST CANCER

AUTHORS	RESPONSE TO TREATMENT		P
COCCONI (1979)	CMF 17/41 (41%)	CMF+TAM 21/29 (72%)	0.02
MOURIDSEN (1980)	CMF 32/68 (47%)	CMF+TAM 46/69 (67%)	0.03
TORMEY (1980)	DA 20/55 (36%)	DA+TAM 37/67 (55%)	0.004

C = Cyclophosphamide ; M = Methotrexate ; F = Fluorouracil
D = Dibromodulcitor   ; A = Adriamycin   ; Tam = Tamoxifen

TABLE 4

OVARIECTOMY IN METASTATIC BREAST CANCER
IN PRE-MENOPAUSE

AUTHOR	RESPONSE	%
Treves (1958)	32/122	43
Block (1960)	9/26	35
Dao (1962)	28/84	32
Taylor (1962)	113/381	30
Fracchia (1969)	140/442	32
Veronesi (1975)	162/550	29
Falkson (1979)	7/38	18
Dao (1980)	21/55	38
Onnis-Fiorentino (1984)	49/143	34

TABLE 5

METASTATIC BREAST CANCER IN PRE-MENOPAUSE

(230 METASTATIC SITES EXAMINED IN 143 PATIENTS)

OVARIECTOMY PLUS

TREATMENT	SOFT TISSUE		BONE		VISCERAL	
	metastatic sites	response (CR+PR)	metastatic sites	response (CR+PR)	metastatic sites	response (CR+PR)
CHEMOTHERAPY	50	15(30%)	27	8(29.6%)	28	7(25%)
HORMONOTHERAPY	23	13(56.5%)	24	10(41.6%)	8	6(75%)
CHEMO-HORMONOTHERAPY	25	8(32%)	29	7(24.1)	16	4(25%)
TOTAL METASTATIC SITES	98	36(36.7%)	80	25(31.2%)	52	17(32.6%)

REFERENCES

1. Allegra, J.C., Lippman, M.E., Thompson, E.B., Simon, R., Barlock, A., Green, L., Huff, K.K., Do, H.M.T., Aitken, S.C. and Warren, R., Estrogen receptors status is the most important prognostic variable in predicting response to endocrine therapy in metastatic breast cancer. Europ. J. Cancer, 16, 323-331, 1980.

2. Breast Cancer Study Group, Identification of breast cancer patients with high risk of early recurrence after radical mastectomy. Cancer, 42: 2809-2826, 1978.

3. Ciocca, D.R., Adam, D.J., Edwards, O.P., Bjercke, R. Jr and Mc Guire, W.L., Distribution of an estrogen induced protein with a molecular weight of 24.000 in normal and malignant cells. Cancer Res., 43, 1204-1210, 1983.

4. Cocconi, G., De Lisi, V., Boni, C., Amadori, D., Poletti, T. and Bertusi, M., Proceedings of the American Association for Cancer Research and the American Society of Clinical Oncology, 20, 302, 1979, (abstract).

5. Croghan, G., Papsidero, L., Valenzuela, L. and Nemoto, T. Tissue distribution of an epithelial and tumor associated antigen recognized by monoclonal antibody F 36/22. Cancer Res. 43, 4980-4988, 1983.

6. De Lena, M. and Volonterio, A., Efficacy of Tamoxifen in Metastatic Breast Cancer. The experience of the National Cancer Institute of Milan. In: The role of Tamoxifen in Breast Cancer, S. Iacobelli, M.E. Lippman, G. Robustelli, eds, Raven Press, New York, 1982, pp. 65-72.

7. Engelsman, E., Mouridsen, H.T., Palshof, T. and Sylvester,R CMF versus CMF plus Tamoxifen in advanced breast cancer in postmenopausal women: an EORTC study, Reviews on Endocrine Related Cancer, Suppl. 9, 427-436, 1981.

8. Fisher, E.R., Gregorio, R.M., Fisher, B., The pathology of invasive breast cancer. A syllabus derived from findings of the National Surgical Adjuvant Breast Project (protocol N°4) Cancer 36, 1-85, 1975.

9. Galasco, C.S.B., Screening for the potentially curable patients. In: Breast Cancer Management. Early and Late. B.A. Stoll, ed, W. Heineman, London, 1977, pp. 15-23

10. Maehle,B.O. and Jarven, R.S.K., Prediction of prognosis in axillary lymph-node positive breast cancer. Brit. J. Surg., 71: 459-462, 1984.

11. Mouridsen, H.T., Breast Cancer: Experimental and Clinical Aspects. Proceedings second EORTC Breast Cancer Working Conference Copenhagen, May 1979, Mouridsen, H.T. and Palshof, T., eds, Pergamon Press, Oxford, 1980, pp. 119-123.

12. Nardelli, G.B., Lamaina, V., Mozzanega, B. and Becagli, L. Steroid receptors in breast cancer. In: Proceedings of International Meeting of Gynaecological Oncology. A. Onnis, et. S.O.G., Padua, 1985, pp. 340-344.

13. Osborne, C.K., Yochmowitz, M.G., Knight, W.A. and Mc Guire, W.L., The value of the estrogen and progesterone receptors in the treatment of breast value. Cancer, 46, 2884-2888, 1980.

14. Patterson, J.S., Battersby, L.A. and Edwards, O.G., Review of the clinical pharmacology and international experience with Tamoxifen in advanced breast cancer. In: The role of Tamoxifen in breast cancer., S. Iacobelli, M.E. Lippman, and G. Robustelli, eds. Raven Press, New York, 1982, p.17-33.

15. Rasmussen, B.B., Hilkens, J., Hilgers, J., Nielsen, H.H., Thorpe, S.M. and Rose, C. Monoclonal antibodies applied to primary human breast carcinoma relationship to menopausal status, lymph node status and steroid hormonereceptor content. Breast Cancer Res. Treat. 2, 401-405, 1982.

16. Roberts, J.G., Gravelle, I.H., Baum, M., Bligh, A.S., Leach, K.G. and Hughes, L.E., Evaluation of radiographic and isotopic scintigraphy for detecting skelet Lancet, i, 237-239, 1976. metastasis

17. Rosen, P.P., Menendez-Botet, C.J., Urban, J.A., Fracchia, A. and Schwartz, M.K., Estrogen receptor protein in multiple tumor specimens from individual patients with breast cancer. Cancer, 39, 2194-2200, 1977.

18. Samaan, N.A., Buzdar, A.U., Aldinger, K.A., Schultz, P.N., Yang, K., Romsdahl, M.M. and Martin, R. Estrogen receptors: a prognostic factor in breast cancer. Cancer, 47, 554-560, 1981.

19. Stenkvist, B., Bengtsson, E., Dahlquist, B., Eklund, G., Eriksson, O., Jarkans, T. and Nordin, B. Predicting breast cancer recurrence. Cancer, 50, 2884-2893, 1982.

20. Tormey, D.C., Selected aspects of Tamoxifen containing combination therapies. Reviews on endocrine related cancer. Suppl. 8: 37, 1981.

21. Umsawasdi, T., Vogel, C.L., Voigt, W. and Thomasen, J. Breast, Disease of the Breast, 7: 26-29, 1981.

22. Webster, D.J.T., Bronn, D.G. and Minton, J.P., Estrogen receptor levels in multiple biopsies from patients with breast cancer. Am. J. Surg. 136, 337-401, 1978.

CHEMOTHERAPY FOR BREAST CANCERS

L. ISRAEL

Department of Cancerology at Université Paris XIII
Centre Hospitalier Universitaire Avicenne
93000 Bobigny, France.

INTRODUCTION

Breast cancers are among the types of neoplasm with the highest sensitivity to currently available chemotherapy, at least in terms of rates of response and regression. Unfortunately, this does not mean that chemotherapy is completely able to eradicate detectable or occult metastases of these cancers and therefore permanently cure a significant number of them. This point still remains to be demonstrated, as can easily be understood if we look at the list of theoretical and practical limitations encountered in antineoplastic chemotherapy.

LIMITATIONS OF CHEMOTHERAPY

The first limitation consists of toxicity to healthy cells, which means that maximum tolerated doses are often lower than optimal doses.

Another limitation resides in the presence of cells that are resistant to currently available chemotherapy due to resistance to one or more drugs as a result of the development of selected clones with double or triple resistance or even pleiotropic resistance to a large number of drugs because of alterations in membrane permeability and very marked active efflux. These types of resistance have a genetic basis: mutations, rearrangements and gene amplification (Curt et al. 1984).

Kinetic resistance is encountered when a drug attains effective blood levels but not all of the cells are in cycle or, if in cycle, they are not in the phase susceptible to the action of a particular drug.

The repair of DNA lesions induced by cytostatic agents can be a very active phenomenon which, according to estimations, can affect 4 out of 5 cells.

Finally, a malignant cell population should be visualized as possessing considerable genetic instability resulting in very marked adaptability to the environment: hence, the permanent emergence of more aggressive and more resistant clones.

CHEMOTHERAPY OF METASTATIC BREAST CANCERS

Chemotherapeutic regimens, such as CAF (Cyclophosphamide, Adriamycin, Fluorouracil) or CFMVP (Cyclophosphamide, Fluorouracil, Methotrexate, Vincristine, Prednisone), are reported to elicit a positive response in up to 85% of cases with maintenance of the response for 12 to 18 months. We have reported response rates of 90% with a mean survival of 3 years with very high doses of Cyclophosphamide and Fluorouracil. These results, obtained during initial treatment and in the absence of any previous chemotherapy, are fairly satisfactory. IO to 20% of patients with metastases survive for more than 5 years (Legha et al., 1979; Cummings et al., 1985; Israel et al. 1984).

In the case of second line treatment, following failure of the above regimens, results are less encouraging. However, in this difficult "salvage" situation, we have obtained response rates of 60% with survival for over 12 months in 80% of these cases, with the use of Platinum, Adriamycin and Bleomycin (Breau et al. 1986).

Very encouraging trials are currently under way with these same drugs administered continuously for 7 to 14 days per cycle.

ROUTINE CHEMOTHERAPY OF INVISIBLE METASTASES

All of the post-operative statistics indicate that occult metastases are already present at the time of surgery in 90% of breast carcinoma with lymph node involvement (N+) and in 60% of breast carcinoma without lymph node involvement (N-). Simulations performed by means of a mathematical model recently developed by Markovitch, in association with the present author, indicate that, by the time the tumour is discovered, there are already a large number of viable metastases (IO to 300) containing several thousand cells which have mutated towards resistance. In addition, a significant number of metastases are derived from already resistant cells (Mouridsen and Palshof, 1983; Consensus Conference on Adjuvant chemotherapy for breast cancer, 1985).

These theoretical considerations, together with concrete analysis of the results of various trials with adjuvant treatments, demonstrate that:

1. Routine chemotherapeutic treatment should not be reserved exclusively for cases with lymph node involvement. It should also be used in cases without nodal involvement but with high nuclear grades and susceptibility to recurrence.

2. "Moderate-dose" treatment, employed on the pretext that only a small number of residual cells are present, fails. Postoperative adjuvant treatment of breast cancers should be administered with the same intensity as for metastatic cancers

in order to achieve eradication or quasi-eradication.

3. A 6-month treatment is inadequate to obtain eradication of occult metastases.

HOW CAN CHEMOTHERAPEUTIC RESULTS BE IMPROVED?

We believe that it is possible to improve the results of current chemotherapy by observing the following procedure:

a) use of maximally tolerated doses,

b) in the form of continuous rather than intermittent chemotherapy,

c) for prolonged periods of time.

We probably also need to use products capable of altering the permeability of cancer cells to cytostatic agents, such as Verapamil and calcium modulators.

Finally, the routine addition of anti-hormones and differentiation-inducing agents produces an effect on cells that are minimally sensitive to cytostatic agents because they are already differentiated.

CONCLUSION

Chemotherapy has provided satisfactory short-term results but is still only minimally effective in the long term. Results could be considerably improved, however, through controlled innovative trials.

REFERENCES

1. Curt,G.A., Clendeninn, N.J. and Chabner B.A.: Drug resistance in cancer. Cancer Treat.Rep., 68: 87-99, 1984.

2. Legha, S.S., Buzdar, A.U. and Smith, T.L. et al., Complete remissions in metastatic breast cancer treated with combination drug therapy. Ann. Intern. Med, 91: 847-852, 1979.

3. Cummings, F.J., Gelman, R. and Horton, J. Comparison of CAF versus CMFP in metastatic breast cancer. Analysis of prognostic factors. J. Clin. Oncol. 3: 932-940, 1985.

4. Israel, L., Breau, J.L. and Aguilera, J.: High-dose cyclophosphamide and high dose 5 fluorouracil. A new first-line regimen for advanced breast cancer. Cancer, 53: 1655-1659, 1984.

5. Breau, J.L., Israel, L., Morère, J.F. and Aguilera, J.:
   Second-line treatment of advanced breast cancer resistant
   to cyclophosphamide, methotrexate, 5 fluorouracil (CMF)
   with bleomycin, adriamycin and cisplatinum (BAP) combination chemotherapy. Proceedings of ASCO, 1986, (in press).

6. Mouridsen, H.T. and Palshof, T.: Adjuvant systemic therapy
   in breast cancer; a review. Eur. J. Cancer Clin. Oncol. 19:
   1753-1770, 1983.

7. Consensus Conference. Adjuvant chemotherapy for breast
   cancer. JAMA, 254: 3461-3463, 1985.

SURGICAL APPROACH TO THE AXILLA IN BREAST CANCER

J. REYNIER, R. VILLET and F. SAFA

Department of Surgery, Hôpital Boucicaut, Paris, France.

Twenty years ago, surgery involved radical mastectomy with excision of the axillary lymph nodes including the subclavicular nodes. The number of lymph nodes examined was considered the best criterion for judging the surgical procedure. Lymphedema was a common occurrence and was aggravated when surgery was combined with radiotherapy, a general strategy in the presence of metastatic nodal invasion. At times, the radiotherapists systematically irradiated the axilla and the cancerous breast and obtained in some cases sterilization of the cancer, but often with serious functional drawbacks; in other cases, the disease recurred in the axilla or the chest wall after a lapse of time.

Nowadays, there has been a fundamental change in the therapeutic approach to local and regional lesions, and over the past 15 years, the surgical procedures for breast cancer have narrowed down. Tumorectomy is regarded by many surgeons as the treatment of choice, provided the procedure is justified by the size and location of the tumor and not contra-indicated by the morphology of the breast. The current attitude with respect to the axillary nodes is even more restrictive since some French surgeons make a point of stating that nodes should only be removed in Berg's stage I (Berg, 1971) or Adair's first level lesions.

This reduced surgical approach is directly related both to the effectiveness of modern radiotherapy which has few or no after-effects and to a better understanding of the systemic nature of the cancer disease. Moreover, although occult lymph nodes metastases are present in 25% of patients with no clinical signs of axillary involvement (Foster, 1984), it is now universally recognized that systematic removal of the axillary lymph nodes does not reduce the incidence of metastases. According to Crile (1967) neither lymphadenectomy performed at the time of mastectomy nor excision by second intention of axillary node metastases has any effect on the survival rate. Our own results and those of Bosworth and Ghossein (1984), who studied the same number of patients (150 and 143, respectively), indicate in node-negative cases a comparable 10-year recurrence rate, i.e., 1.5%, either after systematic radiotherapy or surgery alone.

One important role of surgery, however, is to yield
material for histologic examination, providing prognostic
informations. Thus, the pathologist can pinpoint the number
and sites of metastasized nodes and the degree of tumoral
invasion which may range from a single embolus to
penetration of the capsule with infiltration of the
surrounding tissues. He can also determine the reactions
encountered in the draining lymph nodes regardless of
whether they are due to metastasis or not. The immunological
significance of these reactions must not be overlooked. As a
result of the histopathologic study, it is possible to adopt
a rational approach to systemic treatment, such as
chemotherapy or immunotherapy, administered alone or
combined, as a supplement to local and regional surgery.

In this respect, axillary lymphadenectomy is regarded
as essential, but must be correctly performed and free of
sequelae. The external mammary lymphatics and nodes draining
the breast are supported by an anatomically defined sheet of
fat tissue which lies against the thorax opposite the first
five intercostal spaces. An adequate surgical approach is
achieved by maintaining intact the lymphatic trunks at the
upper axilla which run parallel to the axillary blood
vessels and the nerves of the brachial plexus. The upper
extension of the fat tissue sheet with the external mammary
lymphatics needs also to be left in place (fig. 1 to 5).
This procedure avoids interrupting the lymphatic drainage of
the arm and subsequent lymphedema.

A well conducted lymphadenectomy does not need to be
supplemented with irradiation of the upper axilla and the
sub- and supraclavicular region. In fact, despite the
accuracy of present-day radiation dosimetry, the risk of
lymphedema as a result of sclerosis induced by combined
treatment is all too common, and the recurrence rate of
lymph node involvement following external mammary
lymphadenectomy is not reduced by supplementary radiotherapy.

Thus, best therapeutic approach to the axilla in breast
cancer is external mammary lymphadenectomy resting on firm
anatomical grounds and combined with systemic treatment.
This strategy makes it easier to establish prognostic
parameters and thereby select the most suitable course of
treatment to be followed. If the histologic examination of
the nodes fails to show evidence of metastatic invasion, the
surgical procedure does not affect the immune response of
the body which has developed long before emergence of
clinical signs of a tumor. Axillary lymphadenectomy provides
important immunological informations which direct the
further planning of treatment.

REFERENCES

Berg, J.W., Morphological evidence for immune response to breast cancer, Cancer, 1971, 28, 1453-1456.

Bosworth, J.L. and Ghossein, N.A., Limited surgery and radiotherapy in the treatment of localized breast cancer. Symposium on breast cancer, 1984, 64, 1115-1123.

Crile G., A biologic consideration of treatment of breast cancer, Ch. C. Thomas, Springfield, 1967

Foster R., Surgery and radiotherapy for primary breast cancer. Symposium on breast cancer, 1984, 64, 1125-1144.

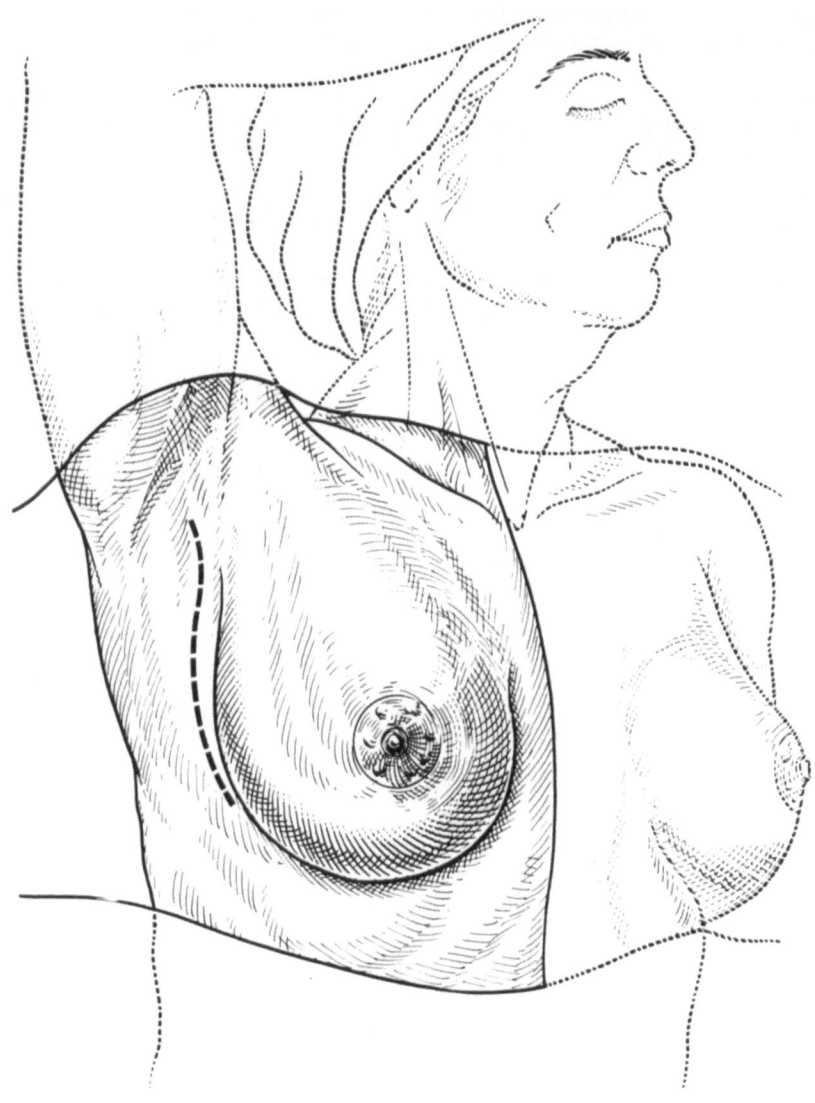

Fig.1 Skin incision for removal of the axillary lymph-nodes

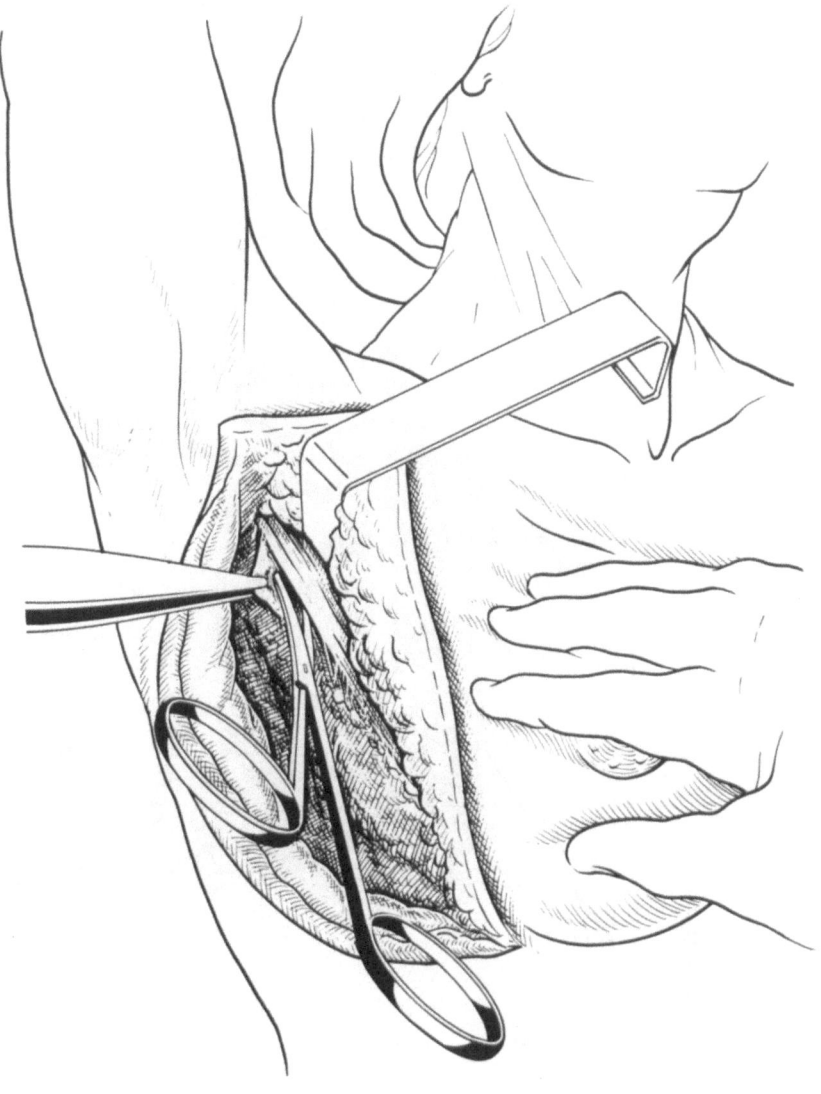

Fig.2 Beginning the dissection of the adipo-lymphatic
sheet

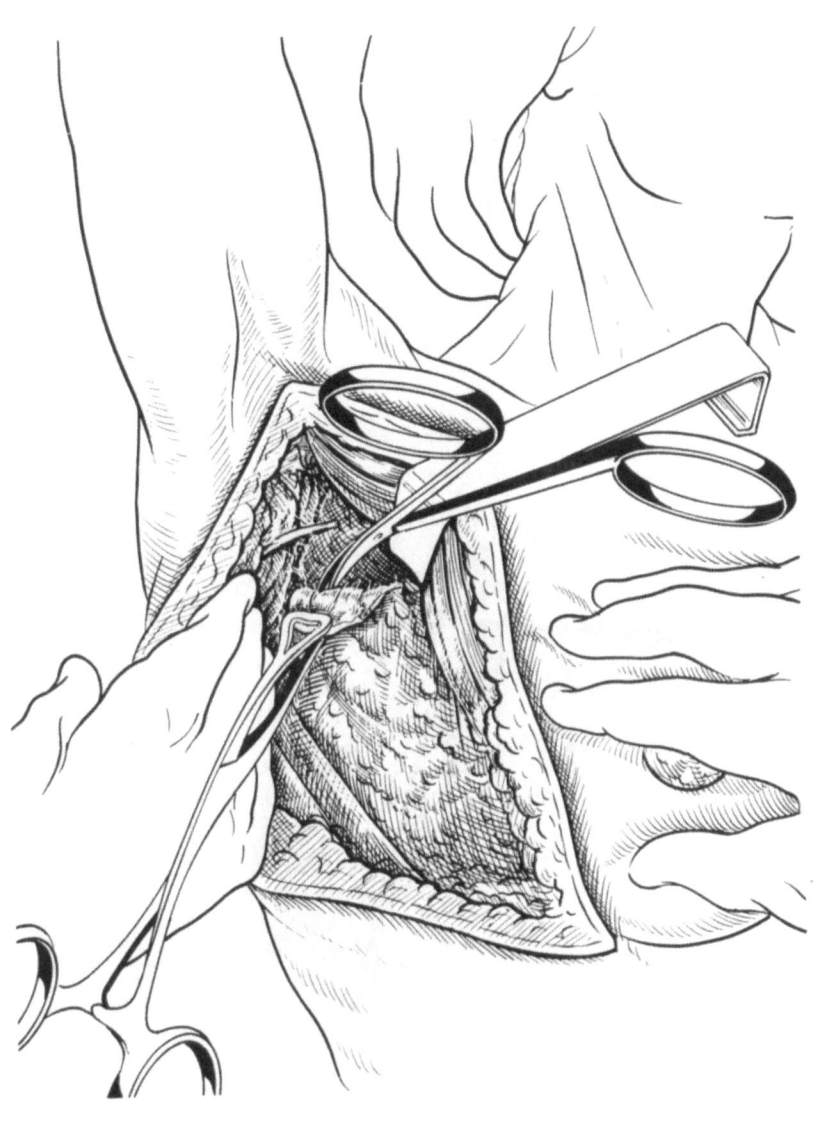

Fig.3 Downward dissection of the adipo-lymphatic sheet

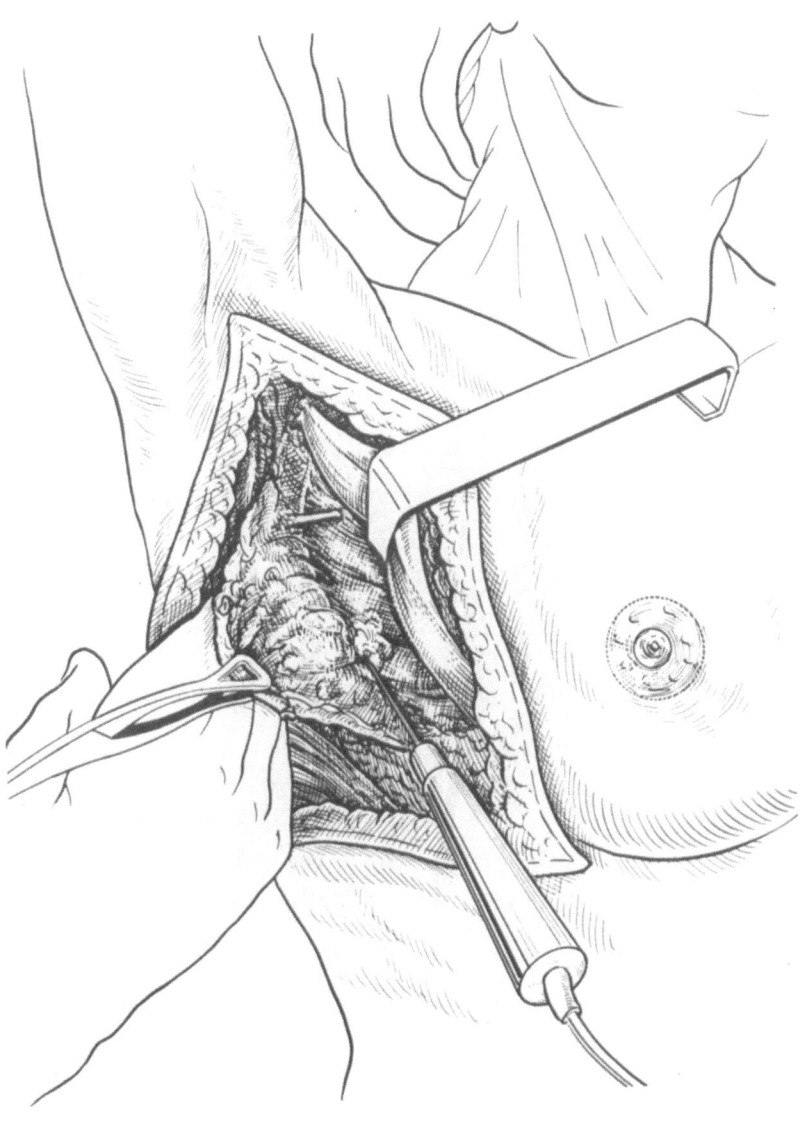

Fig.4 Separation of the sheet from the serratus muscle

392

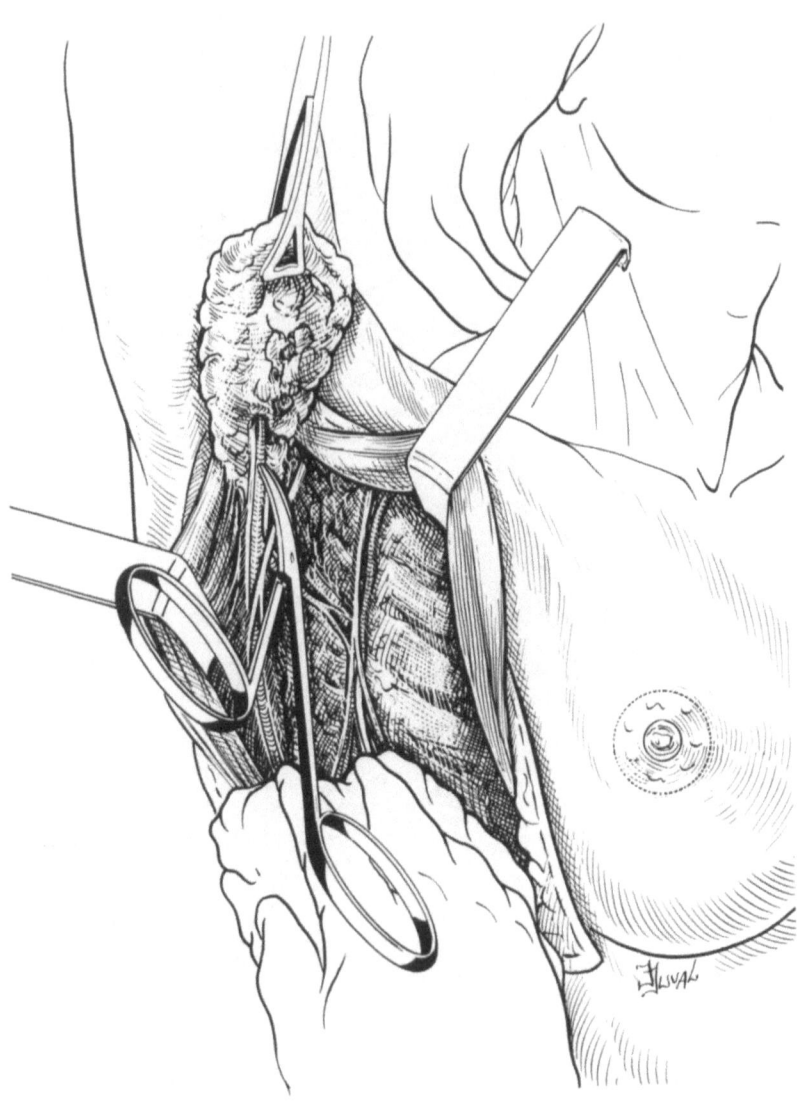

Fig.5 Dissection of the subscapular vessels

SURGICAL MANAGEMENT OF PULMONARY METASTASES OF CARCINOMA

OF THE BREAST

J.F. REGNARD, J. MARZELLE, D. SILBERT, J.M. VERLEY and
M. MERLIER

Centre Chirurgical Marie Lannelongue, 133, avenue de la
Résistance, 92350 Le Plessis Robinson, France.

INTRODUCTION

Surgical resection of lung metastases of several primary tumors is an effective and well-established treatment. (McCormack and Martini, 1979; Mountain et al., 1984; Regnard et al., 1985; Takita et al., 1981).

The role of surgery in lung metastases of breast carcinoma is still difficult to evaluate since these metastases may follow a slow spontaneous course.

As shown by Kreismann et al. (1983) in a prospective study, lung metastases of breast carcinoma are rarely considered for resection. These authors observed that thoracic involvement occurred in about 20 % of patients with mammary carcinoma. In 90% of the cases, involvement was diffuse (pleuropulmonary carcinosis, carcinomatous lymphangitis, extensive mediastinal involvement) and in only 10% was it localized (solitary mediastinal adenopathy or parenchymal metastasis).

The present study is a review of our experience with surgical management of pulmonary metastases of carcinoma of the breast. Prognostic factors were analyzed in order to define better criteria for selecting patients for surgery.

MATERIALS AND METHODS

Sixty-three patients surgically treated for pulmonary metastasis of breast carcinoma, at the Centre Chirurgical Marie Lannelongue, from 1959 to 1983, were selected for this study. The criteria for selection were:
1. Treated carcinoma of the breast, without evidence of residual or recurrent disease.
2. No demonstrable metastasis to other parts of the body,
3. Removal of all neoplastic tissue deemed possible,
4. Amount of functional lung tissue remaining after surgery providing the patient with sufficient pulmonary parenchymal reserve,
5. Histologically confirmed pulmonary metastasis.

Patients undergoing only biopsy or palliative surgery (surgical pleural symphysis for carcinosis) and patients with metastasis of breast sarcoma were excluded from the study. Of the 63 patients, 62 were female and 1 male. Ages ranged from 28 to 69 with a median of 53 years.

In 75% of the cases, the patients were asymptomatic and the metastasis was discovered on routine follow-up chest roentgenograms. In 25% of the patients there were symptoms (chest pain, cough, hemoptysis) leading to the discovery of metastasis. The disease-free interval between the primary tumor and pulmonary metastasis ranged from 1 to 16 years with a median interval of 5.4 years.

Clinically most of the lesions appeared to be solitary (74%). Multiple lesions occurred either unilaterally (13%) or bilaterally (13%). Bronchoscopy was positive in 21% of the cases, showing endobronchial tumor or stenosis more often than compression. In 7 cases (12%), it resulted in a preoperative histologic diagnosis.

Surgery was unilateral in 57 patients (90%) and bilateral in 6 (10%). Bilateral resections were performed 4 times in a single stage and twice in two stages within a 3-week period. In addition, 2 subsequent resections were performed, one for ipsilateral recurrence and one for recurrence in the opposite lung. Total resection was performed in 48 patients (76%) and palliative resection with gross evidence of residual neoplastic tissue in 15 patients (24%) (Table 1).

TYPE OF SURGICAL PROCEDURE

Wedge resection	12
Multiple wedge resection	16
Lobectomy	18
Pneumonectomy	4
Biopsy	13
Complete resection	48
Palliative procedure (biopsy or tumor reduction)	15

TABLE 1

Complete follow-up data were available for all but two foreign patients, with a minimum follow-up of 18 months. Results were analyzed by life-time methods, showing the actuarial survival rates of 61 patients.

RESULTS

In most cases, the post-operative course of the 63 patients was uneventful: there was no operative death and only one severe post-operative complication (empyema).

The actuarial survival rate of the 61 patients followed (curative and palliative resection) is indicated in fig. 1. The survival rate at five years was 28% (14 patients alive more than five years after thoracotomy, and at seven years,

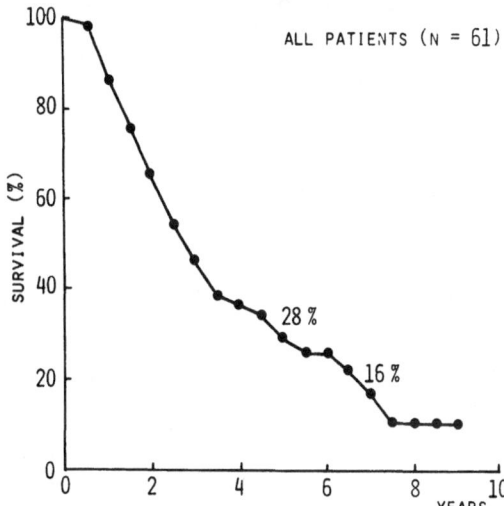

Figure 1.

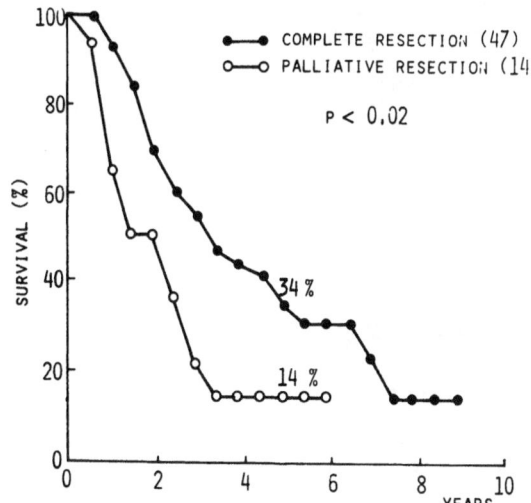

Figure 2.

16%. One patient is alive nine years after surgery without
evidence of recurrence. Patients undergoing total resection
had a 5 year survival of 34% (Fig. 2).

We compared these survival rates to those of two large
groups of patients with pulmonary metastases of other primary
sites (colorectal cancers and osteogenic sarcomas) operated on
at our Institute (Merlier et al., 1985; Regnard et al., 1985)
and found no statistical difference (Fig. 3).

The cause of death was known in 70% of the patients.
In 50% of the cases, the death was related to the onset of
metastases to other organs (bone, brain,..), in 45% to a thoracic recurrence with or without systemic metastatic spread-
out and in 5% to intercurrent diseases.

Prognostic factors

The main predictive factor of long-term survival was complete resection, as shown on Fig. 2: a comparison of survival
rates of patients undergoing curative resection and of those
subjected to palliative surgery shows a very significative sta-
tiscal difference (p< 0.02). All the patients treated by palliative surgery died within seven years.

Lymph node involvement, whether pedicular or mediastinal,
severely influenced the outcome. Fig. 4 shows survival rates
according to the positivity of lymph node mapping. Life expectancy was statistically higher when there was no evidence of
lymph node involvement: 32% at 5 years versus 16% (p< 0.02).

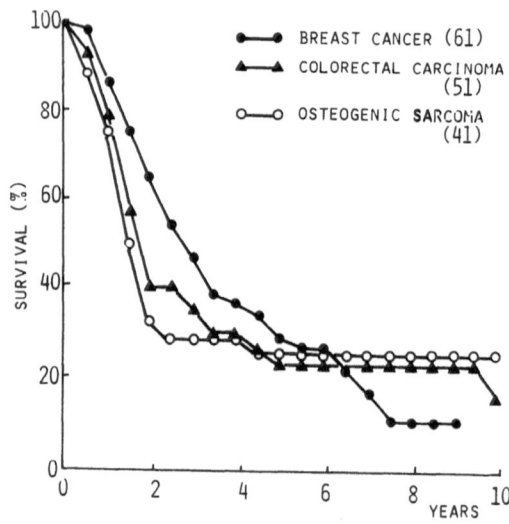

Figure 3.

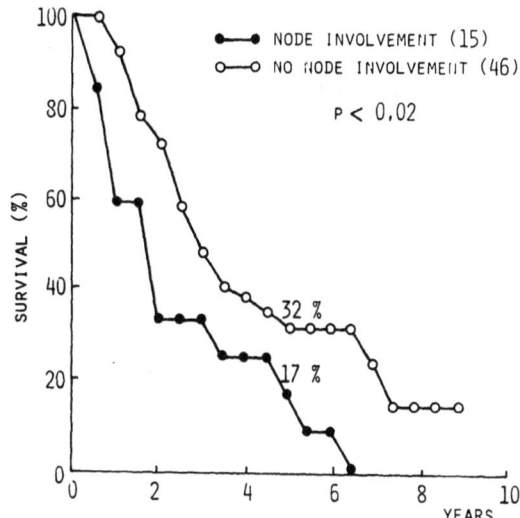

Figure 4.

Patients who were asymptomatic at the time pulmonary metastases were detected, seemed to fare better. Fig. 5 shows the survival rate of patients correlated to the onset of symptoms: asymptomatic patients had a slightly better statistical prognosis ($0.05 < p < 0.10$).

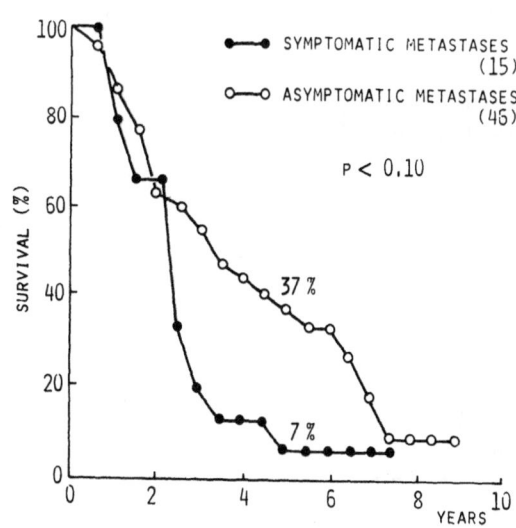

Figure 5.

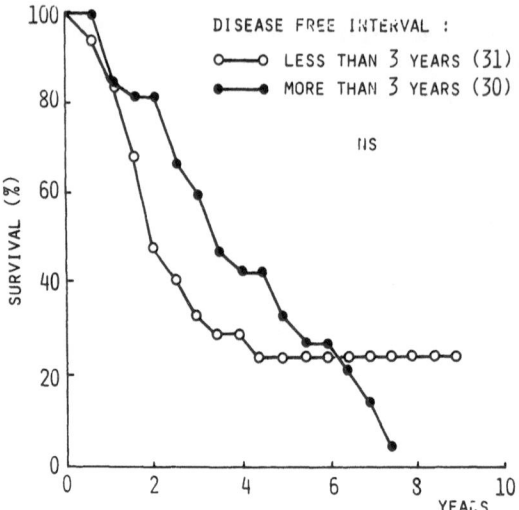

Figure 6.

On the other hand, the interval between primary treatment and detection of pulmonary metastasis apparently had no influence on the outcome. Fig. 6 shows there was no difference in the survival rates of patients whose disease-free interval was greater or less than 3 years.

Statistically, the degree of disease involvement did not influence survival rates: Fig. 7 shows the latter were similar for patients presenting with either solitary or multiple lesions.

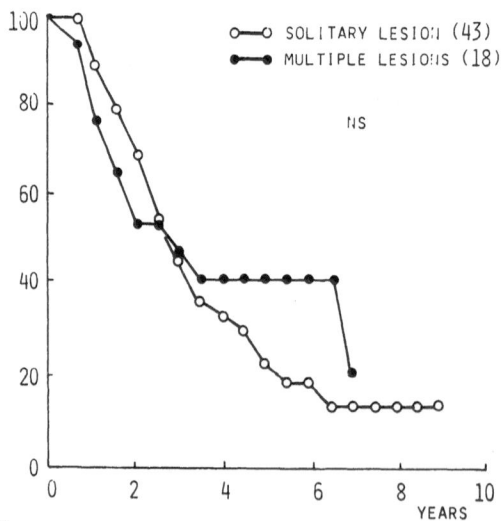

Figure 7.

TABLE II
TYPE OF SURGICAL PROCEDURE

	Actuarial 3 year survival	Actuarial 5 year survival
Wedge resection n = 12	58%	35%
Multiple wedge resections n = 16	45%	45%
Lobectomy n = 18	50%	30%
Extensive pneumonectomy n = 4	50%	0%

Finally, the procedure performed did not seem to affect survival rates, as may be seen in table II. Survival rates at 3 and 5 years were similar, whether patients underwent single wedge resection or multiple wedge resection or lobectomy. Four patients subjected to extensive pneumonectomy died within five years. However, this group was too small to rule out use of this type of procedure.

DISCUSSION

In patients undergoing total resection, the actuarial survival rate at five years was 34%. These results compare favorably to those reported in the literature (Mountain et al., 1984) and are encouraging, insofar as there were no surgical deaths. They incite us to pursue an aggressive surgical approach as part of a multimodal therapy of pulmonary metastases of breast cancer.

With the advent of improved chemotherapy, surgery assumes a new role (McCormack and Martini, 1979; Regnard et al., 1985; Takita et al., 1981). Some metastases may be cured or at any rate vanish as a result of chemotherapy and thus are not considered for surgery. On the other hand, more and more patients are considered for surgery when the lesions fail to respond completely or only partially to chemotherapy. Lastly, surgery may be considered in order to "reclassify" a patient, i.e., if in spite of a dramatic response to chemotherapy, X-rays show evidence of a residual nodule. Is this a case of persisting neoplastic tissue, or a fibrous or necrotic scar? As a result of resection, histologic analysis can determine whether to terminate or change the type of chemotherapy used.

The study of the cause of death showed that half of the patients died from metastases to other organs, mainly bone and

400

brain, without any recurrence in the chest. These findings
emphasize the importance of a meticulous systematic pre-opera-
tive examination for other metastases and the need for post-
operative adjunctive chemotherapy.

It is still difficult to assess pre-operatively the
patients who will benefit maximally from resection of pulmonary metastases of carcinoma of the breast. Criteria for a
favourable outcome are curative resection, no evidence of
lymph node involvement, and asymptomatic metastasis. On the
other hand, the disease-free interval, the number of metastases, and the surgical procedure do not seem to have any
influence on the outcome.

It should be pointed out, however, that our patients
were heterogenous owing to the long period covered by this
study. Furthermore, this was a univariate analysis, which
fails to show links between several criteria.

Can the resection of pulmonary metastasis of breast cancer ensure definitive cure? The answer is difficult to give.
A comparison of the survival rates of patients undergoing
resection for pulmonary metastases of breast cancer, colorectal cancer and osteogenic sarcomas shows no statistical difference. Post resection survival rates of colorectal cancers and
osteogenic sarcomas, however, remain stable after four to ten
years, showing that some patients may be cured of their metastatic disease. In contrast, there is no stabilization of the
survival curve in breast cancer, indicating persistent cancer-
related mortality for periods over five years. The results,
consequently, as far as complete resection is concerned, are
less clearcut.

At all events, our experience showing a long-term survival after curative surgery, in agreement with other reports in
the literature (Kreisman et al., 1983; Mountain et al., 1984)
supports the approach of surgical excision of lung metastases
of breast carcinoma.

REFERENCES

1. Kreisman, H., Wolkove, N., Schwartz Finkelstein, H.,
   Cohen, C., Margolese R., and Franck H.: Breast cancer and
   thoracic metastases; review of 119 patients.
   Thorax 1983, 38, 175-179.

2. Mc Cormack, P.M. and Martini, N.: The changing role of surgery for pulmonary metastases.
   Ann. Thorac. Surg., 1979, 28, 139-145.

3. Merlier, M., Silbert, D. and Regnard, J.F.: Chirurgie des
   métastases pulmonaires.
   Nouvelle Presse méd. 1985, 14, 1907-1908.

4. Mountain, C.F., Mc Murtrey, M.J. and Hermes, K.E.: Surgery for pulmonary metastases; a 20 years experience.
Ann. Thorac. Surg. 1984, 38, 323-330.

5. Regnard, J.F., Marzelle, J., Cerrina, J., Silbert, D. and Merlier, M.: Chirurgie des métastases pulmonaires.
Chirurgie 1985, 111, 512-522.

6. Takita, H., Karakousis, C. and Vincent, R.G.: Surgical management of metastases to the lungs.
Surg. Gynecol. Obstet., 1981, 152, 191-194.

SELECTED FREE PAPERS

LYMPHOSCINTIGRAM IN BREAST CANCER: A SUPERIMPOSED TECHNIQUE

SHOJI TERUI, NOBORU TAIRA, TAKESHI NANASAWA and HIRISHI YAMAMOTO

Department of Nuclear Medecine and Surgery,
National Cancer Center Hospital, Tokyo, Japan.

INTRODUCTION

A lymphoscintigram is a simple and non-invasive means of visualizing regional lymph nodes in cancer patients. Real contributions have been made in breast cancer with lymphoscintigrams (Agwunobi, 1978; Ege, 1976; Hultborn, 1955) but the images show only the accumulation of radioactive colloid in the form of hot spots which are transcribed on a roughly sketched hand drawn anatomical background. As a result, it is difficult to diagnose the exact location of these lymph nodes.

In order to locate regional lymph nodes in breast cancer, more accurately, we applied a new technique in which lymphoscintigraphic results were superimposed on the patient's chest roentgenogram. With the resulting superimposed image, it was possible to visualize the spread of the disease to the regional lymph nodes, especially the internal mammary nodes, as well as to evaluate the correlation between hot nodes and metastasis.

MATERIALS AND METHODS

Lymphoscintigrams were made in 17 preoperative patients with breast cancer at the National Cancer Center Hospital in Tokyo. In 13 of the 17 patients, the internal mammary lymph nodes were surgically removed (Table 1).

Lymphoscintigrams were obtained after injection of Tc-99m Rhenium colloid (Tc-99m-Re) (Pecking, 1978). Altogether, five mCi of Tc-99m-Re in 2ml solution were injected, one day before surgery, into the periosteum of the 4th and 5th right and left ribs. The injection was administered just on the inner side of the tumor in the affected breast and, as a control, on the mid-clavicular line of the contralateral breast. Pressure was exerted on the skin over the rib with the free hand while a 23-gauge needle was inserted vertically into the skin. The needle transversed the mammary gland and the pectoralis muscles to attain the periosteum of the ribs. 0.5 ml of Tc-99m-Re was then injected. The procedure was always attended by some pain which, unfortunately, could not be avoided. Images were then taken under the gamma camera, with the patient in a supine position. The injection sites were covered with lead plates to protect against high radioactivity. A life-sized antero-posterior lymphoscintigram was made 3 hours after the injection. The ster-

PATIENTS EXAMINED AND MODALITY OF SURGERY

	Number of patients
Radical mastectomy,	
- With internal mammary node dissection.....	13
- Without internal mammary node dissection..	4
	Total : 17

Age : 33 to 68 (Average : 51.4)

TABLE 1

nal notch was marked on the film (Fig. 1). In order to locate the lymph nodes accurately, the life-sized lymphoscintigram was superimposed upon a postero-anterior roentgenogram of the chest (Fig. 2). Then the ribs, clavicles and contours of the breasts were transposed with indelible ink onto the lymphoscintigram: this is what we refer to as a superimposed image (SI image) (Fig. 3) from which the location and number of visualized nodes were assessed.

After surgery, the lymph nodes were dissected and classified anatomically. After dissection, the hot nodes were determined by scintigraphy (Fig. 4). Dissected nodes were thus studied histologically and an attempt was made to correlate the hot nodes and metastatic foci.

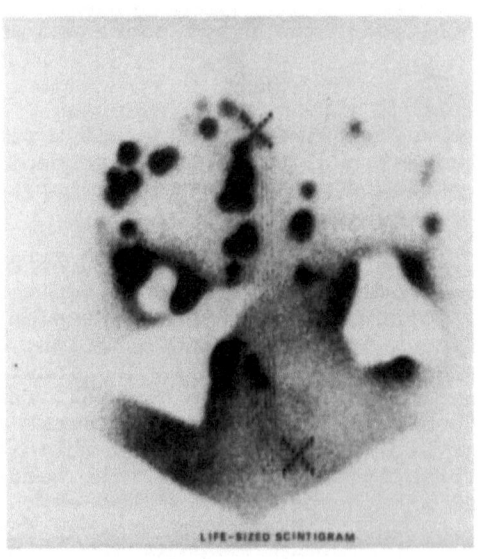

LIFE-SIZED SCINTIGRAM

Fig. 1. Life-sized lymphoscintigram. Left side with involvement.

RESULTS

After injection of Tc-99m-Re into the periosteum of the ribs, the internal mammary lymph nodes could be visualized on the superimposed images in all 17 patients. In 13 of these patients, the internal mammary nodes in addition to the axillary nodes were removed. A total of 47 mammary nodes were excised, 40 of which (85%) were identified on the superimposed image. The rate of axillary node visualization was 13.7%, with a failure of visualization of axillary nodes in 2 cases. The lymph node visualization rate is indicated in Table 2 and Fig. 5. The internal mammary nodes could be visualized from the supraclavicular to the fifth intercostal space. The second intercostal space was most frequently visualized on the images.

Table 3 shows the average number of the visualized internal mammary nodes per person. According to histological findings, the patients could be divided into two groups, i.e., those with and without lymph node metastasis. Distribution in

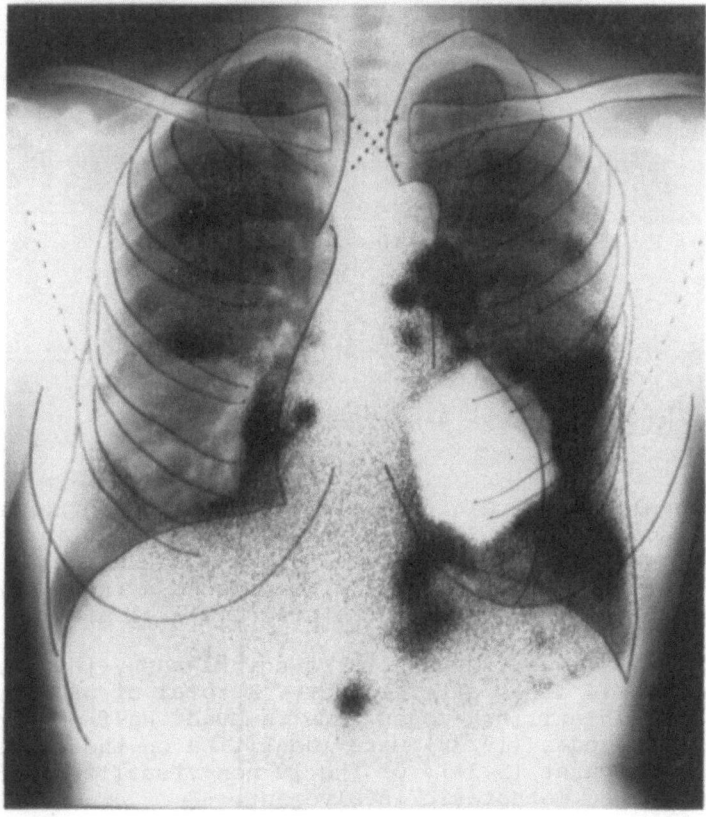

Fig. 2. Life-sized lymphoscintigram superimposed on the chest roentgenogram.

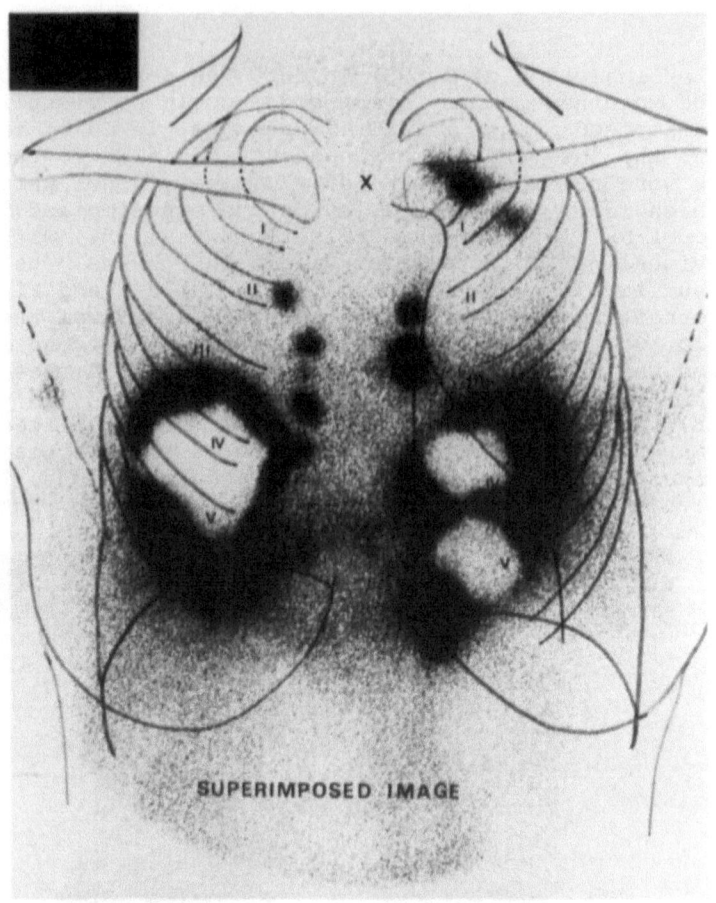

Fig. 3. SI image, left side with involvement.

the uninvolved contralateral side was considered normal and
served as a control. In patients with lymph node metastasis,
the average number of visualized nodes was 2.8 and no statis-
cal correlation could be established between these patients and
the normal data recorded in the contralateral side.

Table 4 shows the results of scintigraphy in specimens
obtained in 14 cases after surgery. A total of 38 internal mammary and 275 axillary nodes were removed. Half of the internal mammary nodes (19/38) were identified on the scintigram.
One was malignant (5.3%). Of the 19 non-visualized nodes, two
(10.5%) showed metastatic involvement.

DISTRIBUTION OF Tc-99m-Re IN REGIONAL LYMPH NODES IN
13 PATIENTS IN WHOM INTERNAL MAMMARY NODES WERE EXCISED

	Internal Mammary	Axillary	total
Total number of lymph nodes dissected.............	47	292	339
Visualized on the scintigram..................	40 (85%)	40 (13.7%)	80

TABLE 2

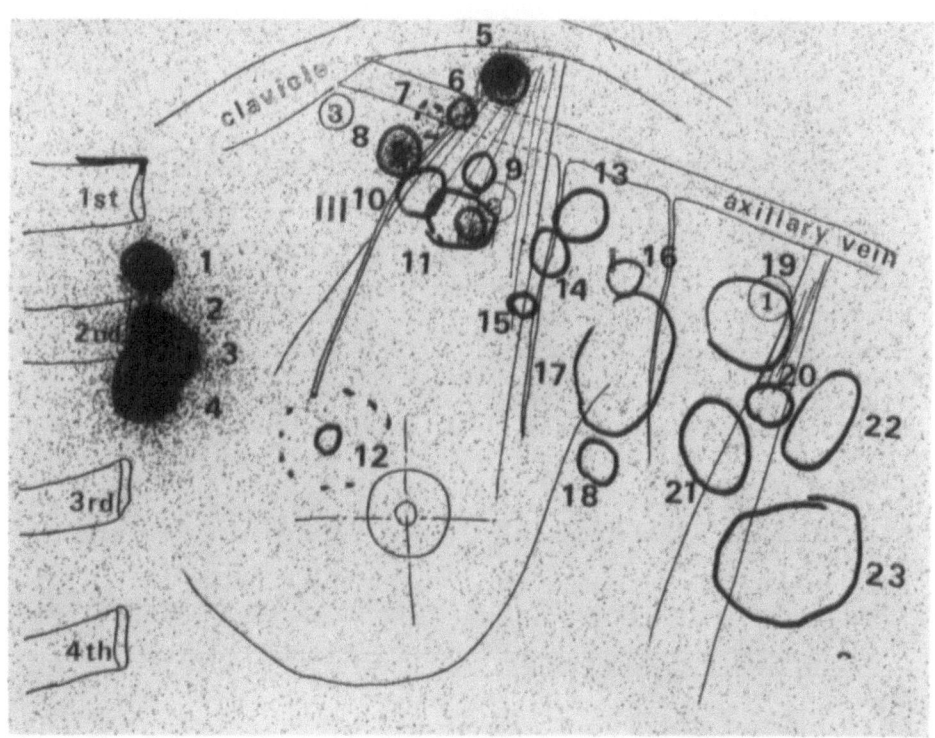

Fig. 4. Scintigram of Fig. 3.

AVERAGE NUMBER OF VISUALIZED LYMPH NODES
PER PERSON IN THE INTERNAL MAMMARY REGION

	Patients with Metastasis	Patients without Metastasis	Contralateral breast
Supraclavicular	1	2	1.8
Intercostal I	1	2	2.5
II	1.6	2.1	2
III	1.6	1.7	1.5
IV	1	0	2.3
V	0	0	2.5
Average	2.8	3.8	4.7

TABLE 3

DISTRIBUTION OF Tc-99m-Re IN REGIONAL
NODES IN 14 PATIENTS WITH BREAST CANCER

	Internal mammary	Axillary
Total number of lymph nodes dissected	38	275
Visualized on the scintigram	19	39
Histologically malignant	1(5.3%)	5(13.5%)
Impossible to visualize on the scintigram	19	238
Histologically malignant	2(10.5%)	34(14.3%)
Total number of malignant lymph nodes	3	39

TABLE 4

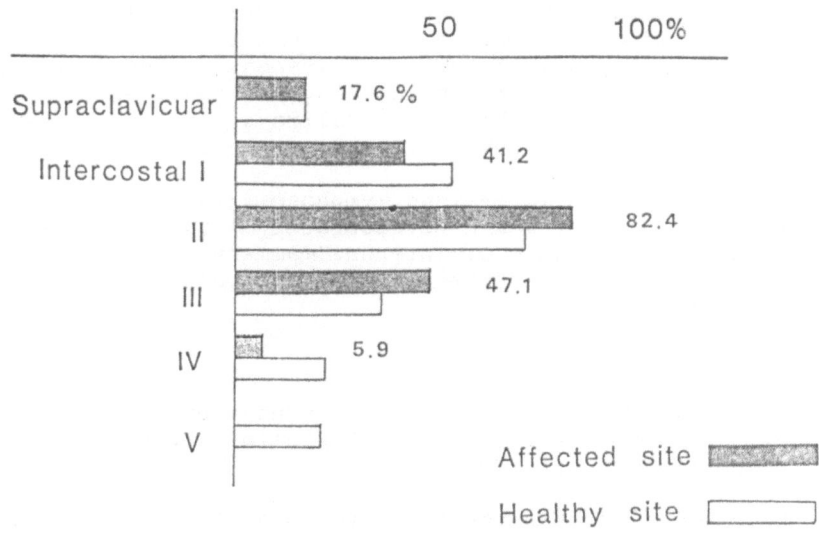

Fig. 5. Rate of internal mammary node visualization in 17
patients.

DISCUSSION

     In order to study the spread of cancer to the lymph nodes,
using lymphoscintigraphy, a radioactive colloid must be injected near the primary site of the tumor, along the same lymphatic drainage as the cancer cells (Terui, 1982). Part of the
lymph from the mammary glands is transported by the lymphatic
system through the pectoralis major muscle and intercostal spaces, then flows along the internal mammary vessels (Turner-
Warwick, 1959). Lymphatic drainage may therefore be used to
achieve visualization of the internal mammary nodes. The injection of Tc-99m-Re into the periosteum of the ribs is a simple
and reliable technique for visualizing regional lymph nodes in
breast cancer. In this study, visualization was obtained in 85%
(40/47) of the internal mammary nodes (Table 2). Since the rate
of axillary node visualization was only 13.7%, our injection
technique opened up a predominantly clear passage to the internal mammary region as compared with the axillary region.

     Lymph nodes with cancerous invasion are usually depicted
as cold. Seaman (1955) observed by autoradiography, that radioactive colloidal gold was found in the remaining lymphoid tissue
(and not on the cancerous spread of metastasized axillary lymph
nodes in breast cancer. In Seaman's study, from 356 nodes removed from 12 patients, 143 (40.2%) were radioactive. Metastases
were found in 63 of the 356 nodes. The incidence of the radioactive nodes with cancer was 14% (20/143), and that of the nonra-
dioactive nodes with cancer was 20.2% (43/213).

In our study, 50% of the nodes (19/38) including one with cancer, could be identified on the scintigrams. Of the other 50%, two displayed metastatic involvement but could not be visualized (Table 4). Our findings suggest that, with a proper technique, it is possible to visualize a certain number of lymph nodes affected by metastasis.

Superimposing life-sized lymphoscintigrams on chest-roentgenogram is an easy means of accurately locating lymph nodes, especially in the case of internal mammary nodes in breast cancer. This technique has been shown to be useful in locating metastatic nodes.

REFERENCES

1. Agwunobi, T.C.: Diagnosis of malignant breast disease by axillary lymphoscintigraphy: A preliminary report. Br. J. Surg., 65: 379-383, 1978.

2. Ege, G.N.; Internal mammary lymphoscintigraphy. The rationale, technique, interpretation and clinical application: A review based on 848 cases. Radiology, 118: 101-107, 1976.

3. Hultborn, K.A.: The lymph drainage from the breast to the axillary and parasternal lymph nodes, studied with the aid of colloidal Au-198. Acta Radiol, 43: 52-64, 1955.

4. Pecking, A.: Résultats préliminaires de l'essai d'un nouveau composé pour lymphographies isotopiques: Le sulfure de rhénium colloidal marqué par du technétium-99m. J. Fr. Biophys. Med. Nucl., 2: 117-120, 1978.

5. Seaman, W.B.: Studies on the distribution of radioactive colloidal gold in regional lymph nodes containing cancer. Cancer, 8: 1044-1046, 1955.

6. Terui, S.: An evaluation of the mediastinal lymphoscintigram for carcinoma of the esophagus studied with Tc-99m rhenium sulfur colloid.Eur. J. Nucl. Med., 7: 99-101, 1982.

7. Turner-Warwick, R.T.: The lymphatics of the breast. Brit. J. Surg., 46: 574-582, 1959.

BILATERALITY IN BREAST CANCER. CLINICAL AND PATHOLOGICAL ASPECTS

Hiroshi YAMAMOTO[1] and Teruyuki HIROTA[2]
1. Department of Surgery
2. Department of Pathology
National Cancer Center Hospital, Tokyo, Japan.

During the 23-year period from 1962 to 1984, 3,326 patients with breast carcinoma were surgically treated at the National Cancer Center Hospital (NCCH) of Tokyo. Of the total, there were 131 cases (3.9%) of bilateral breast carcinoma. In 103 of these patients (3.1%), the disease developed metachronously and in 28 (0.8%), synchronously, during the period studied (Table 1). In this category, were included patients who had received treatment for the initial carcinoma in other hospitals before 1962.

The age distribution of the patients at the time the first primary and the second primary breast carcinomas were diagnosed is given in Table 2. Patients who subsequently developed second primary carcinomas were somewhat younger at the time their initial disease was diagnosed than those with synchronous bilaterality. Clinically, the majority of the synchronous as well as metachronous lesions occurred as mirror images in the upper outer quadrants of both breasts. Early detection of the second primary breast carcinoma through repeated physical examination and diagnostic imaging was difficult and uncertain. There was a heavy predominance of bilateral invasive ductal carcinomas in this series (39.3% were synchronous and 61.9%, metachronous) whereas there were only a few cases of non-invasive contralateral lesions (Tables 3 and 4). Only in 10 patients with synchronous bilateral breast cancer, were the tumors clinically

TABLE 1

BILATERAL BREAST CANCER
(in 3,326 breast cancer patients observed from 1962 to 1984)

Synchronous cancer	28	(0.8%)
Metachronous cancer*	103	(3.1%)
Total :	131	(3.9%)

* Second primary treated at NCC : 40
  First and second primary treated at NCC : 63

AGE DISTRIBUTION

	synchronous	metachronous first primary	second primary
20-29	0	5	0
30-39	1	27 (26.2%)	8 (7.8%)
40-49	3 (10.7%)	43 (41.7%)	33 (32.0%)
50-59	16 (57.1%)	14 (13.6%)	35 (34.0%)
60-69	4 (14.3%)	11 (10.7%)	19 (18.4%)
70-79	4 (14.3%)	3	5
80-	0	0	3
	28	103	103

TABLE 2

classified as TO (non palpable tumor). Lobular carcinoma was infrequently diagnosed.

Correlations were found between the occurrence of bilaterality and hormone influences: abortion, poor lactation, menopause, family history of breast carcinoma. However, these trends were somewhat equivocal. The seventeen-year survival rate was 39.9% in synchronous bilateral breast cancer but 61.9% and 46.0% respectively in patients with metachronous involvement who were a) treated bilaterally at the NCCH or b) treated at other hospitals for the initial carcinomas before being referred to the NCCH for second primary cancers (Table 5). There were no statistically significant differences between the three survival rates. There was a 6.09% risk of a second primary cancer in the opposite breast over a 20-year period (Table 6). Furthermore, it was found that the risk of developing a second primary breast carcinoma was 4.8 times higher than the risk of developing a first primary carcinoma of the breast.

The data of 156 patients with primary breast carcinoma in whom second cancers were diagnosed at our hospital during the period studied were reviewed. The second cancer consisted of contralateral breast cancer in 85 cases, cancer of the uterus in 20 cases, of the stomach in 19, of the large intestine in 6 and others in 26 (Table 7).

In our series, no correlation between the occurrence of a subsequent primary cancer and adjuvant treatments such as radiotherapy and/or chemotherapy was found in a long-term follow up study. The incidence of second primary carcinomas in the pa-

HISTOLOGIC TYPE
(synchronous)

	Duct. Ca. invasive	Duct. Ca. minimal	Lobular Ca. in situ	Mucinous Ca.	Squamous cell. Ca.	Total
Duct. Ca. non-inv.	4	1	0	0	0	5
Duct. Ca. invasive	11 (39.33%)	2	2	2	1	18
Medullary Ca. with lymphoid stroma	2	0	0	0	0	2
Lobular Ca. invasive	2	0	0	0	0	2
Carcinosarcoma	1	0	0	0	0	1
	20	3	2	2	1	28

TABLE 3

HISTOLOGIC TYPE (METACHRONOUS)

	Duct ca. non-inv.	Duct ca. minimal invasion	Duct ca. invasive	Lobular ca.inv.	Mucinous ca.	Paget's disease	Squamous cell ca.	Unknown	Total
Duct ca. non invasive	0	0	2	0	0	0	0	0	2
Duct ca. minimal invasion	0	0	1	0	1	0	0	0	2
Duct ca. invasive	4	4	39 (61.9%)	1	1	1	0	1	51
Lobular ca. invasive	0	0	0	0	0	0	0	0	0
Mucinous ca.	0	0	2	0	0	0	0	0	2
Medullary ca. with lymphoid stroma	0	0	5	0	0	0	0	0	5
So-called carcinoma-sarcoma	0	0	0	0	0	0	1	0	1
	4	4	49	1	2	1	1	1	63

TABLE 4

SURVIVAL IN BILATERAL BREAST CANCER

(KAPLAN-MEIER)

1962-1983

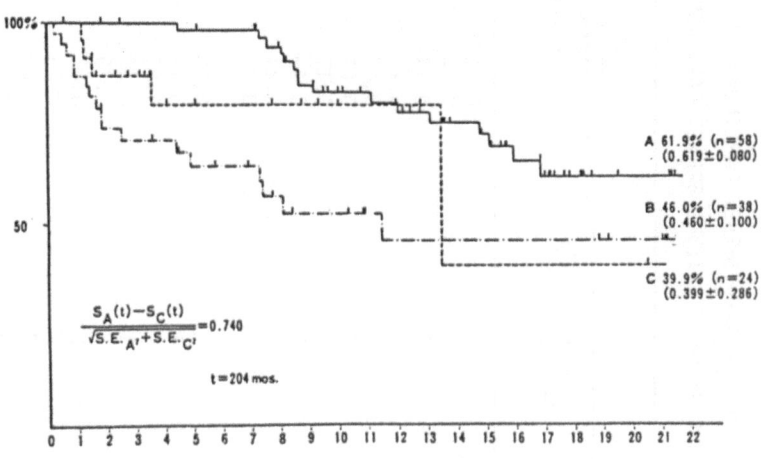

Postoperative Years

A metachronous both treated at NCC
B metachronous, opposite treated at other hospitals
C synchronous

TABLE 5

RATE OF OCCURENCE OF SECOND PRIMARY BREAST CARCINOMA IN 2,547
PATIENTS FOLLOWING SURGERY FOR PREVIOUS BREAST CARCINOMA   (1962-1981)

Years	Number of patients				annual % developping Second Primary	cumulative % with Second Primary
	at risk	died	lost to follow-up	developing Second Primary (per year)		
1	2,547	74	5	4	0.16	0.16
2	2,464	128	165	1	0.04	0.20
3	2,170	107	170	3	0.14	0.34
4	1,890	94	64	4	0.22	0.56
5	1,728	57	23	8	0.47	1.03
6	1,640	48	336	9	0.61	1.63
7	1,247	38	163	2	0.17	1.80
8	1,044	32	32	5	0.49	2.28
9	975	31	6	2	0.21	2.49
10	936	29	13	0	0.00	2.49
11	894	14	350	5	0.70	3.17
12	525	22	23	1	0.19	3.35
13	479	16	16	1	0.21	3.55
14	446	3	19	1	0.23	3.77
15	423	8	90	3	0.79	4.53
16	322	9	173	2	0.85	5.34
17	138	1	24	1	0.79	6.09
18	112	5	35	0	0.00	6.09
19	72	3	40	0	0.00	6.09
20	29	3	7	0	0.00	6.09
		722	1,754	52		

TABLE 6

BREAST CARCINOMA AND SUBSEQUENT MALIGNANCY
(1962-1984)
- 156 patients -

Breast (opposite)		85	(56.7%)
Uterus (cervix	11		
(corpus	7	20	(13.3%)
(unknown	2		
Stomach		19	(12.7%)
Colon and rectum		6	(4.0%)
Thyroid		6	(4.0%)
Ovary		5	
Lung		4	
Pancreas		2	
Esophagus		1	
Gall bladder		1	
Brain		1	
Urinary bladder		2	
Maxilla		1	
Chest wall		2	
Tongue		1	
		156 *	

* Overlap of 6 patients with multiple carcinoma (3 or more tumors) is included.

TABLE 7

tients treated by adjuvant chemotherapy was much lower (1.99%) than in patients treated by surgery alone. It was interesting to note the development of malignant fibrous histiocytoma (MFH) in the chest wall in two irradiated patients. The risk of second primary cancers developing in organs other than the second breast over a 20-year period, was 5.20% (Table 8).

The findings of this study as regards the development of second primary cancers indicate that the risk of a second primary carcinoma developing in the contralateral breast was the highest, particularly in the younger age groups, and early detection of the second primary breast carcinoma was considered essential for effective treatment.

RATE OF OCCURENCE OF SECOND PRIMARY CARCINOMA IN 2,550
PATIENTS FOLLOWING SURGERY FOR PREVIOUS BREAST CARCINOMA   (1962-1981)

Years	Number of patients				annual % developing Second Primary	cumulative % with Second Primary
	at risk	died	lost-to follow-up	developing Second Primary (per year)		
1	2,550	75	4	14	0.55	0.55
2	2,457	131	165	7	0.29	0.84
3	2,154	103	172	5	0.24	1.08
4	1,874	90	65	6	0.33	1.41
5	1,713	57	21	4	0.23	1.64
6	1,631	47	338	4	0.27	1.91
7	1,242	37	162	3	0.26	2.17
8	1,040	34	34	0	0.00	2.17
9	972	31	5	0	0.00	2.17
10	936	29	12	3	0.32	2.48
11	892	14	352	2	0.28	2.75
12	524	22	23	1	0.20	2.94
13	478	14	15	0	0.00	2.94
14	449	4	19	0	0.00	2.94
15	426	8	89	2	0.52	3.44
16	327	9	173	2	0.83	4.24
17	143	1	24	0	0.00	4.24
18	118	5	36	1	0.10	5.20
19	76	3	41	0	0.00	5.20
20	32	3	7	0	0.00	5.20
		717	1,757	54		

REFERENCES

1. Martin, J.K., van Heerden, J.A. and Gaffey, T.A., Synchronous and metachronous carcinoma of the breast. Surgery 91, 12-16, 1982.

2. Mider G.B., Schilling, J.A., Donovan, J. and Rendall, E.S. Multiple cancer. A study of other cancers arising in patients with primary malignant neoplasms of the stomach, uterus, breast, large intestine or hematopoetic system. Cancer 5, 1104-1109, 1952.

3. Rilke, F., Andreola, S., Carbone, A., Clemente, C. and Pilotti, S., The importance of pathology in prognosis and management of breast cancer. Seminars in Oncology 5, 360-372, 1978.

4. Schoenberg, B.S., Greenberg, R.A. and Eisenberg, H., Occurrence of certain multiple primary cancers in females. J. Natl. Cancer Inst., 43, 15-32, 1969.

5. Schottenfeld, D. and Berg, J., Incidence of multiple primary cancers. IV. Cancer of the female breast and genital organs. J. Natl. Cancer Inst., 46, 161-170, 1971.

6. Turco, M.R.D., Ciatto, S., Pergli, G., Borrelli, D., Carcangiu, M.L. and Santucci, M., Bilateral cancer of the breast. Tumori, 68, 155-160, 1982.

7. Urban, J.A., Papachristou, D. and Taylor, J., Bilateral breast cancer. Cancer, 40, 1968-1973, 1977.

8. Wanebo, H.J., Senofsky, G.M., Fechner, R.E., Kaiser, D., Lynn, S. and Paradies, J., Bilateral breast cancer. Risk reduction by contralateral biopsy. Annals. Surg., 201, 667-677, 1985.

BREAST TUMORS IN JORDAN

Y.F. DAJANI[1] and S. AL-JITAWI[2]

1. Consulting Medical Laboratories, P.O. Box 35198, Amman, Jordan.
2. King Hussein Medical Center, Amman, Jordan.

Four hundred and six breast tumors were reviewed from the surgical pathology files of King Hussein Medical Center and the Consulting Medical Laboratories in Amman and the tumors were classified according to the Revised WHO Classification of Breast Tumors (1981).

In this series, 228 tumors were malignant (225 carcinomas and 2 malignant Phyllodes tumors) and 177 were benign (Table).

Breast carcinomas occurred in women in 217 cases (96.4%) and in men in 8 cases (3.6%). Ages ranged from 20 to 85 years with an average of 44 years in women and 70 years in men. In women, the majority of cases occurred during the fertile period of life. Five per cent of the tumors developed before 30years, 23% before 40 and 64% before 50 years. Ten invasive carcinomas (4.5%) were observed during lactation. The age distribution with a peak in the fifth decade reflects the pattern of the general population rather than the natural occurrence of the disease (Dajani and Lipkin, 1985).

The lesions were often discovered in an advanced clinical stage. At diagnosis, the size of the tumors ranged from 1 to 8 cm with an average size of 3.3 cm, without predilection for the left or right breast (ratio 0.96/1). For half of the patients, the mastectomy specimen was available and tumor deposits were found in axillary lymph nodes in 76.4% of these cases, involving 4 nodes or more in 50%.

Histologically, invasive ductal carcinomas were predominant in both males and females, and only one single case of non-invasive ductal carcinoma was found in this series. Accompanying changes included elastosis in 55 of 174 cases (32%), perineural invasion in 16 (9%), tumor necrosis in 12 (7%), lactational changes in 8 (4.5%), mucinous metaplasia in 7 (4%) cases. Paget's disease occurred in 6 cases (3.4%).

HISTOLOGICAL CLASSIFICATION OF 406 BREAST TUMORS (1980-1985)
(according to the revised WHO classification (1981)

I. EPITHELIAL TUMORS

A. Benign

1. Intraductal papilloma	3
2. Adenoma of nipple	2
3. Lactating adenoma	5
4. Benign papillomatosis	1

B. Malignant

__Noninvasive__

1. Ductal	1

__Invasive__

1. Ductal	174 (+ 8 male)
2. Ductal with predominant intraductal	3
Mixed Ductal + lobular	3
3. Lobular	6
4. Mucinous	1
5. Medullary	1
6. Papillary	4
7. Tubular	3
8. Adenoid cystic	1
9. Apocrine	1
10. Metaplastic	
– squamous	4
– spindle cell	2
11. Others	
– undifferentiated	10
– clear cell	2
– osteoclast-like cells in stroma	1

II. MIXED CONJUNCTIVE AND EPITHELIAL TUMORS

A. Fibroadenoma	147
Fibroadenomatous hyperplasia	15
B. Phyllodes tumor	
Benign	4
Malignant	2

One of the malignant Phyllodes tumors showed a fibrosarcomatous stroma,the other an osteosarcoma.

Among the 177 benign tumors, 83% were fibroadenomas , 138 of which being solitary and 9 multiple. The age distribution ranged from 12 to 56 years, with a mean of 27 years, 4 of them occurring in lactating women. The size of the tumors ranged from 0.8 to 6 cm, with an average of 2.9 cm.

Fibroadenomatous hyperplasia was observed in 15 cases. This lesion, often multinodular, is characterized by lobular hyperplasia and fibroadenoma merging together surrounded by an incomplete capsule. It occurred in young women of 16 to 27 years, with an average age of 22 years. Since this condition shows a 5-year-lag behind fibroadenoma a pathogenic link between hyperplasia and fibroadenoma may exist.

In conclusion, breast tumor in Jordan reviewed according to the revised WHO Histologic Classification closely resemble to the histologic pattern reported for other countries. However, there was a predominance of malignant tumors. (Amr, 1986). Generally, tumors were too lately detected, already in an advanced clinical stage (average size 3.3 cm) with metastases to the axillary lymph nodes (76.4%)(Amr, 1986; Tarawneh, 1980).

The lack of screening programs for breast cancer in Jordan and the insufficient level of education among native women are certainly related to this situation.

REFERENCES

1. Amr, S.S., Breast disease in Jordanian females: a study of 1000 cases. Europ. J. Surg. Oncol., in press.

2. Dajani, Y.F. and Lipkin, M., An appraisal of comparative epidemiologic data on colorectal cancer in Jordanians and Americans. Path. Res. Pract., 1985, 180, 261 (abstract).

3. Tarawneh, M.S., Breast cancer in Jordan. A pathological review. J. Kuwaiti Med. Assoc., 1980, 14, 79-86.

4. World Health Organization. Histologic typing of breast tumors. In: International histological classi-fication of tumours, 2nd Ed., World Health Organization, Geneva, 1981.

LOBULAR CARCINOMA "IN SITU" (LOBULAR NEOPLASIA)

A.VIEGAS MENDONCA

Universidade Nova de Lisboa, Faculdade de Ciencias Medicas, Departamento de Anatomia Patologica, 130, Campo de Santana, 1198 Lisboa Codex, Portugal

Lobular carcinoma "in situ" or lobular neoplasia (Haagensen et al., 1978) is a non-palpable tumor which can only be diagnosed under the microscope (fig. 1 and 2). Histologically, the terminolobular units are densely filled with loosely adherent tumor cells which distend the lobules and increase their diameter. The tumor cells are larger than normal cells and their cytoplasmic boundaries are often indistinct. The nuclei are round and of uniform shape and staining intensity.

Since lobular neoplasia has generally a good prognosis, conservative treatment should always be considered as alternative in order to avoid aesthetic and psychological consequences for the patient.

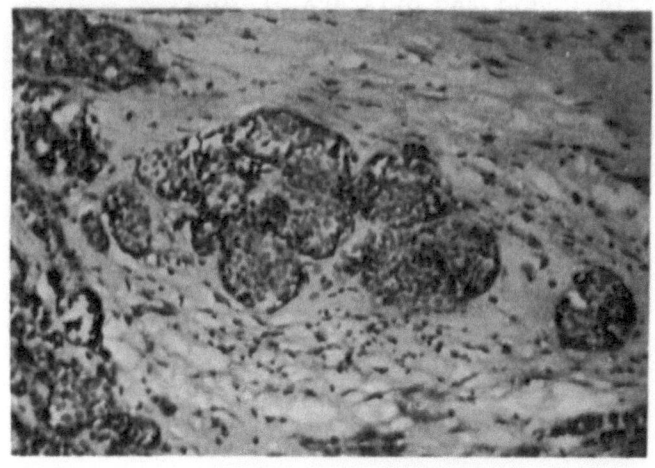

FIGURE 1

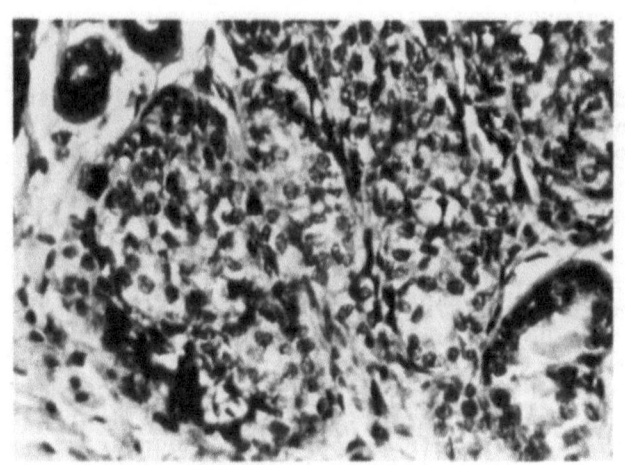

FIGURE 2

        In   our   material   of   1,270   cases   of   benign   breast
lesions, 71 cases (5.5%) of lobular neoplasia were observed.
The   age   distribution ranged from 20 to 59 years, with   an
average   age   of   41.1   years.   52.1% of the patients   were
between   40   and   49 years old. The lesions predominated   in
premenopausal women (97%)(Table   1).   They   were   frequently
multicentric (66%) and bilateral (30%).

AGE OF PATIENTS WITH LOBULAR NEOPLASIA

20-24	2
25-29	6
30-34	3
35-39	14
40-44	15
45-49	21
50-54	7
55-59	1
Not specified	2
	71

TABLE 1

Forty-three of our 71 patients were followed over 1 to 33 years, with an average follow-up of 12,8 years. 18 patients were followed over 2 to 10 years and 25 over more than 10 years (until 33 years). In 38 cases (88.3%), the evolution was followed over more than 5 years (Table 2).

FOLLOW-UP OF PATIENTS WITH LOBULAR NEOPLASIA
(average 12.8 yrs)

Follow-up (in yrs)	Number of Patients
1	0
2	1
3	1
4	3
5	4
6-10	9
11-15	9
16-20	9
21-25	6
26-30	0
31-35	1

TABLE 2

From the 43 patients followed, only 2 women died: one from breast carcinoma with liver metastases, the other from an unrelated disease 21 years after the initial diagnosis. All other patients were alive at the time of this investigation. Eight patients had recurrences, in the same or in the contralateral (3 cases) breast, but all were cured by local excision.

These observations underline the fact that lobular carcinoma in situ has a good prognosis although it has some tendency to recur. Since metastases are almost inexistent, the choice of treatment should be carefully considered. The best treatment of lobular neoplasia is still subject of controversy. Some authors prefer radical mastectomy since the lesions are often multicentric and may lead, in some cases, to cancer. (Carter and Smith, 1977; Ashikari et al., 1977; Rosen, 1980; Hutter, 1984). Other authors advocate a conservative treatment consisting of a close follow-up (Andersen, 1977; Haagensen et al., 1978; Lattes, 1980 and, depending on the cases, Hutter, 1984). Their opinion is based on the slow evolution of the disease, on the low probability of subsequent carcinoma occuring only after many years, on the tendency of the lesion to regress spontaneously after menopause, and on the experience that carcinomas which arise from lobular neoplasia have generally a favourable evolution and can be easily and completely cured by surgery. A final argument is that lobular neoplasia is often multicentric, tending to affect both breasts, and that a logic surgical cure has to be bilateral mastectomy, a procedure which seems to be excessive for a disease with such a slow development and rare tendency to metastasize.

We agree with this opinion and believe that conservative treatment with careful and frequent examinations (every 3 or 4 months, eventually completed by mammography) can be recommanded to those patients who understand the necessity of repeated and regular follow-up.

REFERENCES

1. Andersen, J.A., Lobular carcinoma in situ of the breast. Cancer, 39, 2597-2602, 1977.

2. Ashikari, R., Huvos, A.G., and Snyder, R.E., Prospective study of non-infiltrating carcinoma of the breast. Cancer, 39, 435-439, 1977.

3. Carter, D., and Smith, R.L., Carcinoma in situ of the breast. Cancer, 40, 1189-1193, 1977.

4. Haagensen, C.D., Lane, N., Lattes, R., and Bodian, C., Lobular neoplasia (Lobular carcinoma in situ) of the breast. Cancer, 31, 1553-1560, 1978.

5. Hutter, R.V.P., The management of patients with lobular carcinoma in situ of the breast. Cancer, 53, 798-802, 1984.

6. Lattes, R., Lobular neoplasia (Lobular carcinoma in situ) of the breast. A histological entity of controversial clinical significance. Path. Res. Pract., 166, 415-429, 1980

7. Rosen, P.P., Lobular carcinoma in situ: recent clinicopathologic studies at Memorial Hospital. Path. Res. Pract., 166, 430-455, 1980.

RADIATION INDUCED CHANGES IN NON-NEOPLASTIC BREAST EPITHELIUM.

A POSSIBLE PITFALL IN CYTODIAGNOSIS

J.L. PETERSE and P. VAN HEERDE

Department of Cytology and Pathology,
Netherlands Cancer Institute (Antoni van Leeuwenhoekhuis)
Plesmanlaan 121, 1066 CX Amsterdam, The Netherlands

Less radical treatment is increasingly employed in patients with operable breast cancer. Since 1979 nearly 600 patients have been treated in the Netherlands Cancer Institute according to the breast conserving protocol of the EORTC trial 10801. After tumorectomy and axillary lymph node dissection, external radiotherapy is given up to a dose of 45 Gy in 5 weeks, followed by Iridium implantation to achieve a surdosage of 25 Gy in the tumor area.

All patients are closely followed. Interpretation of palpatory and mammographical examinations may be hampered by fibrosis and fat necrosis, and scars may simulate recurrent carcinoma (Clarke et al. 1983).

Since the introduction in our hospital in 1973, fine needle aspiration is performed of all palpable breast lesions. Giemsa staining is used on air dried, methanol fixed smears. More than 8000 breast aspirations have been performed, preferably by the cytologists, and in more than 2300 a carcinoma was present. There is an increasing number of fine needle aspiration of doubtful breast lesions in patients, who earlier underwent breast conserving treatment.

Surprisingly little is known about morphological changes in non-neoplastic irradiated breast tissue (Fajardo, 1982). In animal studies epithelial linings of ducts and acini proved relatively radioresistant (Turner & Gomez, 1936). Radiation-induced cellular atypia has been recently described in the human terminal duct lobular unit varying in severity from one patient to another (Schnitt et al. 1984). False-positive diagnosis in fine needle aspiration of irradiated breasts has been briefly reported earlier, but is not mentioned as pitfall in leading textbooks.

However, fine needle aspiration may be a source of error in irradiated breast, as the following history shows:

A 45 years old woman underwent, in October 1979, breast conserving treatment in our hospital. An invasive ductal car-

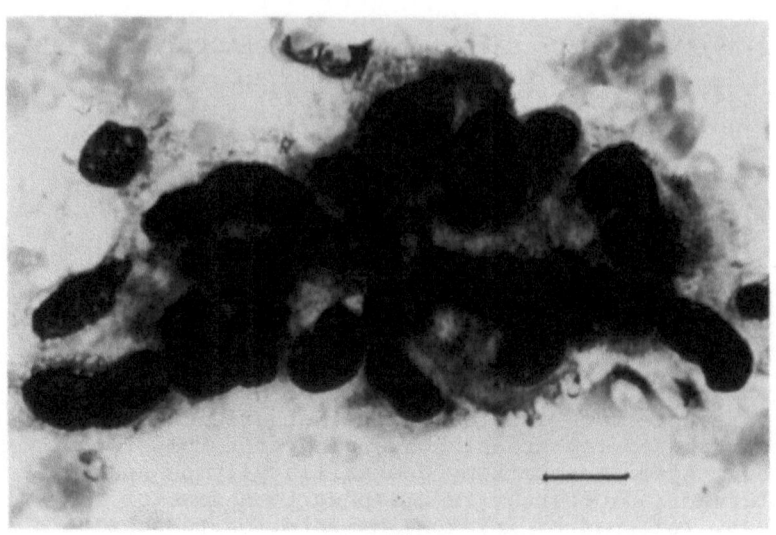

Fig. 1.   Fine needle aspiration cytology ; cluster of atypical
cells, karyolysis, cytoplasmic vacuolisation
(Giemsa, bar = 10 μ).

cinoma n.o.s. was completely removed by lumpectomy. External
radiotherapy was followed by Iridium implantation. After 3
years a painful mass developed in the lumpectomy area, increasing in diameter, clinically difficult to interpret, mammographically doubtful. Fine needle aspiration showed a moderately
cellular smear with atypical cells in clusters, nuclear poly-
morphism, small nucleoli and cytoplasmic vacuoles (Fig. 1 & 2).
The cytological conclusion was : suspicious of malignancy.
A breast ablation was performed. In the specimen only radiation
induced changes were found (Fig. 3).

According to our experience, fine needle aspiration of
non-neoplastic irradiated breast tissue usually yields poorly
to moderately cellular smears. These contain small cell clusters with microacinar arrangements. Although these cells show
anisocytosis and anisonucleosis, their nuclear-cytoplasmic ratio is normal. The smooth borders of well preserved nuclei, the
regular chromatin pattern and especially the naked bipolar
(myoepithelial) nuclei in and around the clusters are cytologi-
cally compatible with a benign lesion (Fig. 2). Unfamiliarity
with the radiation-induced cellular changes like nuclear poly-
morphism, small nucleoli and, probably degenerative, changes as
cytoplasmic vacuolisation and karyolysis may lead to a false-
positive diagnosis (Fig. 1).

Cell dissociation and necrotic cell debris, as often seen

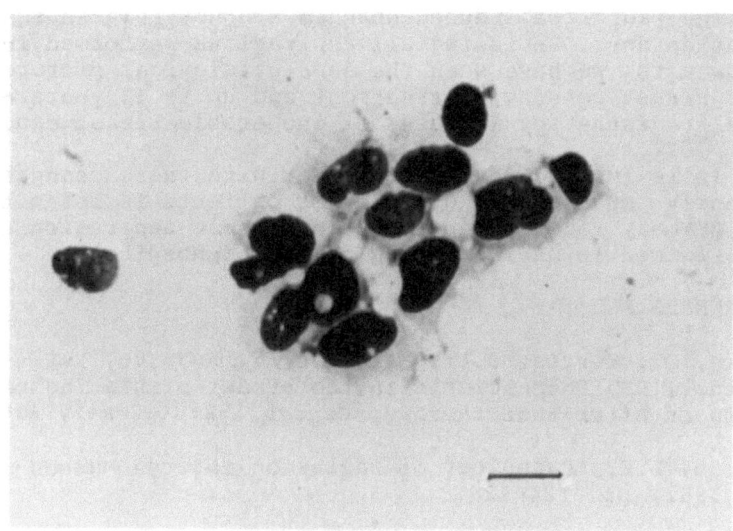

Fig. 2. Fine needle aspiration cytology ; cluster of atypical
cells, microacinar arrangement, bipolar nuclei
(Giemsa, bar = 10 μ).

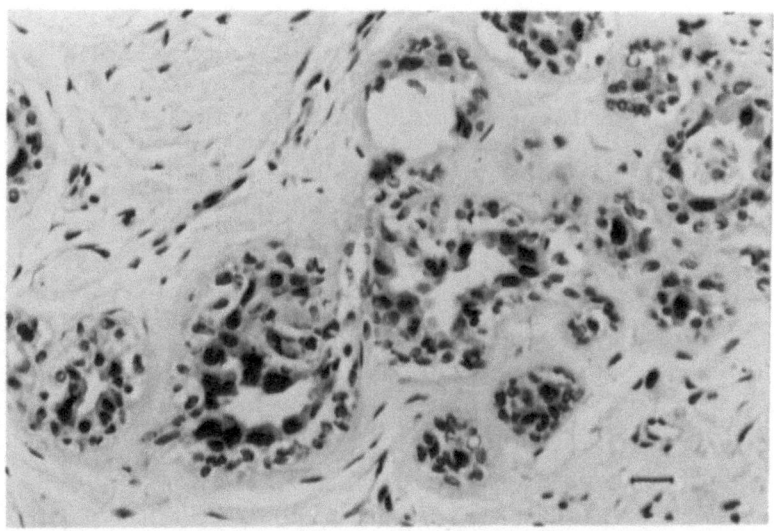

Fig. 3. Terminal duct lobular unit ; radiation induced cell
atypia. (H & E, bar = 20 μ).

in breast cancer smears, were never encountered in fine needle aspiration of irradiated non-neoplastic breasts.

The radiation induced changes are not related to time or radiation dose. Reviewing all aspirations performed in irradiated breasts, we have seen the same cytological picture 3 months after breast conserving treatment and up to 13 years after external radiotherapy in cases of inoperable breast cancer.

It is important to be familiar with these changes since presently an increasing number of patients is being treated with primary radiotherapy and fine needle aspiration cytology is performed in an increasing number of hospitals.

REFERENCES

Clarke, D., Curtis, J.L., Martinez, A., Fajardo, L., and Goffinet, D., Fat necrosis in the breast simulating recurrent carcinoma after radiotherapy. Cancer, 52: 442-445, 1983.

Fajardo, L.F., Pathology of radiation injury, Masson publishing USA, 1982, pp. 124-128.

Schnitt, S.J., Connolly, J.L., Harris, J.R. and Cohen, R.B., Radiation-induced changes in the breast. Hum. Pathol., 15: 545-550, 1984.

Turner, C.W. and Gomez, E.T., Radiosensitivity of cells of mammary gland. Am. J. Roentgenol., 36: 79-93, 1936.

CYTO-HISTOLOGIC CORRELATION IN NODULAR BREAST PATHOLOGY

P. LITTA, A. AZZENA, M. MOLLESENA DEL MONACO, G.L. ONNIS, A. CASCIO, T. MAGGINO, D. MINUCCI, and D. de SALVIA

Department of Gynaecology and Obstetrics, University of Padua, 35100 Padua, Italy.

It has been demonstrated that fine needle aspiration does not induce tumor spread during cytologic sampling (Robbins et al., 1954). Due to its easy and rapid execution, low costs and high diagnostic reliability, this procedure has thus acquired an important position in the diagnostic approach to breast cancer (Bauermeister, 1980; Cornillot et al., 1971, Franzen and Zajicek, 1968). This report further confirms the reliability of cytologic evaluation of fine needle aspirated material in the diagnosis of breast tumors (Azzarelli, 1982; Azzarelli et al., 1981, 1983; Pilotti, 1982; Pilotti et al., 1982).

In the last two years, 985 women with breast disorders were examined at the Breast Pathology Center of the Department of Gynaecology and Obstetrics at the University of Padua. All the patients underwent a thorough investigation consisting of clinical examination, contact thermography, diaphanoscopy and mammography. Solid breast nodules were detected in 107 cases, 103 of which were disposable 20 ml syringes and 22 to 18 G needles, depending on the consistency of the nodules. The aspirated material was smeared on slides, fixed with Merckofix, and stained according to Papanicolaou (Furnival et al., 1975; Kline et al., 1979; Koss, 1980; Zajdela et al., 1975). Reliability of the clinical and cytologic examination, alone and in association, were evaluated, and compared with histologic findings (Hajdu, 1973; Kreusen and Boquoi, 1976; Van Bogaert and Mazy, 1971).

Cytology of aspirates from the 103 patients revealed 19 positive cases with malignant cells, 8 doubtful cases and 71 negative cases. Material was inadequate for evaluation in 5 cases.

Histologic examination of the 19 positive cases confirmed malignancy. Two of the 8 doubtful cases were carcinoma, while the other 6 cases were negative. In the 71 negative cases on cytology, only 1 was histologically

malignant. The 5 cases with inadequate material revealed to
be benign lesions on histology (Table 1). Thus, 22
carcinomas (21.4%) were histologically ascertained in this
series of 103 cases.

Cytologic evaluation was highly sensitive (95%) and
specific (92%), whereas clinical examination showed a good
sensitivity (90%), but a poorer specificity (79%). The
sensitivity and specificity of the above examinations in
association did not substantially modify the results of the
single procedure.

CYTO-HISTOLOGIC CORRELATION IN 103 CASES

| CYTOLOGY | HISTOLOGY | |
	Cancer	No Cancer
Positive	19	–
Doubtful	2	6
Negative	1	70
Inadequate	–	5
TOTAL	22	81

TABLE 1

Thus, fine-needle aspiration cytology is highly useful
in the diagnostic of breast diseases, with a reliability of
100% when findings indicate the presence of malignant tumor
cells. Doubtful cases should be confirmed by histologic
examination. In negative cases, the cytologic examination
should be repeated after a brief interval, or a surgical
biopsy should be performed.

Although our data seem to indicate that clinical
examination does not improve the sensitivity and specificity
of diagnosis, it represents a fundamental step in detecting
the presence of neoformations in the breast, and guides the
physician in the choice of further examinations.

REFERENCES

1. Azzarelli, A., Di Pietro, S. and Pilotti, S.: L'agoaspirazione nella diagnosi del carcinoma mammario. Argomenti di oncologia, 2: 29-40, 1981.

2. Azzarelli, A.: Indicazioni ed applicabilità della biopsia
   per agoaspirazione. In: Il carcinoma della mammella. Diagnosi e tarapia.Ambrosiana, Milano 1982.

3. Azzarelli, A., Guzzon, A., Pilotti, S., Quagliuolo, V.,
   Bono, A. and Di Pietro, S.: Accuracy of breast cancer diagnosis by physical, radiologic and cytologic combined examinations. Tumori, 69; 137-141, 1983.

4. Bauermeister, D.E.: The role and limitations of frozen section and needle aspiration biopsy in breast cancer diagnosis.
   Cancer, 46: 947-949, 1980.

5. Cornillot, M., Verhaeghe, M., Cappelaere, P. and Clay, A.:
   Place de la cytologie par ponction dans le diagnostic des
   tumeurs du sein (2267 examens cytologiques), Lille Méd.,
   16: 1027-1031, 1971.

6. Franzen, S. and Zajicek, J.: Aspiration biopsy in diagnosis
   of palpable lesions of the breast. Critical review of 3479
   consecutive biopsies. Acta Radiol., 7: 241, 1968.

7. Furnival, C.M., Hughes, H.E., Hocking, M.A., Reid, M.M.W.
   and Blumgart, L.H.: Aspiration Cytology in breast cancer.
   Its relevance to diagnosis. Lancet, 2: 446, 1975.

8. Hajdu, S.I. and Melamed, M.R.: The diagnostic value of aspiration smears. Am. J. Clin. Pathol., 59: 350, 1973.

9. Kline, T.S., Joshi, L.P. and Neal, H.S.: Fine needle aspiration of the breast: diagnosis and pitfalls. A review of
   3545 cases. Cancer, 44: 1458, 1979.

10. Koss, L.G.: Editorial. Thin needle aspiration biopsy. Acta
    Cytol., 24, 1, 1980.

11. Kreuzer, G. and Boquoi, E.: Aspiration biopsy cytology,
    mammography and clinical exploration. A modern set up in
    diagnosis of tumours of the breast. Acta Cytol. 20: 319-
    323, 1976.

12. Pilotti, S.: Sensibilità e valore predittivo della citolo-
    gia da agoaspirato. In: Il carcinoma della mammella. Dia-
    gnosi et terapia. Ambrosiana, Milano 1982.

13. Pilotti, S., Rilke, F., Delpiano, C., Di Pietro, S. and
    Guzzon, A.: Problems in fine needle aspiration biopsy

cytology of clinically or mammographically uncertain breast tumors. Tumor, 68: 407-412, 1982.

14. Robbins, G.F., Brothers, J.H. III, Eberhart, W.F. and Quan, S.: Is aspiration biopsy of breast cancer dangerous to the patient? Cancer, 7: 774-778, 1954.

15. Van Bogaert, L.J. and Mazy, G.: Reliability of the cyto-radio-clinical triplet in breast pathology diagnosis. Acta Méd., 16: 1027-1031, 1971.

16. Zajdela, A., Ghossein, N.A., Pilleron, J.P. and Ennuyer, A.: The value of aspiration cytology in the diagnosis of breast cancer: experience at the Fondation Curie. Cancer, 35: 499-506, 1975.

LIST OF INVITED SPEAKERS

BUSSOLATI, G., Dept. of Human Oncology, Istituto di Anatomia e Istologia Patologica, Via Santena, 7, 10126 - Torino, Italy

COOPER, G.M., Dana-Farber Cancer Institute and Dept. of Pathology, Harvard Medical School, Boston, MA 02115, USA

EUSEBI, V., Istituto di Anatomia e Istologia Patologica, Policlinico s. Orsola, 40138 - Bologna, Italy

GULLINO, P.M., Istituto di Anatomia e Istologia Patologica, University of Torino, Via Santena, 7, 10126 - Torino, Italy

HAGMAR, B., Dept. of Pathology, Faculty of Medicine, Kuwait University, P.O. Box 24, 923 - Safat, Kuwait

HARTVEIT, F., Dept. of Pathology, The Gade Institute, University of Bergen, 5000 - Bergen, Norway

HOLLMANN, K.H., Dept. of Pathology and Oncology, Hopital Marie Lannelongue, 92350 - Le Plessis Robinson, France

ISRAEL, L., Dept. of Cancerology, Hopital Avicenne, University Paris XIII, 93000 - Bobigny, France

KATAYAMA, I., Dept. of Pathology, Saitama Medical School, Saitama 350-04 , Japan

LECLERCQ, G., Laboratoire de Cancerologie Mammaire, Service de Medecine, Institut J. Bordet, 1000 - Bruxelles, Belgium

LYNCH, H.T., Dept. of Preventive Medicine, Creighton University School of Medicine, Omaha, Nebraska 68178, USA

MAREEL, M., Laboratory of Experimental Cancerology, Dept. of Radiotherapy and Nuclear Medicine, University Hospital, De Pintelaan, 185, 9000 - Ghent, Belgium

MOORE, D.H., Dept. of Microbiology and Immunology, Hahnemann University, School of Medicine, Philadelphia, PA 19102, USA

MORNEX, F., Dept. of Radiology, Centre Leon Berard, 69000 - Lyon, France

438

ONNIS, A., Institute of Gynecology and Obstetrics, University of Padua, 35100 - Padua, Italy

OZZELLO, L., Arthur Purdy Stout Laboratory of Surgical Pathology, Columbia University, College of Physicians and Surgeons, New York, NY 10032, USA

PINOTTI, J.A., Dept. of Obstetrics and Gynecology, Faculty of Medical Sciences, State University of Campinas, UNICAMP, 13.100 - Campinas, Brazil

REGNARD, J.F., Dept.of Surgery, Hopital Louis Mourier, 92700 - Colombes, France

REYNIER, J., Dept. of Surgery, Hopital Boucicaut, 75015 - Paris, France

TARIN, D., Nuffield Dept. of Pathology, University of Oxford, John Radcliffe Hospital, Oxford OX3 9DU, England

VERLEY, J.M., Dept. of Pathology, Hopital Marie Lannelongue, 92350 - Le Plessis Robinson, France

WAELTI, E., Dept. of Pathology, University of Bern, Freiburgstrasse 30, 3010 - Bern, Switzerland

SUBJECT INDEX